Praise for HEART 411

"From the warning signs of an impending heart attack to the cardiac effects of red wine, this book has it all. Gillinov and Nissen engage you with their friendly tone and their patients' stories *and* give you the critical information you need to ensure your heart health. *Heart 411* is a must-read."
—**TOBY COSGROVE, M.D.**, CEO and president, Cleveland Clinic

"It's rare a book so vital to health is also such an engaging and entertaining read. *Heart 411* is an invaluable resource, and one that I would recommend everyone add to their reading list."
—**MARY JOE FERNANDEZ**, two-time Olympic Gold Medalist and ESPN and CBS Commentator

"As a heart disease survivor, I look for the best information I can find, and I've found it in *Heart 411*. It is essential reading for patients like me, as well as those who want to keep their heart healthy. In a world filled with conflicting information, Drs. Gillinov and Nissen separate fact from fiction, providing patients and their families with easy-to-use tools to understand heart disease and find the best possible care. It has become my go-to book!"
—**LARRY KING**, CNN talk-show host; founder of the Larry King Cardiac Foundation

"Every one of us, no matter how good we feel, faces a risk of heart disease. *Heart 411* reveals the secrets you *must* know to ensure your heart health."
—**TED DANSON**, Emmy Award– and Golden Globe Award– winning performer

"A useful and—dare I say—fun masterpiece. Reading *Heart 411* is like having your own personal consultation with two of the most skilled and compassionate heart doctors on the planet. Gillinov and Nissen provide a delightful blend of the latest research, moving experiences with patients at the renowned Cleveland Clinic, and warmth and humor to show each of us how to live a longer, healthier, and happier life."

—**ROBERT SUTTON**, Stanford professor and author of the *New York Times* bestsellers *Good Boss, Bad Boss* and *The No Asshole Rule*

"In the 21st century, we are held to the expectation that health care be safe, effective, patient-centered, timely, efficient, and equitable. Achieving these goals requires the free flow of unbiased information to allow for informed and shared decision-making. With this book, Drs. Gillinov and Nissen provide patients and their families a balanced, evidence-based, and practical view of the diagnosis, treatment, and prevention of common cardiovascular diseases. Readers will find it a trustworthy reference to help focus their understanding and navigate the maze of information overload that surrounds us."

—**PATRICK T. O'GARA, M.D.**, director, Clinical Cardiology, Brigham and Women's Hospital; professor, Harvard Medical School

"Preventative care for your cardiac plumbing, and steps to rectify what has gone amiss . . . With an affable thoroughness, the authors inform readers about the world of coronary heart disease. . . . The text is designed so readers can either drop in on a specific topic or extend their understanding by reading the entire chapter to gain the broad, contextual picture. This book is like the doctor of old—white coat, black bag, stethoscope—ready to counsel from broad experience. So listen and act."

—*KIRKUS REVIEWS*

"I commend your dedicated research of the heart. May you continue helping the young and old with this most important study."

—Comedian **DON RICKLES**

"Read *Heart 411* and you may never have to call 911."

—**STEVE LAWRENCE** and **EYDIE GORMÉ**, Emmy- and Grammy-winning performers

Marc Gillinov, M.D., and Steven Nissen, M.D.

HEART 411

*The Only Guide to
Heart Health You'll Ever Need*

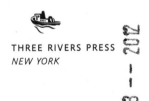

THREE RIVERS PRESS
NEW YORK

This book contains general information and advice relating to heart disease. It is not intended to replace personalized medical advice and should be used to inform patients and supplement the regular care of a physician. We strongly recommend that you consult with your doctor about questions and concerns specific to your heart health. The authors and publisher expressly disclaim responsibility for any adverse effects that may result from the use or application of the information contained in this book.

Copyright © 2012 by Steven Nissen, M.D., and A. Marc Gillinov, M.D.

Published in the United States by Three Rivers Press, an imprint of the Crown Publishing Group, a division of Random House, Inc., New York.
www.crownpublishing.com

Three Rivers Press and the Tugboat design are registered trademarks of Random House, Inc.

Library of Congress Cataloging-in-Publication Data
Gillinov, Marc.
    Heart 411 : the only guide to heart health you'll ever need / Marc Gillinov and Steven Nissen. —
1st ed.
        p. cm.
    1. Coronary heart disease—Popular works. 2. Coronary heart disease—Treatment—Popular works. 3. Coronary heart disease—Prevention—Popular works. I. Nissen, Steven E. II. Title.
    RC685.C6G49 2012
    616.1'2—dc23   2011034576

ISBN 978-0-307-71990-4
eISBN 978-0-307-71992-8

Printed in the United States of America

Book design by Elina Nudelman
Cover design by Jen O'Connor

10 9 8 7 6 5 4 3 2 1

First Edition

*To my parents, Dr. Sheldon Gillinov and Lynda Gillinov,
who provided the guidance, love, and support that enabled me to
become a doctor.
And to my wonderful wife, Lisa, who does it all.*
—Marc Gillinov, M.D.

*To my colleagues in the department of cardiovascular medicine
at the Cleveland Clinic, from whom I have learned so much about
the science and art of medicine.*
—Steven Nissen, M.D.

CONTENTS

HEART 411

HEART HEALTH AND DISEASE: THE BASICS THAT YOU MUST KNOW

CHAPTER 1

SAVING YOUR LIFE

"Why me?"

We've heard those words thousands of times, repeated again and again by our heart patients over the years.

Lying in the hospital bed staring at the white ceiling of his cubicle in the Cleveland Clinic coronary care unit, the forty-eight-year-old man didn't have time for a heart attack. He needed to finish a few things at work before leaving to take his son on a whirlwind college tour, planning to hit seven schools in nine days. He had a schedule, but another wave of chest pain brought him back to today's reality. Looking with dread at his already thick hospital chart with our names—Nissen and Gillinov—emblazoned on the spine, he realized that he was having a heart attack. His plans with his son would have to wait. We had a radically different plan for him.

Had he been able to peer around the corner from his room, he would have seen us, his cardiologist and heart surgeon, conferring. The coronary care unit (CCU) is where we meet. Twenty feet from the bedside, we studied a computer screen that displayed images of the patient's coronary arteries.

Steve and I easily identified the problem—severe blockages of all three coronary arteries, meaning a trip to the operating room was imperative.

Sleep-deprived and responsible for a twenty-four-bed ICU filled with every manner of complex heart patient, Steve was clearly pleased to have a quick disposition in this case. The treatment plan was clear, and success was almost certain. He could move on to the next bed, which served as a temporary home to yet another patient with a life-threatening cardiac condition.

Meanwhile, I needed to figure out how to fit another surgery into an already full OR schedule. Making my way past the busy nurses, technicians, and doctors, I called the operating room and told them to cancel a scheduled elective surgery to make room for the emergency. The nurses had an OR ready, and the anesthesia team would be down to pick him up in fifteen minutes.

The bypass surgery went well, and our patient was discharged from the hospital in six days with a good prognosis. We never learned what happened with his son's college trip. By the time the forty-eight-year-old heart attack victim left the hospital, Steve had seen fifty new patients in the CCU, and I had operated on ten more. Together, we focused on that case for a grand total of only a few hours and then moved on to the next one. It was a monumental event for our patient and his family, but for us, it was a routine part of a hectic day on the cardiac service at the Cleveland Clinic.

Between the two of us, working separately or together, we have cared for more than 10,000 cardiac patients. Over the last twenty years we have successfully made use of EKGs, stress tests, and cardiac catheterizations to diagnose heart problems, and medicines, angioplasty, and heart surgery to treat the diseases we have discovered. Along the way, we have helped thousands of patients and saved thousands of lives. We have basked in the warm and flattering glow created by successful procedures and grateful families. The rewards of a career in heart medicine have been tremendous.

But over time, we have come to recognize a key limitation to the way we practice medicine. Our experience with the forty-eight-year-old heart attack victim plays out over and over. We hurry from one patient to the next, doing our best to treat their diseased hearts. But we see our patients too late, after they already have heart disease or established risk factors for developing it—toxic diets, abandoned exercise programs, dangerous supplements, ill-advised combinations of prescription medicines, and failure to manage emotional stress are among the notations we record in patients' charts again and again. There seems no end to the flow of patients who require complex procedures to fix their hearts—not to mention the ones who show up year after year for another bypass operation, or one more stent. Like the mythological Sisyphus condemned to spend eternity pushing a boulder up a mountain only to have it roll back down every night, we feel the frustration associated with trying to prevent a monumental, recurring problem. But unlike Sisyphus, as doctors, we have the opportunity to achieve success.

The solution to our dilemma becomes clear when we revisit the classic ideal of the physician from generations past. You know the type: the kindly, unhurried, gray-haired gentleman with a white coat, a black bag, and a stethoscope. Decades ago, doctors could not imagine peering into the body with real-time, three-dimensional MRI scanners or dream of preventing heart attacks by propping open the heart's two-millimeter-wide arteries with tiny metallic stents. With limited technology, what did these physicians do? *They communicated with their patients.*

Doctors of old took the time to listen and to talk. When they came to a hospital bed, they saw whole patients, often surrounded by generations of people whom they had also treated. In today's whirlwind of technological marvels and breakthrough cures, these aspects of medicine have all but disappeared. We heart doctors tend to "fix" the plumbing problem of the moment and then move on rapidly to the next one. All too often, patients become "cases" ("Can you check on the 80 percent left main coronary artery obstruction in cath lab number 4?") rather than people in desperate need of advice and counseling.

The fact that we are missing an important piece of the puzzle really hit home a few years ago as we prepared to do some cardiac plumbing on our fourth patient from a single family. Periodically, we treat two or three members of the same family, and we have even performed his-and-hers heart surgeries for married couples. But the Whelton family's cardiac problems were like an annuity for heart doctors. Their story forced us to reexamine our long-held assumptions of what it means to be a successful doctor.

THE WHELTONS: A FAMILY PLAN FOR HEART DISEASE

This time it was Jim Whelton's turn. Sitting in the consultation room with Jim were his father, Sam (triple bypass surgery, 1998), brother, Rick (quadruple bypass, 2007), sister Noreen (two coronary artery stents, 2005), and sister Susan (no cardiac procedures to date). Their mother had died of a heart attack four years earlier. When we entered the room, it was a warm reunion. Sam, Rick, and Noreen enthusiastically reported that they were all feeling great and doing well. Jim, on the other hand, did not look particularly thrilled: he was facing his turn with coronary artery bypass surgery.

We talked about the procedure, explaining how we would open his chest and reroute the blood flow around his heart's blocked arteries. With each detail, Jim lost a bit more color; he would soon blend in perfectly with the white hospital walls. His brother and father tried to cheer him up. They assured Jim that it would be a piece of cake. He would do fine.

And he did—technically, Jim's surgery was a success. But a conversation with his younger sister, Susan, the day before Jim left the hospital made us realize that it was also a failure. Susan cornered us in the hall outside Jim's room, fidgety and obviously worried. Picking up on her distress, we assured her that everything was fine. Jim's EKG and echocardiogram revealed that his heart had weathered the surgery well, and he would be going home within twenty-four hours. For doctors, a patient's hospital discharge after heart surgery always represents a victory.

As Susan talked, though, we quickly realized that we had missed the point completely. She was glad Jim had done well, but *his* health wasn't what was keeping her up at night. She was the only member of the family who had not yet developed heart disease. Wasn't there some way to avoid it? Should she try coenzyme Q_{10}, chelation therapy, or one of the antioxidants she read about on the Internet? Maybe she should add blueberries, Cheerios, and POM Wonderful to her diet? Wouldn't these keep her arteries clean? At first we were amazed. How could she not know that coronary heart disease is preventable? Wasn't everybody conversant with its risk factors, including diets too rich in calories and saturated fat, high blood pressure, elevated cholesterol, smoking, family history and all the other usual suspects? But then we turned the question back on ourselves. Where could she get the information she needed to avoid a trip to the cardiac cath lab or operating room? The answer was obvious: from us.

The next question followed quickly, though it was not one that we really wanted to dwell upon. We had been taking care of the Whelton family for more than a decade, seeing them through operations and writing endless prescriptions for aspirin, Lipitor, and Plavix. We had talked to them at length about these how these medical therapies can help with coronary heart disease. But had we failed to give them the relevant information they needed to manage their heart health and even prevent heart disease in the first place? Painfully, we concluded that our efforts had fallen short.

Susan and the rest of the Whelton family did not see us as failures. We had fixed their hearts! But our follow-through was too limited, and our plumbing efforts came too late, at a stage when they already had severe cardiac problems that required high-tech and invasive solutions.

Susan wanted information, not an operation. Realizing that we could not tell her everything she needed to know in a three-minute discussion outside her brother's hospital room, she asked us to point her to the best website. Googling "heart disease" the night before had presented her with more health information than is contained in all of the world's medical libraries put together. Surely one of these sites had it all, including plans for prevention for her and disease management for her family. We promised to look into this and get back to her.

We checked, and checked again, and found no such resource. The volume of available material was tremendous, but no single site or book contained all of the critical information. Many websites contained recommendations that were shockingly wrong and even dangerous, touting ultra-low-fat diets and unregulated supplements that promised to make artery-clogging plaque melt away. Sensational headlines and unrealistic promises abounded, but sound advice was elusive. So we decided to provide that advice. That's the reason we wrote this book.

EVIDENCE-BASED ANSWERS VERSUS UNFILTERED INFORMATION

As a society, we crave medical information. Eight out of ten Internet users search the Web for health information. We are hungry for the facts and for a to-do list that will make us healthy. But most available information is unvalidated and unsorted. Even when the information is correct, how can you determine how to use it? A website may describe a new medical study extolling the virtues of aspirin for heart attack prevention and conclude that an aspirin a day is generally good for most people. But are you "most people"? Do *you* need an aspirin a day?

Adding to the confusion and anxiety, pharmaceutical-company-sponsored Internet sites try to brand medical conditions and convince people they are suffering from them. We're all familiar with this approach. An animation shows blood clots forming in the heart. Ringing with authority, a deep voice proclaims, "This could be happening in *your* chest right now!" The solution—run out and "ask your doctor" about taking Plavix. As a consequence of this tactic and the huge volume of information on the Web, we have developed a new medical condition, cyberchondria—hypochondria fostered by too much time spent on medical websites. Search any symptom and you will wade through medical jargon and conflicting recommendations, encountering nightmare scenarios involving people who seemingly had exactly the same problem as you.

Susan Whelton, her family, and just about all of us—both heart patients and those who want to avoid becoming heart patients—need reliable information we can act on. The challenge of filling this gap created an opportunity to expand our definition of what it means to be a good doctor. It gave us a chance to move beyond fixing cardiac plumbing that is already broken to arming people with the critical information that will enable them to care for their hearts and perhaps avoid seeing us altogether.

We approached this project much the same way that we manage a patient with heart disease. Medical decision making should be evidence-based. When we treat a patient, we choose only those therapies that are supported by the scientific data. But such rigor is lacking in much of the medical content on the Internet or the overflowing shelves in the health section of your local bookstore. Weekly health headlines skim the surface of the medical ocean—take fish oil, pass on heart scans, throw away your aspirin—but what do the studies *really* say? What is the message for you and your heart? We decided to explore the science behind the headlines and to explain clearly but completely the evidence supporting our plan for your heart health.

WHY NOW?

The threat has never been more dire, the need for action never so urgent. After decades of progress, a new tidal wave of heart disease is building. Look around you. Fast food and supersized meals have replaced healthy choices and appropriate portions. Video games and iPods have edged out exercise as sources of entertainment. Smoking remains stubbornly entrenched, and our waistlines are expanding at an alarming rate. Today two-thirds of us are overweight or obese, and nearly everybody harbors one or more risk factors for heart disease.

The statistics concerning cardiovascular disease in general and heart disease in particular are staggering. Eighty-two million American adults have cardiovascular disease, a broad group of disorders that includes coronary heart disease, stroke, high blood pressure, heart failure, and cholesterol abnormalities. Each year, 800,000 Americans will have a new heart attack, while 500,000 will suffer a second (or third, or fourth) one. This amounts to a heart attack every twenty-five seconds. When we combine the two most serious cardiovascular problems—coronary heart disease and stroke—we find that these conditions account for one of every three deaths in the United States. If we could eliminate all forms of cardiovascular disease, life expectancy would increase by seven years. In comparison, eliminating cancer would add only three years.

When it comes to heart disease, ignorance and complacency are the enemies. Countless recent media reports reiterated an important but potentially misleading statistic from the American Heart Association: "From 1997 to 2007, the death rate from cardiovascular disease declined 27.8 percent." Good news, but how does that help the million-plus people who will have a heart attack this year and the 900,000 who will die from cardiovascular disease? We can be gratified by the progress, but we should not be satisfied. When we are operating on somebody's heart, we don't relax when we have merely slowed the bleeding. We keep working until we have it completely stopped.

People affected by heart disease come from all strata of society, from celebrities such as Robin Williams, Barbara Walters, David Letterman, and Bill Clinton to teachers, firefighters, athletes, and even heart doctors. It is the proverbial elephant in the living room: heart disease can attack anybody—young and old, male and female—and its prevention must begin early.

Therefore, one of our key initiatives addresses the causes of cardiovascular disease. Heart disease is not like breast cancer and prostate cancer, which often seem to strike unfairly and indiscriminately. We know what causes heart disease, and you do, too: high blood pressure, smoking, elevated cholesterol, diabetes, obesity, and family history. Except for family history, each of these factors is modifiable—meaning that to a very great extent, you can control it. Right now we are doing a poor job of managing our risk factors. Much of the problem stems from what seems to be our society's motto: eat more, exercise less.

This society-wide increase in cardiac risk factors is shifting the ground beneath us, preparing to create a tsunami of cardiovascular disease. The number of cardiovascular operations and procedures done annually—attempts to fix the plumbing damaged by our unhealthy lifestyles—has increased from 5.4 million to 6.8 million over the last decade. Our society can't afford to pay for this. The economy and health care budgets are buckling under the strain of a $167 billion annual price tag to treat cardiovascular disease and an additional $119 billion in lost productivity caused by the illness. If we don't make headway, these costs will triple by 2020, dragging down the economic well-being of every American.

The solutions are not all that complicated. We know how to prevent cardiovascular disease and better treat existing heart problems. The government cannot solve the problem with legislation, and your employer can't fix it by removing soda from the vending machines at work. Solutions must begin on an individual level—with you. Once you learn how to help yourself, you can rescue your family and friends from a future diminished by cardiovascular disease.

CARDIOVASCULAR DISEASE IN MUMMIES

Atherosclerosis, or hardening of the arteries, is pervasive today, but disease-causing, cholesterol-filled plaques have actually been around for a long, long time. Scientists recently reported the results of high-tech, whole-body CT scanning on twenty-two mummies in the Museum of Egyptian Antiquities in Cairo, Egypt. While the "patients" were not waiting for their test results, the medical community was curious. In fact, the results generated so much interest that they were reported in the *Journal of the American Medical Association*, a leading medical journal, and a few days later in the *New York Times*.

Of sixteen mummies who lived between 1981 BCE and 334 BCE, the CT scans showed that nine had either definite or probable atherosclerosis. The most ancient mummy with arterial disease was Lady Rai, nursemaid to Queen Nefertari, who died in approximately 1530 BCE. One of the study authors quipped, "She went in a relic. She came out a patient."

This intriguing study demonstrates that the history of cardiovascular disease extends thousands of years into the past. Our plan is to limit its impact on our future.

What if you have moved beyond the risk factor stage and already have coronary heart disease? We have critically important information for you, too. There is good news from the front lines for the millions of Americans who have existing cardiovascular problems. In addition to increasing our understanding of the risk factors for heart disease, our pills and procedures for diagnosing and treating it have never been better. But there is a catch—you must ensure that you receive the *right* treatments.

When it comes to medicines for high blood pressure and high cholesterol, strategies to open blocked arteries and urgent measures to manage heart attacks, the difference between an okay treatment and the best treatment can mean the difference between life and death. Coronary heart disease and its management are not mysterious. The obstacle faced by Susan Whelton and millions of others is simply their lack of good information. Which brings us back to our mission.

MAKING A PLAN

Whether you are young or old, male or female, already a parent or planning to start a family, you need to understand how to keep your heart and your family's hearts healthy. Our plan to ensure your heart health is simple. We will cover it all—from how factors such as cholesterol and genetics cause coronary heart disease to the role of high-tech procedures such as CT scans and even heart transplants. Explaining the science and the studies behind today's headlines, we will provide you with the tools you need to judge for yourself the next time the media report on "a startling new medical breakthrough." You will be able to distinguish fact from fiction and understand what the new information means for your health. Armed with the right information and sound, scientifically validated strategies, you, the intelligent and motivated reader, can grow from a passive patient into an active partner in your heart health.

CHAPTER 2

CORONARY HEART DISEASE: THE RISK FACTORS YOU KNOW AND THOSE YOU DON'T

THE BIG PICTURE

Coronary heart disease (also called coronary artery disease or coronary atherosclerosis) is characterized by cholesterol-filled plaques that block arteries and can cause chest pain (angina) or heart attacks. As with every medical condition, the development of coronary heart disease depends upon the presence of predisposing conditions or behaviors, known as risk factors. The more risk factors that you have, the greater the likelihood that you will end up in our office with chest pain or a heart attack. On the other hand, if you recognize these risk factors and reduce them as much as possible, you may never have to meet us professionally.

While some basic risk factors are beyond your control—advancing age, a family history of heart disease—others are completely up to you. Most people are aware of the usual suspects leading to coronary heart disease: high blood pressure, diabetes, obesity, tobacco use, lack of exercise, and abnormal cholesterol levels. Managing these risk factors can go a long way toward reducing your risk of developing heart disease.

In the last few years, scientists have extended our understanding of the genesis of heart disease. We now recognize a host of factors and conditions with previously unsuspected links to heart disease, including inflammatory diseases (such as rheumatoid arthritis), migraine headaches, and even living near a highway. In this chapter, we will look at heart disease from this wider perspective.

IT'S YOUR HEART, NOT YOUR ARTHRITIS

Sally Robinson was no stranger to doctors. Now fifty-one years old, she had been seeing her rheumatologist regularly for nearly thirty years, as he constantly adjusted Sally's medicines to treat the rheumatoid arthritis that threatened to take control of her life. For the most part, Dr. Frazier had been successful. Although constant low-grade knee pain made it hard to exercise, Sally could do almost anything she wanted and was only a few pounds overweight. Sally took her arthritis medicines religiously and suffered few side effects, although the steroids she needed to take caused slight elevations in her blood pressure and blood sugar.

One Sunday afternoon, Sally developed pain in her back and left shoulder, which she blamed on her arthritis. Although shoulder pain was new for Sally, she just increased her arthritis medications, which seemed to work. During the next week, the pain in the front of her left shoulder waxed and waned. By Friday, it was such a nuisance that she finally called Dr. Frazier, who gave her an appointment for the following Monday and advised her to take it easy over the weekend. When Dr. Frazier saw Sally, he pushed and prodded her shoulder but could not reproduce the pain. During his standard examination of Sally's lungs, Dr. Frazier suddenly grew serious. He told Sally that he wanted to get a chest X-ray to check things out, and walked her down the hallway to the radiology suite. Nervously, Sally watched as Dr. Frazier silently examined the chest X-ray and then asked his assistant to perform an EKG.

Dr. Frazier finally told Sally that he had heard "crackles" when listening to her lungs. These crackles, which sound like Rice Krispies when you pour in the milk, indicated a possible buildup of fluid in Sally's lungs, and the chest X-ray confirmed his suspicion. Although rheumatoid arthritis *can* cause lung problems, the combination of her left shoulder pain and the new lung findings pointed toward a problem with Sally's heart. Comparing her new EKG to a previous one done years earlier, Dr. Frazier saw changes indicating that Sally had suffered a heart attack, probably beginning at the onset of her left shoulder pain.

Sally was stunned. She believed that only older women, not those her age, developed heart disease. When Sally came to us to treat her heart problems, we told her that young women *can* develop heart disease, especially when they have risk factors. We explained that people with rheumatoid arthritis, which is characterized by whole-body inflammation, actually face an increased risk of coronary heart disease. Had Sally known this earlier, she might not have ignored her shoulder pain.

Fortunately, Sally's heart was not severely impaired. The damage was minor, and her cardiac catheterization showed that only a single small artery was blocked. She did not need surgery or stents—but she did require aggressive measures to manage her other risk factors, including her slightly elevated blood pressure and blood sugar and her extra weight. Today, Sally remains healthy and active, and neither her joints nor her heart slows her down.

HOW CORONARY HEART DISEASE BECAME OUR NUMBER ONE HEALTH PROBLEM

Coronary heart disease (CHD) currently looms as the greatest health threat to Americans. The rise of coronary heart disease to the top of our medical "to-do list" is relatively recent. In 1900, pneumonia was the leading cause of death in the United States, and the average life expectancy was only forty-seven. During the first half of the twentieth century, doctors and scientists focused on treating infectious diseases—for example, developing new drugs to cure pneumonia and virtually eradicate tuberculosis. These dramatic advances enabled people to live longer—and inadvertently opened the door to coronary heart disease.

By 1930, average life expectancy in America had risen to about sixty, and heart disease had become the number one cause of death. These statistics reflect an important feature of CHD: the incidence of the disease increases strikingly with age. Longer life means more time for arterial plaques to develop and cause problems. The risk of an eighty-five-year-old man having a heart attack is twenty-five times that of a forty-five-year-old.

Longer life does not by itself cause CHD, but the combination of longer life and damaging lifestyles increases the risk of developing coronary heart disease. Contemporary lifestyles have created a minefield of risk factors for CHD. Liberated from the grip of infectious diseases, too many of us fill our extra years of life with smoking, eating, and many excuses not to exercise.

THE BATTLE FOR YOUR ARTERIES' HEALTH: THE GENESIS OF CHD

Before we examine the risk factors for coronary heart disease, let's focus on your arteries and the mechanisms by which plaques form. The process begins with damage to the endothelium, a smooth, tile-like layer of specialized cells lining the inner walls of blood vessels through which blood flows on its way to our organs. More than simply a watertight seal to keep the blood inside the artery, the endothelial lining is biologically active, producing chemicals that prevent blood from clotting at its surface. In addition, the endothelium acts as a barrier to prevent toxic substances from entering the blood vessel's wall.

Many of the risk factors for CHD initiate and accelerate disease by damaging the endothelium. Smoking and air pollution increase levels of carbon monoxide and other toxic chemicals in the blood, triggering chemical reactions that assault and damage the endothelium. High blood pressure causes the blood to act like a battering ram, attacking and disrupting the endothelium.

Over the last few years, scientists have recognized that inflammation also damages endothelial cells and contributes to plaque formation. The term *inflammation* is derived from the Latin meaning "to set on fire." Inflammation is not always bad; it actually represents the body's normal response to injury and infection, and in the appropriate setting it restores health. But when it occurs inside blood vessels, inflammation can initiate plaque formation.

Regardless of the source of injury, when the endothelium is damaged, LDL cholesterol can breach its defenses and enter the artery wall. When LDL molecules oxidize—that is, when they combine with oxygen in the blood—they become particularly hazardous. (See page 45 to learn more about LDL cholesterol.) As oxidized LDL makes its way past the damaged endothelium and enters the artery wall, the body misinterprets the event and responds as it would to an infection, sending white blood cells called macrophages to the area. The macrophages ingest the oxidized LDL, which augments the inflammatory reaction and causes more damage to the endothelial lining. The cycle continues, and over time, the collection of white blood cells, cholesterol, and inflammatory proteins forms a large plaque within the artery wall.

Breaking this cycle by removing the sources of inflammation and endothelial damage allows the artery to heal, and we have the tools to make this happen. Statins can help by reducing the concentration of LDL, and they also inhibit inflammation. Treating high blood pressure prevents further damage to the endothelium. Quitting smoking lowers blood levels of carbon monoxide and other harmful chemicals, preventing these noxious substances from damaging the endothelium.

The battle for your arteries' health begins early in life. Plaques form in the walls of the coronary arteries over the years, initially causing no signs or symptoms to signal their presence. Although people rarely suffer heart attacks in their twenties and thirties, the plaques are already present. Autopsies performed on young soldiers who died during the Korean and Vietnam wars revealed early plaque buildup in many of their arteries. Similar studies by Cleveland Clinic physicians uncovered plaques in the coronary arteries of young trauma victims—by age thirty, more than half of them had measurable atherosclerotic plaques in their coronary arteries.

Does this mean that we should go looking for these early plaques in young people? Probably not. Detecting coronary plaques during their silent phase can be very difficult. Some physicians advocate a test known as calcium scanning to try to detect the early development of CHD, but there are many downsides to this procedure (including radiation exposure and false positive results), and we don't recommend it. Instead, we believe that the best approach is to gather intelligence by screening patients for the risk factors that cause CHD and then aggressively treating those risk factors to prevent the disease from developing or progressing.

Notice that many of the most important risk factors for coronary heart disease are modifiable, meaning they are under your control. Several recent studies suggest that up to 90 percent of CHD could be prevented by addressing these treatable risk factors! The most important modifiable risk factors are increased cholesterol, high blood pressure, smoking, diabetes, abdominal obesity, and absence of regular physical activity.

Risk Factors for Development of Coronary Heart Disease

RISK FACTOR	STRENGTH OF EVIDENCE FOR AN ASSOCIATION*	CAN YOU CHANGE IT?
The Usual Suspects		
Family history	++++	No
Advanced age	++++	No
High blood pressure	++++	Yes
Diabetes	++++	Yes[†]
Cholesterol/lipid abnormalities	++++	Yes
Tobacco use	++++	Yes
Obesity	+++	Yes
More Recently Identified Risk Factors		
Inflammatory diseases		
Rheumatoid arthritis	+++	No
Psoriasis	++	No
Lupus	++	No
Sleep apnea	++	Yes
Periodontal/gum disease	++	Yes
Air pollution	++	Yes
Emotional stress	++	Yes
Migraine headaches	+	No

*++++ Conclusive evidence

+++ Strong evidence

++ Moderate evidence

+ Weak evidence

[†] Type 2 diabetes can be treated with lifestyle changes in many patients

THE RISK FACTORS YOU KNOW

Cholesterol

We cover the problem of high cholesterol and its treatment thoroughly in Chapter 3. Although the science is complicated, the key message is clear:

a combination of diet and drugs can treat high cholesterol in nearly all affected individuals. Yet despite the wide range of effective options available, we still see many patients with a first heart attack who didn't know they had an elevated cholesterol level. Some of these individuals had a strong family history of premature CHD and yet chose not to have a cholesterol test. We cannot emphasize enough: you *must* know your cholesterol levels.

Every adult should have a cholesterol test (lipid panel) in his or her twenties. If this initial blood test reveals normal cholesterol levels, repeat it every five to ten years, because cholesterol tends to rise with age. Don't make the mistake of assuming that a normal lipid panel at age twenty-five comes with a fifty-year guarantee. On the other hand, we don't agree with those pediatricians who advocate cholesterol screening in all children. We prefer a selective and thoughtful approach, testing children only if they suffer from obesity or have a strong family history of early CHD. Finding a high cholesterol level in a child or young adult does not necessarily lead to drug therapy, but it should always serve as a wake-up call leading to significant lifestyle changes. Achieving normal cholesterol levels dramatically reduces the likelihood of a first heart attack or stroke.

When discussing cholesterol with our patients, we focus on LDL cholesterol. As you'll learn in Chapter 3, the lower the LDL, the lower the risk of heart attack and stroke. There is no threshold or LDL value that is too low: like the old adage that you can be never be too rich or too thin, you can never have too low an LDL. We also measure HDL, which is *inversely* related to the risk of CHD—that is, the higher your HDL, the lower your risk of heart disease. However, the relationship between CHD and low levels of HDL is not as strong as the relationship with high LDL levels. Finally, triglycerides appear to be weakly associated with an increased risk of CHD, but the relationship is controversial because people with high triglycerides also tend to have low HDL, making it difficult to prove that triglyceride levels are the actual culprit. Because of the weaker evidence for relationships between CHD and HDL or triglycerides, these lipids are considered secondary, not primary, targets for treatment.

Some doctors routinely order advanced cholesterol tests that measure the levels of apolipoprotein B (also called ApoB), a protein associated with LDL, and apolipoprotein A (or ApoA), a protein associated with HDL. While some suggest that these measurements help to determine the risk of developing CHD, we don't find them particularly useful in most people. Similarly, fancy tests that measure the size of LDL particles have become very popular, but they are expensive and add little to the risk factor picture.

If you know your LDL, HDL, and total cholesterol levels, you have most of the information you need to accurately assess your risk for CHD and track your treatment progress.

High Blood Pressure

High blood pressure (hypertension) is a powerful and modifiable risk factor for development of CHD. We divide hypertension into two categories: primary and secondary. More than 90 percent of patients have primary hypertension, which means that we cannot identify a specific medical cause for the increased blood pressure. In the early years of the twentieth century, physicians thought it was normal for blood pressure to rise with aging, but now we know they were wrong. Hypertension isn't a normal part of aging, and it can be deadly.

Secondary hypertension accounts for only 5–10 percent of cases, but it is very important because in these patients the elevated blood pressure is caused by some other medical disorder. Treating the underlying condition can return the blood pressure to normal. Certain hormonal imbalances can cause secondary hypertension, but kidney problems are the most common culprit. When atherosclerotic plaques narrow kidney arteries, reducing blood flow to the kidneys, these organs attempt to counteract it by releasing a hormone that triggers blood vessels to tighten, thereby raising blood pressure. For cases of blocked kidney arteries, stenting or surgery can dramatically lower blood pressure. Rarely the kidney itself is abnormal, rather than its artery; in such cases, surgical removal of the affected kidney may be necessary to control blood pressure.

If you have high blood pressure, do you need to worry that it might be caused by an uncommon kidney issue or a rare hormonal imbalance? Probably not. But if your blood pressure is very high and multiple medicines fail to control it, you and your doctor should consider blood tests and scans to look further.

What is a normal blood pressure? For many years, physicians were taught that anything lower than 160/90 mm Hg was acceptable. However, careful randomized clinical trials demonstrated that this threshold was too high, so doctors adopted 140/90 as the cutoff for normal blood pressure. Alas, they were wrong again, as new evidence suggested that 140/90 is still too high, leaving people at increased risk for heart attack and stroke. To arrive at the truth, scientists studied non-industrialized populations, where diets were low in salt and primarily vegetarian, and people were always active and not obese. Most of these people had a blood pressure less than 120/80, which remains our "normal" value today. If your blood pressure is between 120/80 and 140/90, you are considered prehypertensive. Although you probably don't need to begin taking blood-pressure-lowering medicines, you should lower your salt intake, follow a special diet (the DASH diet; see Chapter 5), and lose weight. With these steps, blood pressure often returns to normal.

The number of people with hypertension in developed countries is staggering and increases sharply as the population ages. According to the American Heart Association, more than 76 million Americans have high blood pressure. The rate of hypertension reaches 50 percent for individuals ages fifty-five to sixty-four, rising to more than 70 percent by age seventy-five. The incidence of hypertension is substantially higher in certain subgroups, especially African Americans and people with diabetes, indicating the need for closer vigilance. Hypertension has even reached our schools, where obese children are developing high blood pressure at alarming rates.

A key challenge to lessening the toll from hypertension is early recognition. Like high cholesterol levels, hypertension generally manifests no symptoms until it causes a major problem such as a heart attack or stroke. You should know your blood pressure and ensure that every member of your family has his or her blood pressure checked. We have excellent medicines and strategies to treat high blood pressure, but we are less effective at repairing the damage it can cause.

While the relationship between blood pressure and the risk of heart attack is strong, the link between high blood pressure and stroke risk is even more dramatic. In both cases, the systolic pressure (the top number) exerts the strongest impact on the risk. High-quality randomized trials show that a five-point reduction in systolic blood pressure can reduce heart attacks by 15 to 20 percent and strokes by 25 to 30 percent. Current guidelines suggest reducing blood pressure to less than 140/90 for most patients and less than 130/80 for diabetics. However, the exact target levels for systolic blood pressure remain controversial, because many studies do not show benefit from reducing blood pressure substantially below 140/90. Unlike LDL cholesterol, where there is no lower threshold for benefit (lower is always better), blood pressure reduction has a definite range in which benefit occurs. In fact, too low a blood pressure can actually harm certain patients. Fear of complications related to low blood pressure may be one explanation for the finding that physicians are frequently not aggressive enough, often

BLOOD PRESSURE AND THE BARBER

African American men have the highest death rate from hypertension of any group in the United States. Compared to a white man, an African American man faces a threefold increase in the risk of dying from hypertension. As scientists have examined this threatening situation, they have discovered that diagnosis and medical access are the key problems. This realization sent Texas researchers straight to the barbershop.

Because the barbershop presents a comfortable and nonthreatening environment, doctors reasoned that African American men might allow barbers to take their blood pressure and might follow their recommendations if the barbers informed them it was too high and a visit to the doctor was in order.

In a randomized, controlled clinical trial in seventeen black-owned barbershops in Dallas County, Texas, barbers were trained to take blood pressure readings, and screened their clients when they came in for a haircut. The barbers identified 1,300 men with hypertension. Half of the hypertensive men received pamphlets about blood pressure control while the other half received more intensive intervention, including blood pressure checks with every haircut and physician referrals when hypertension was detected.

The barbers did a great job. Average blood pressure fell in both groups, with a slightly larger decrease among those who had more intense screening and treatment. Next up: hairdressers for women.

tolerating unacceptably high blood pressure levels. The optimal blood pressure in the elderly remains controversial because overly aggressive lowering can cause adverse consequences.

Therapy for hypertension always starts with lifestyle modifications (reduced salt intake, exercise, and weight loss) but often progresses to drugs. For patients with severe hypertension (blood pressure greater than 160/100) many physicians will start with two drugs, because a single drug is unlikely to adequately lower blood pressure. You may not feel well when you start medical therapy, but don't be too quick to abandon your pills; as your body adjusts to a lower blood pressure, symptoms such as dizziness tend to resolve. And don't let yourself run out of your blood pressure medications. Suddenly stopping anti-hypertensive drugs can cause a sudden rebound in which blood pressure spikes to dangerous levels.

For patients with hypertension, purchasing an automated blood pressure cuff is a great investment. These simple instruments typically cost less than $100 and provide accurate blood pressure measurements. Always take your blood pressure in the same position (usually sitting) after a few minutes of relaxation. Keep a log of your blood pressure and share it with your doctor.

Diabetes

Diabetes mellitus is an important potentially modifiable risk factor for CHD, but reducing the influence of diabetes on heart disease is not always simple.

Insulin is needed by all the body's tissues to metabolize sugar (glucose). In type 1 diabetes (formerly known as juvenile diabetes), which accounts for about 10 percent of cases, specialized cells in the pancreas fail to produce enough insulin. This can lead to an abrupt rise in blood glucose levels, which can be fatal if not recognized and treated promptly. Although people with the far more common form known as type 2 diabetes (previously called adult-onset diabetes) do have elevated blood sugar levels, their problem is not inadequate insulin production. Rather, their problem is insulin resistance—the pancreas produces sufficient insulin, but the body's tissues do not respond properly, allowing sugar to build up in the bloodstream. Although the pancreas initially compensates by producing more insulin, eventually, blood sugar rises. The current obesity epidemic in the United States and other developed countries has produced a corresponding explosion of type 2 diabetes.

Patients with insulin resistance who have not yet exhausted the ability of the pancreas to respond (by making more insulin) are considered "prediabetic." Remarkably, if the causes of insulin resistance—obesity and a sedentary lifestyle—are recognized and corrected early enough, full-blown diabetes can be prevented. In one study, a program of intensive weight loss and increased physical activity reduced the incidence of type 2 diabetes by more than two-thirds, while the medication metformin reduced diabetes incidence by only about one-third. The earlier that weight loss is initiated, the more likely this strategy will prevent the development of type 2 diabetes. Even in patients who already have the disease, weight loss brings their blood glucose levels under better control and may enable them to reduce the amount of medication required or even eliminate the need for insulin injections. If recognized early, the equation for prevention of type 2 diabetes is clear:

Diabetes affects nearly every organ in the body, from the kidneys to the eyes to the heart. Patients with either type of diabetes are much more likely to develop coronary heart disease than their non-diabetic counterparts. The increase in CHD risk for diabetics depends upon the duration of the diabetes (longer is worse), with most studies indicating that long-term diabetics face an approximate doubling of the rate of CHD. Heart attack or stroke is the cause of death in approximately 65 percent of diabetics.

GASTRIC BYPASS CAN REVERSE DIABETES

Gastric bypass surgery is proven to cause substantial weight loss in extremely obese people. Now the International Diabetes Federation advocates this therapy for certain obese diabetics. When obese diabetic patients undergo gastric bypass surgery, blood sugar often begins to drop within hours to days of the operation, well before actual weight loss sets in. In some cases, patients requiring 100 units of insulin per day no longer require any insulin at all by the time of hospital discharge. While the precise mechanism for this rapid benefit is not completely clear, it appears to relate to changes in blood levels of certain chemicals produced by the intestine. This therapy shows promise, but physicians advise caution, favoring weight loss through lifestyle changes as the initial step to try to reverse type 2 diabetes.

How does diabetes cause or accelerate CHD? We don't yet completely understand the precise mechanisms, but we have identified several factors that play important roles. Patients with diabetes typically have lower levels of HDL and higher triglyceride levels than non-diabetics. In addition, as we discussed above, a very strong association exists between diabetes and hypertension. Diabetics also have increased blood levels of markers of inflammation, suggesting an important role for inflammation in their CHD.

It would be natural to assume that good control of blood sugar would lower the risk of CHD in diabetics, but it turns out that this is only a small part of the answer. We assess long-term blood sugar control by using a blood test called HbA1c (commonly called A1c), which measures how much of the blood's hemoglobin contains glucose. Normal HbA1c levels are less than 6 percent, and diabetes is usually defined as a level greater than 6.5 percent. There is a moderate relationship between the A1c level and the risk of developing coronary heart disease, but it's not nearly as strong as the relationships for other common risk factors, such as LDL cholesterol or high blood pressure. Lowering blood sugar levels only modestly reduces the risk of CHD. But good glucose control is still very important, because it reduces the risk of other diabetic complications such as kidney failure, nerve damage, and blindness.

If controlling blood sugar is not the key to CHD prevention in diabetics, what are the most effective strategies? High-quality trials demonstrate that blood pressure control has a dramatic effect on rates of CHD in diabetics. In fact, the national guidelines for hypertension set a more aggressive target for blood pressure levels in diabetics (130/80) compared with nondiabetics (140/90). Use of statins to lower LDL cholesterol also confers substantial benefit in diabetics, even when they have normal LDL levels. Therefore, many practitioners believe that *all* patients with diabetes, regardless of cholesterol level, should take a statin.

Despite all our knowledge and corresponding treatment targets, study after study demonstrates that most diabetics don't achieve optimal LDL, blood pressure, and glucose levels. Know your goals and partner closely with your doctor to achieve these targets. For most people with diabetes, these are reasonable targets:

• LDL cholesterol	100 mg/dL or less
• Blood pressure	Lower than 130/80
• A1c	7.0–7.5 percent or lower

Smoking

Despite more than fifty years of warnings, smoking remains a depressingly common cause of CHD. Make no mistake: people who smoke double their risk of developing coronary heart disease and cut their life expectancy by an average of eight to eleven years. Smoking exhibits a dose-response effect: the more cigarettes you smoke and the more years you smoke, the greater your risk.

Smoking causes heart disease by multiple mechanisms, but the most important factor appears to be damage to the endothelium that lines the insides of our arteries. Remember, endothelial cells protect against the entry of cholesterol into the blood vessel wall. Carbon monoxide and other chemicals in tobacco smoke damage the endothelium, breaking the barrier and enabling plaque-forming oxidized LDL to penetrate the arteries. The effect of tobacco is so powerful that even exposure to secondhand smoke by living or working near a smoker elevates the risk of developing CHD. And don't fool yourself into thinking that smokeless tobacco represents a safe alternative; it too increases the risk of coronary heart disease.

Despite these well-known risks, 50 million American adults (21 percent of the population) continue to smoke. These sorry statistics actually represent progress. The number of smokers increased dramatically during and immediately after World War II, reaching a peak of 42 percent of the population in 1965. We have cut the percentage of smokers in half, but we still have a long way to go.

People continue to smoke, despite extensive health warnings and graphic images of what smoking can do, because nicotine is addictive. Within seconds of taking a drag on a cigarette, nicotine reaches the smoker's brain, triggering a cascade of chemical reactions that produce relaxation and euphoria. Addiction experts place nicotine's addictive strength in the same class as illicit drugs such as cocaine and heroin. As with those drugs, addiction has economic implications, meaning that there is money to be made from selling it. Consequently, tobacco companies have a history of manipulating the nicotine content of cigarettes to promote and maintain addiction.

We see the powerful and tragic effects of tobacco addiction in our daily practice. Almost every cardiologist has had some version of this poignant exchange when interviewing a patient the day after a heart attack:

> *Physician:* "Do you smoke?"
> PATIENT: "No."
>
> *Physician:* "Did you ever smoke?"
> PATIENT: "Yes."
>
> *Physician:* "When did you quit?"
> PATIENT: "Last night."

With the crushing pain and terror of the heart attack fresh in his memory, the patient has decided to quit, convincing himself that he is no longer a smoker. But in many cases, this situation changes shortly after hospital discharge. We see many patients who resume smoking soon after returning home from a hospital stay, even after suffering a heart attack or undergoing heart surgery. You might expect that someone who has just experienced the discomfort and stress of open heart surgery would be scared straight, frightened by the very idea of resuming smoking. Unfortunately, the power of the addiction drives people to light up "just one more" cigarette. We do our best to help them understand that the stakes are high, while the benefits of quitting are real and occur quickly.

The cardiac damage caused by smoking does not need to be permanent. Remarkably, the risk of developing coronary heart disease in smokers declines quickly once a patient stops smoking. About half of the excess CHD risk disappears within one year of quitting, and the risk continues to fall over time; after ten years of tobacco abstinence, the ex-smoker has a risk virtually identical to that of a non-smoker. However, as any former (or trying-to-be-former) smoker will tell you, quitting is extremely difficult. As Mark Twain said, "Quitting smoking is easy. I've done it hundreds of times."

Today's smoker has more options available to help than did Twain. While we recognize that people are different and no single strategy works for everyone, one strategy is nearly always doomed to failure: resolving to cut down gradually. Studies demonstrate that nearly all smokers can relatively easily reduce the number of cigarettes they consume, and at first blush that finding sounds promising. However, when measuring the urine concentration of nicotine breakdown products, scientists found that they actually remain constant in patients even as they reduce their cigarette consumption. How can this be? The question was answered when researchers realized that smokers who cut down on the number of cigarettes they smoked actually worked harder to get more out of each one: they inhaled more deeply, held the smoke in their lungs longer, and smoked more of the length of each cigarette, unconsciously maximizing their nicotine intake from each cigarette.

Many people need a little pharmacologic help to quit smoking, and we think that is just fine. Nicotine replacement therapy using gum or skin patches significantly increases your chances of quitting. Once you stop smoking, it is usually not too difficult to gradually reduce the use of the nicotine gum or patches. A new drug called varenicline (Chantix) also helps some patients. With chemical effects similar to those of nicotine, varenicline reduces the craving for cigarettes. Studies confirm its effectiveness at helping motivated patients to quit. However, the drug is controversial because it causes some patients to experience serious psychological side effects, including anxiety, anger, and suicidal thoughts. The antidepressant bupropion, rebranded as a smoking cessation drug (Zyban), also helps some patients quit. However, bupropion can increase blood pressure and may also cause behavioral changes and, rarely, seizures. Regardless of whether or not you use these drugs or therapies to help yourself quit, it is essential that you keep trying. Successful quitters often report many failed attempts before achieving long-term success.

Obesity and Its Friends: Metabolic Syndrome

While daily news reports warn that obesity (particularly abdominal obesity) is the single most important modifiable risk factor for CHD, the real threat probably comes from the bad company that obesity keeps. People with abdominal obesity frequently develop a constellation of risk factors that includes high blood pressure, low HDL cholesterol, elevated triglycerides, diabetes, and increased waist circumference. If a person has three or more of these risk factors in tandem, he or she is said to have metabolic syndrome. This is a controversial subject among physicians, with some doctors claiming that it is nothing more than a cluster of individual risk factors. Other doctors contend that these factors are synergistic in their impact on the development of coronary heart disease, meaning that their combination poses a greater threat to the patient than the sum of the individual conditions.

Why should increased waist circumference be a criterion for metabolic syndrome? Isn't all fat equally bad? When it comes to obesity, most scientific data show differences in health risks for patients with the "apple" and "pear" body shapes. People who carry their extra weight around the stomach (apple shape) face a greater risk of developing heart disease than do those people with large buttocks and thighs (pear shape). Although some new studies have cast doubt on this distinction, asserting that all body fat, no matter where it is distributed, is equally dangerous, we believe that such a distinction exists. Fat cells that accumulate in the abdomen are metabolically more active than those in other parts of the body, causing insulin resistance (the hallmark of type 2 diabetes) and producing substances that increase inflammation. This explains why women with large thighs (a pear shape) but not a particularly large waistline are not as likely to develop CHD as women with an apple shape. To their misfortune, men tend to gain weight in their abdomen, the pattern more strongly associated with CHD.

If you carry excess pounds—no matter where they reside—we urge you to follow a sensible weight loss plan. Most fad diets don't work in the long term. A program of moderate calorie restriction coupled with exercise remains the best strategy for sustained weight loss.

Age

Although you can modify most of the classic CHD risk factors, you can't turn back the clock and change your age. The incidence of coronary heart disease increases with age. As we noted earlier, heart attacks rarely occur in men younger than thirty-five or women younger than forty-five. For both genders, heart risk increases steeply with age, but women have a lower overall incidence of heart disease than do men—that is, until menopause, after which they slowly catch up with their male counterparts. You don't need a blood test or the latest scan to assess this risk factor. Keep your heart healthy at all ages, and be especially vigilant as you reach middle age.

Family History

Family history remains one of the most important non-modifiable factors to assess your risk of developing coronary heart disease. If either of your parents or a sibling developed CHD before age fifty-five, your risk of CHD is increased approximately one and a half to two times. This increased risk associated with family history is independent of other risk factors, such as smoking, diabetes, cholesterol, or hypertension.

The precise link between family history and CHD is a subject of intense scientific investigation. There is no single "heart disease gene," although many genes appear to contribute to its development. If you have a strong family history of CHD, stay tuned, as we may someday have a genetic test that screens for the genes that contribute to CHD.

Our advice for individuals with a strong family history of heart disease is always the same: do everything possible to reduce the risk factors that you *can* modify. We recommend more aggressive preventive treatment in patients with a strong family history—for example, favoring the use of statins in patients who might otherwise be considered borderline candidates for cholesterol-lowering treatments. With vigilance and proper management, a family history of heart disease is not a death sentence. While there may not be anything you can do about the red hair or freckles you inherited from your father's side of the family, you *can* significantly alter your prognosis for heart health.

THE NEW KIDS ON THE BLOCK: RISK FACTORS YOU MAY NOT KNOW

Rheumatoid Arthritis and Coronary Heart Disease

We know that inflammation contributes to the development of artery-blocking plaque. Therefore, we are not surprised that scientists have established links between a variety of inflammatory diseases and coronary heart disease, including rheumatoid arthritis, psoriasis, inflammatory bowel disease, certain muscle disorders, and systemic lupus erythematosus. Of these, we have the strongest evidence supporting and explaining the association between rheumatoid arthritis and coronary heart disease.

Rheumatoid arthritis develops when the body makes a mistake and the immune system attacks the joints and surrounding tissues, causing inflammation, pain, and limited mobility. The disease usually strikes people over forty, and women are affected more often than men. More than 1 million Americans currently suffer from rheumatoid arthritis. Although these patients and their doctors focus on the complex medical management of their painful joints, they must not forget their hearts.

Like Sally Robinson, whom you met earlier in this chapter, people with rheumatoid arthritis face an increased risk of cardiovascular disease, including strokes and heart attacks. While scientists used to think that this risk became apparent only after years of fighting the disease, new research shows that increased heart and cardiovascular problems occur early: the risk of heart attack increases by 50 percent within one year of the diagnosis of rheumatoid arthritis. Because people often develop rheumatoid arthritis in their forties, cardiac vigilance must start early.

How do rheumatoid arthritis and other inflammatory conditions affect heart health? We don't know the precise mechanisms, but the link between inflammation and blood vessel damage is strong. The inflammation associated with rheumatoid arthritis causes the release of proteins and activated cells into the blood; these can damage the inner lining of arteries and contribute to plaque formation.

What should the person with rheumatoid arthritis do about her heart?

We have two concrete steps to take: manage your other cardiac risk factors and be vigilant about any indicators of potential heart problems. Johns Hopkins researchers have suggested that the increased risk of heart problems is greatest in those patients who have both rheumatoid arthritis *and* traditional risk factors. Don't let yourself gain weight. Put down the salt-shaker. Don't smoke. Take your statin as prescribed. Ask your physical therapist for an exercise program compatible with your joints and your heart. And if you do develop symptoms that could be from your heart—pain in the chest, shoulder, neck, or back, shortness of breath, new fatigue—don't assume it's your arthritis.

Brush Your Teeth

Dentists (and parents) remind us to brush and floss at least twice a day. A clean mouth is a healthy mouth. If you take care of your teeth, you can avoid the high-pitched whine of the dental drill. But if you listen to your dentist, you'll enjoy an additional benefit—good dental hygiene may also help keep you out of our cardiac catheterization laboratory and operating room.

Large observational studies suggest that inflammation and infection of the gums increase the risk of developing coronary heart disease by 20 to 40 percent. About 25 percent of Americans have some periodontal (gum) disease, while 1 percent, or 3 million people, have severe inflammation and infection of the gums. As with most cardiac risk factors, the worse the gum disease, the greater the cardiac toll. In one widely publicized observational study, people who rarely or never brushed their teeth faced a 70 percent increase in their risk of suffering a heart attack or other serious cardiac event over an eight-year period. We suspect they also had really bad breath.

As with rheumatoid arthritis, inflammation is the likely link between gum disease and arterial disease. Gum disease is actually the most common chronic inflammatory condition in the world. In an interesting study using positron emission tomography scans to detect inflammation, Harvard researchers found that when the mouth "lit up" on the scan, the carotid arteries in the neck were also affected, indicating simultaneous inflammation in both parts of the body. Studies also demonstrate that people with periodontal disease have elevated blood levels of C-reactive protein, an indicator of inflammation linked to coronary heart disease. Perhaps as a consequence of inflammation, patients with gum disease display other unfavorable cardiac characteristics, including abnormal function of arteries and an increased tendency for blood to clot.

In addition to increasing inflammation, periodontal disease tends to "travel" with other conventional risk factors. People with poor dental hygiene often smoke cigarettes, eat junk food, and avoid exercise. In such patients, gum problems are just one part of the heart-attack-causing package. Of course, fixing these unfavorable behaviors enhances heart health. But can you help your arteries simply through better dental hygiene?

A preliminary report published in the *New England Journal of Medicine* answers yes to this question. In that study, 120 patients with periodontitis were randomly assigned to receive either usual or intensive gum care. Patients in both groups ended the six-month study with better oral hygiene and reduced inflammation in their bodies, but only those receiving intensive treatment enjoyed the added benefit of improved blood vessel function. The study's message is intriguing: treating gum disease may have a positive influence on your arteries.

Still, some scientists argue that we have not firmly established causality. Proof of a cause-and-effect relationship would require a study in which we randomly assigned people to twice-daily brushing and flossing or to no dental hygiene or care for a year or more. We don't think we would find too many people who would be anxious to sign up for this study, which also raises serious ethical issues. Based upon the data that we have right now, we think that the evidence is strong enough to follow the American Heart Association's recommendation: don't smoke, eat right, and brush your teeth. And while you are in the bathroom, don't forget to floss!

Hold Your Breath: Air Pollution and Your Heart

Scientists first recognized the health risks of air pollution in the 1930s. Exhaust produced by cars and factories contains hundreds of potentially harmful substances. Most people fear that air pollution will hurt their lungs, but it turns out that their hearts also face an increased risk.

Fossil fuel combustion from traffic, industry, and power generation releases particles of different sizes into the air. The smallest among them—tiny, invisible particles less than 2.5 microns in diameter, just a fraction of the width of a human hair—seem to pose a cardiovascular risk. Observational studies have suggested an association between high concentrations of these particles and unfavorable cardiovascular changes.

IS GOING TO THE DENTIST *RISKY* FOR YOUR HEART?

Most of us don't like going to the dentist, and a recent report published in the *Annals of Internal Medicine* claims that invasive treatments for gum disease actually increase the risks of heart attack and stroke. Analyzing records of 32,000 Medicaid patients, researchers identified a weak linkage between cardiovascular events and having had a dental procedure in the preceding four weeks. They suggested that the temporary inflammation associated with the dental procedures could explain the association. Previous studies confirm that dental work causes a brief inflammatory response. In theory, this response could cause a tiny, brief increase in the risk of cardiovascular problems. But the long-term benefits of good dental hygiene far outweigh this short-term effect.

A second possible culprit that might connect dental procedures to heart problems is the common practice of stopping aspirin before dental procedures. In patients with preexisting cardiovascular disease, interrupting aspirin therapy could increase the risks of heart attack and stroke.

A trip to the dentist does pose a potential risk for certain heart valve patients. During dental procedures—whether a simple cleaning or a complex root canal—bacteria enter the bloodstream. These bacteria have a tendency to infect artificial heart valves. A single dose of prophylactic antibiotics before the procedure can prevent this devastating complication in people who've had heart valve surgery.

What should you do if you are a heart patient and you need dental work? Tell your dentist if you have undergone heart valve surgery so that you can receive an antibiotic. If you take aspirin, don't stop taking it without asking your doctor first. But don't let unsubstantiated fears of cardiovascular harm cause you to avoid a needed visit to the dentist. In the long run, it will be good for your smile *and* good for your heart.

Los Angeles residents who live within 100 yards of a highway tend to have abnormal arteries compared to those with homes farther away. On the other side of the country, Bostonians who live closer to highways are more likely to have significant coronary heart disease than those who reside near smaller roads. In a study using air quality data from the Environmental Protection Agency, scientists correlated poor air quality with a 10 percent increase in the risk of cardiac arrest in New York City. Other observational studies suggest that the fumes (and possibly the frustration) of a rush hour traffic jam trigger 7 percent of all heart attacks.

NOISE POLLUTION

We can't sense the tiny particles in the air that enter our lungs and assault our arteries. But we can certainly hear loud and often irritating noises transmitted through the air as sound waves. Recent observational studies suggest that like air pollution, noise pollution may have adverse cardiovascular consequences for some people.

While living near a highway produces multiple cardiovascular challenges, including particulate air pollution, clusters of fast-food restaurants, and a paucity of parks and places for outdoor exercise, a Danish observational study adds traffic noise to this list of risk factors, suggesting that the louder the traffic, the greater the risk of stroke. Along similar lines, studies from England and Switzerland correlate living under an airplane flight path with an increased risk of dying from a heart attack. Analogously, people who work in noisy environments such as factories are more likely to suffer from cardiovascular problems than people with quiet workplaces.

In the United States, 22 million people work in environments with a potentially dangerous noise level. Does this noise predispose them to cardiovascular disease? We don't know for sure, but we suspect that any excessive cardiovascular risk associated with noise is modest. Concurring with this conclusion, Canadian researcher Hugh Davies stated, "If this [noise] affects you, you could think about moving somewhere quieter. But you'd probably find equal heart benefit if you stopped smoking, ate a healthier diet, or exercised more."

How do tiny particles entering the lungs exert an effect upon the heart? As is the case with many of these unconventional risk factors, scientists have not yet pieced together the entire puzzle. Some believe that the particles are so small that they actually cross from the airways to the bloodstream, which then carries them to the heart's arteries, where they can cause damage. Experimental evidence supports the direct effects of air pollution on the cardiovascular system. Animal studies demonstrate that exposure to fine particulate air pollution can both initiate and accelerate atherosclerosis. It increases blood pressure, constricts blood vessels, and diminishes blood vessel function in addition to increasing blood clotting and inflammation and contributing to the development of abnormal heart rhythms.

In a given individual, the increased cardiovascular risk posed by air

PLASTIC, BPA, AND YOUR HEART

A 2008 publication in the *Journal of the American Medical Association* worried doctors and stunned consumers with its conclusion that bisphenol-A, or BPA, is linked to heart disease. A ubiquitous component of polycarbonate plastic items such as baby bottles, food packaging, and the lining of food cans, BPA can contaminate the food stored in these containers.

Health experts and the FDA have long recognized potential neurologic toxicity from BPA exposure in babies. A published report extended this concern, suggesting that higher levels of BPA exposure in adults increase the risk of developing cardiovascular disease. A 2010 update of the study suggested a similar association.

While the media created a sensation from these reports, the scientific evidence that BPA actually causes heart disease is relatively weak. It's impossible to avoid BPA completely, but if you are worried, you can limit your exposure with a few simple steps:

- Avoid plastic containers with the number seven in the recycling symbol on the bottom, as these are most likely to contain BPA.
- Don't microwave polycarbonate plastic food containers.
- Avoid canned foods.

pollution is actually quite small: exposure to severe air pollution increases the odds of having a heart attack by less than 5 percent (by comparison, cocaine use increases the risk 230 percent). But when we consider the enormous number of people who regularly inhale polluted air, the overall impact is potentially huge. Taking all of the health consequences into consideration, the World Health Organization estimates that air pollution contributes to 800,000 premature deaths per year, making it the thirteenth-leading cause of worldwide mortality.

We agree with the American Heart Association's conclusion that fine particulate matter may be a modifiable risk factor that can contribute to cardiovascular disease. What can you do about it? If possible, try not to travel during rush hour. You can determine your local air quality by visiting the website www.airnow.gov: when the air quality index for particulate matter is in the unhealthy range, limit your outdoor activity, and try to schedule your outdoor workouts away from rush hour traffic.

FIREPLACES AND WOOD-BURNING STOVES

When considering air pollution and heart health, we focus on fossil fuel combustion by cars and factories. But could your fireplace or wood-burning stove pose a similar risk? It may, but the magnitude of this potential risk is small.

Smoke produced by a fireplace or wood-burning stove causes measurable changes in blood vessel function and inflammation. While we don't have conclusive evidence that these changes are severe enough to lead to heart disease, they are similar to the changes that we see with regular air pollution. But there is an important difference between these two scenarios. While you can't clean the air of New York City, you *can* treat the air in your home.

A standard HEPA filter removes about two-thirds of the particles produced by wood-burning stoves, reducing the negative impact on your blood vessels. You don't have to give up the comfort of curling up in front of the fireplace with a good book on a winter night, but first make sure that the flue is working properly, and consider using an air filter to ensure that you enjoy the warmth without stressing your heart.

Get a Good Night's Sleep: Rest for the Heart

Over the last fifty years, the average American's nightly sleep has been cut by two hours. More and more of us have problems getting to sleep and staying asleep. Scientists estimate that 50 million to 75 million Americans suffer from a chronic sleep disorder. The consequences of this problem may extend beyond daytime fatigue and grouchiness. Sleep disturbances are associated with heart problems.

The links between sleep and heart health occur on many levels, ranging from the quantity and quality of sleep to the cardiovascular impact of obstructive sleep apnea, a potentially serious medical condition that affects about 10 percent of adults, though it is more common in men. In obstructive sleep apnea, periods of sleep are interrupted when the muscles of the throat and airway relax enough to narrow or even block the upper airway. The person struggles to draw a breath through the narrowed airway, and breathing temporarily halts (apnea). He gasps, draws a breath, and awakens briefly, although he usually has no memory of the incident. Over the course of the night, the pattern can repeat itself dozens of times.

Ultimately, the patient awakens feeling exhausted, unaware that he or she has actually had disturbed sleep during the night.

Fatigue is not the only consequence of the condition. Periods of airway obstruction are stressful and can cause increases in blood pressure (up to 240 systolic). Although individual episodes are short-lived, their cumulative effects can be long-lasting: insulin resistance, susceptibility to abnormal heart rhythms, increased blood clotting, and inflammation. People with obstructive sleep apnea appear to face increased risks of coronary heart disease, heart attack, stroke, high blood pressure, and arrhythmias.

A medical sleep study can confirm the diagnosis, allowing for successful treatment of the problem. Many people with obstructive sleep apnea are overweight; in such cases, weight loss can make the problem disappear with the pounds. Avoiding alcohol and sedatives near bedtime also helps. Continuous positive airway pressure (CPAP) delivered via a tight-fitting mask eliminates the episodes of apnea in most people. In a randomized controlled trial of heart failure patients with obstructive sleep apnea, CPAP produced cardiovascular benefits including reduced blood pressure, lower heart rate, and stabilization of heart rhythm; other studies demonstrate that CPAP can improve heart function in these patients. The take-home message here: if you are tired all the time and snore loudly, see a specialist. Treatment of obstructive sleep apnea will make you feel better during the day and may provide welcome relief to your cardiovascular system (not to mention to your spouse).

In the absence of obstructive sleep apnea, how much nightly sleep does your heart need to stay healthy? The answer probably varies from person to person. A normal night's sleep varies widely but averages approximately seven and a half hours. We all know people who appear to function well on five hours a night, while others require nine hours in order to feel good. How does your heart "feel" about this? Observational studies suggest that people with a poor quality of sleep as well as people with inadequate sleep duration may face an increased risk of coronary heart disease. Those who sleep six hours per night or less appear particularly vulnerable to coronary heart disease. Other studies suggest a similar effect in people who spend more than eight hours per night in bed. And those people who work the night shift or rotating shifts that alter normal sleep patterns exhibit changes in blood pressure and blood sugar that can adversely influence cardiovascular health.

People who don't get enough sleep are prone to excess inflammation, and they tend to accumulate other cardiovascular risk factors, including obesity and diabetes. Short sleep reduces the production of hormones that suppress appetite, and this may contribute to weight gain. These associations may explain the increased burden of cardiovascular disease in short sleepers. (Another possible explanation for heart disease in long sleepers: they may stay in bed for more hours because they are already unwell.)

When it comes to monitoring your sleep, make sure that you don't have sleep apnea and do your best to get enough sleep, which should be no less than seven hours per night for most of us. Ask yourself two questions: Do you feel tired during the day? Do you snore loudly? If the answer to both questions is yes, ask your doctor to evaluate you for sleep apnea. Meanwhile, take standard measures to improve your sleep, including avoiding caffeinated drinks near bedtime, limiting alcohol, and finding time to exercise during the day. Also, turn off the computer, cell phone, BlackBerry, and television at least half an hour before going to sleep—studies have shown that the mental stimulation from these devices makes it harder to fall asleep and stay asleep. By taking these steps, you'll feel better, sleep better, and be doing your heart a favor.

RELAX IN THE HOT TUB OR SAUNA

Next to almost every hot tub or sauna you see a sign that reads, "Hot tubs and saunas may pose a risk to heart patients" or "If you are a heart patient, consult with your doctor before using a hot tub or sauna." Unless your doctor is with you at that moment, you are going to have trouble getting a permission slip from her. But you can get it from us.

Staying in a hot tub or sauna for too long can certainly cause severe dehydration and dangerous fluid and electrolyte problems. But a ten-minute session in the hot tub or sauna will not hurt you or your heart. Hot tubs and saunas do not cause heart attacks or heart problems or interfere with cardiac pacemakers. As you enter the sauna or immerse yourself in the hot tub, blood vessels near the skin dilate (enlarge), causing a slight drop in blood pressure; this is rarely dangerous. You can minimize the impact of this blood pressure change by getting in and out slowly, which gives your body a moment to adjust to the temperature change. Be careful as you approach the hot tub or sauna: your greatest risk is slipping on the wet tile as you get in or out. Watch your feet, but don't worry about your heart.

The Monday Morning Heart Attack

We all have internal clocks, or circadian rhythms, that direct many of our body's processes. These can exert important influences on cardiovascular function and cardiovascular risk.

Cardiac-wise, mornings are the worst time of day. Heart attacks, strokes, and blood clots in coronary artery stents occur most often in the morning. Many scientists blame this on variations in blood pressure, which tends to drop as you sleep and then increase upon awakening, reaching its highest level at midmorning. The high blood pressure associated with this time of day batters away at plaques in coronary arteries, increasing the chances the plaques will rupture and trigger a heart attack. In the mornings we also have an increased heart rate (which increases the heart's workload), increased blood viscosity (thickness) related to overnight dehydration, and an increased tendency for blood to clot. Together, these changes increase the potential for a heart attack.

Morning heart attacks tend to be large. A team of Spanish researchers recently reported that heart attacks occurring between 6:00 a.m. and noon caused 20 percent more heart damage than those that struck later in the day. The heart patient who likes to exercise first thing in the morning may face particular risk. If you exercise in the morning, hydrate yourself before beginning your workout, and give yourself a slow warm-up to prepare your heart for the stress of exercise.

If mornings are the most dangerous time of day, Monday mornings are the most dangerous time of the week. Doctors have long noted what they call "Monday morning heart attack syndrome," having observed that the risk of heart attack is increased by 20 percent on Monday. What's the problem with Mondays? Poor sleep is probably a factor. Many people sleep in over the weekend, which makes it difficult for them to fall asleep Sunday night; they begin their week with a short and restless sleep. And then there's work. Stresses associated with returning to work can exacerbate the normal morning increases in blood pressure and heart rate, adding to the load on the heart. Don't succumb to temptation and sleep in until noon on Sunday; if you get up at a reasonable hour, you'll be able to go to sleep at your usual time.

Emotion and the Heart

In Chapter 8 we provide an in-depth analysis of the fascinating and complex links between emotions, stress, and your heart. Depression, anxiety, and anger are associated with the development of coronary heart disease. Although the exact cause-and-effect mechanism is not yet established, strong emotions (such as intense anger) and stressful situations can trigger heart attacks in susceptible individuals. Scientists are just beginning to produce data suggesting that stress reduction techniques such as yoga, cognitive behavioral therapy, and even transcendental meditation can ease cardiovascular problems in some heart patients. Exercise also reduces stress, while improving traditional cardiac risk factors. Managing your emotional health is an important component of your personal cardiac program.

Headache and Heartache:
Migraines and the Heart

Recently there has been great media interest in scientific studies reporting a potential link between migraine headaches and heart disease. Because abnormal blood vessel function is one cause of migraine headaches, an association between migraines and other cardiovascular issues seems plausible. For the 28 million Americans who suffer from migraines, this is a critically important issue. Do they need to worry about heart attacks and strokes, too?

A recent observational study of nearly 20,000 people from Iceland sought to answer this question. Researchers found that compared to people without migraines, over a twenty-five-year period people who suffered migraines with aura had modest increases in their risks of dying from coronary heart disease or stroke. (Migraine with aura refers to migraine headaches preceded by visual or other sensory symptoms, which can include flashing lights, blind spots and tunnel vision.) Based upon their observations, the study authors concluded that migraine with aura is a possible marker for cardiovascular mortality, but it is weaker than other established risk factors such as high blood pressure, smoking, and diabetes.

At this point, we don't know if successful treatment of the symptoms of migraines reduces the cardiovascular risk associated with them. Therefore, our cardiac message for migraine sufferers is to focus on the usual suspects in order to ensure your heart health.

EDUCATION, MONEY, AND YOUR HEART

Health behaviors and cardiovascular outcomes are linked to education, social status, and money. Studies examining the impact of education find that the longer you stay in school, the better your cardiovascular health. Specifically, higher levels of education—from high school to college and beyond—correlate with reduced risks of diabetes, high blood pressure, and heart disease. On average, the person who attended graduate school has a blood pressure that is three points lower than that of the high school dropout. Studies suggest that the link between higher educational attainment and a healthy cardiovascular system is a healthier lifestyle.

Like education, income and social standing correlate with heart health. Across the United States and around the world, the poorest people have the greatest risk of cardiovascular disease. Those engaged in manual trades have a fourfold increase in the risk of dying from heart disease when compared to management. Once again, behaviors explain the gap. Exercise, a good diet, and general health consciousness tend to be more prevalent among managers and administrators. The solution is not to aim for advancement at work in order to protect your heart; rather, adopt the right behaviors as you climb the corporate ladder, so that you reach the top with a healthy heart.

RX: CORONARY HEART DISEASE RISK FACTORS

Manage the usual suspects:

Cholesterol

High blood pressure

Diabetes

Smoking

Obesity

Recognize additional risk factors:

Inflammatory diseases (rheumatoid arthritis, psoriasis, lupus)

Gum disease

Air pollution

Sleep apnea

Emotional stress

Migraine

CHAPTER 3

CHOLESTEROL: FRIEND *AND* FOE

THE BIG PICTURE

Everybody knows of the link between cholesterol and coronary heart disease, and scientists have spent decades studying this relationship. New discoveries have changed our thinking and our recommendations concerning cholesterol and heart health. In this chapter we will address the critical questions, including: What are the right cholesterol numbers? Which is more important, total cholesterol or LDL? Does a high level of HDL (good) cholesterol make up for a high level of LDL (bad) cholesterol? How important is diet in determining cholesterol levels? Can medicines fix the problem—or, put another way, does a statin pill cancel out the effect of a Big Mac? While scientists argue about the fine points, we do have some big-picture answers. For your heart's sake, you need to know your cholesterol levels, what they mean, and how to change them if they spell danger.

CHOLESTEROL: ALL IN THE FAMILY

Several years ago, a colleague stopped by our office to discuss a patient who had him stumped. Irene Robins was only thirty-eight years old, but she had already suffered a heart attack (at age thirty-three) and undergone bypass surgery (at age thirty-six). Our colleague was concerned because he could not get her cholesterol down, and he was worried about the continuing impact of her elevated cholesterol on her heart. We always like a good medical challenge, so we looked forward to tackling this one. Reviewing her records before her appointment, we well understood our colleague's concern. Although she was taking the maximum daily dosage of atorvastatin (Lipitor), Irene's total cholesterol hovered at 230 mg/dL, with an LDL cholesterol of 162—way too high.

Irene's threatening numbers signaled an ongoing assault on her arteries. In high-risk patients such as Irene, we want to reduce LDL to a value of less than 70. What could we do to get her LDL into the right range? Part of the problem was that Irene's high LDL was not caused by the usual suspects—too many french fries paired with too little exercise. In Irene's case, her genes were to blame. Like 1 out of every 500 Americans, she had an inherited form of high cholesterol known as familial hypercholesterolemia. Treatment would not be easy.

Irene did not look like most of the people who visit our office—she was young and relatively trim. She got right to the point: how were we going to fix her cholesterol? We immediately assured her that we could manage her cholesterol, but we followed that with an important question, one that no doctor had previously asked: did she have kids? She told us she had three teenage children. We explained that we suspected she had familial hypercholesterolemia, and if she did have it, her children might be similarly affected. Each of her children stood a 50 percent chance of inheriting the problem. We needed to know their cholesterol values now, *before* they developed heart disease. Irene agreed to bring her three kids in for blood tests.

When we met in the office two weeks later, the kids appeared entirely normal, with all of the spunk and vigor of modern teenagers. Laboratory technicians drew their blood, and within a few hours we had our answer. All three of Irene's children had the markedly elevated cholesterol levels typical of familial hypercholesterolemia.

Irene was understandably distraught. She'd come to us to get help with her own cholesterol, and we'd saddled her with the knowledge that her kids faced a future that might be dominated by heart disease. Irene had already experienced a heart attack and bypass surgery. Would her children have the same fate?

Thankfully, we were able to reassure her. We had diagnosed her kids early enough to delay or prevent significant cardiac consequences. We laid out a plan for cholesterol management that would control the LDL levels of the entire family. Explaining the role of a good diet (low in saturated fats, high in fiber and whole grains), we also·emphasized the importance of exercise. Most important, we immediately began all three children on a regimen of statin drugs. Initially Irene protested, worried about giving her kids such medicines. We convinced her that with her children's cholesterol levels so high, a statin could be lifesaving.

We kept our promise to treat Irene's cholesterol levels, and her family's future is bright. Irene always takes her medicines (a cocktail based primarily on a high-dose statin), and her LDL hovers near 100, an acceptable although not optimal value. The kids *usually* take their medicines (they're teenagers, after all), and their cholesterol levels, too, have come under better control. One small pill each day may well keep them out of our catheterization laboratories and cardiac operating rooms. We think that's a pretty good trade-off.

Familial hypercholesterolemia (Irene's disorder) has taught us much about the important role of cholesterol in the development of coronary heart disease. But most people who suffer the cardiovascular consequences of elevated cholesterol do not have this genetic condition and the strong family history that enable early detection and treatment. For the rest of us, vigilance is imperative. Cholesterol remains an important silent killer

High cholesterol has no symptoms; every day, we see patients who learn about their high cholesterol only *after* they arrive in the coronary care unit with a heart attack. Avoid this scenario. Have your cholesterol tested. If the results suggest you are at risk, review the information in the next few pages. It might just save your life.

CHOLESTEROL: WHY DO WE HAVE IT AND HOW DO WE MEASURE IT?

Cholesterol's Functions

What is cholesterol and what does it do? A waxy, yellowish white substance, cholesterol was first isolated by an eighteenth-century French chemist who was studying gallstones. This first identification of cholesterol suggested that its primary roles centered on illness and disease, but subsequent research proved this theory incorrect. It turns out that every cell in your body contains cholesterol, and you can't live without it.

Cholesterol is a key component of the cell membrane, the outer barrier between the cell and the rest of the body. Within the membrane, cholesterol molecules act like tollbooths, helping to regulate the passage of materials into and out of the cell. Cholesterol also serves as a building block for many important hormones, including estrogen, testosterone, and cortisone. Your body even needs cholesterol to manufacture vitamin D from sunlight.

When we talk about cholesterol, we are usually referring to cholesterol in the blood. The blood carries cholesterol to our cells and tissues, where it can be used to synthesize needed chemicals and hormones, broken down and removed from the body, or, under certain conditions, cause damage to the blood vessels themselves. When cholesterol travels in the blood, it is carried in packages of molecules called lipoproteins. We generally focus on two types of blood-borne cholesterol, which are distinguished by their attached lipoproteins: low-density lipoproteins (LDL) and high-density lipoproteins (HDL).

LDL is the major carrier of cholesterol in the blood. High levels of LDL or "bad" cholesterol are associated with development of plaques in arteries. Oxidation of LDL cholesterol in the blood enables it to enter the walls of arteries, leading to the buildup of plaques.

HDL or "good" cholesterol works in an opposite fashion, removing cholesterol from the arteries and returning it to the liver, where it is either broken down or removed from the body. By this mechanism, HDL retards the formation of artery-blocking plaques. Contemporary research demonstrates that some forms of HDL can actually clear the arteries, reducing the burden of plaque. Naturally occurring high levels of HDL are clearly associated with protection from heart disease.

If you want to influence cholesterol levels, you first need to know where it comes from. For the most part, you make it. Eighty percent of the body's cholesterol is made by the liver. While most people think that diet is the most important factor in determining cholesterol levels, this is a myth. Only 20 percent of your cholesterol comes from your diet, which explains why it is so difficult to reduce blood cholesterol levels via dietary interventions alone. Theoretically, if you completely eliminated all cholesterol from your diet, you might reduce your total cholesterol level by 20 percent. In reality, dietary modifications are usually even less effective because the liver responds to reduced dietary cholesterol intake by increasing cholesterol synthesis.

Understanding the limitations of dietary interventions often helps people with high cholesterol levels accept the fact that they need to take cholesterol-lowering drugs. If your cholesterol level is 50 percent higher than normal, you are simply not going to reach your cholesterol goals by diet alone. In such a case, you need to combine a good diet with the right medication.

Measuring Cholesterol

When physicians want to determine cholesterol levels in patients, we obtain a laboratory test known as a lipid panel. Your lipid panel will include four important numbers: total cholesterol, LDL, HDL, and triglycerides. Many patients who come to us can recite only one of these numbers, the total cholesterol. But of the four numbers, total cholesterol is often the least important.

When it comes to predicting heart disease, the LDL level is the most useful. Study after study has confirmed the strong relationship between high levels of LDL and heart disease. In contrast, high HDL levels reduce the risk of cardiac events. Because these two forms of cholesterol have opposite effects on risk, total cholesterol has major limitations as a predictor of heart disease. For example, consider a healthy young woman with a very high HDL level (85) and a normal LDL level (125). Although her total cholesterol is elevated (above 200), that is mainly as a consequence of high HDL. In this case, we deem this a favorable lipid profile.

Similarly, we usually do not rely on the ratios of the different lipids to guide our treatment. We want to know the individual values, not their ratio; these are the numbers most closely tied to treatment and prognosis.

What are normal levels of LDL, HDL, total cholesterol, and triglycerides? That's a surprisingly difficult question to answer. "Normal" cholesterol levels have been a moving target throughout the years. In the

1960s, American physicians decided that a total cholesterol of less than 300 was normal. A decade or two later, we changed our minds, deeming levels less than 240 acceptable. Most recently, experts have settled on the value of 200 as the upper limit of normal for total cholesterol. Why can't we decide?

The problem relates to our diets and our habits. Beginning after World War II, cholesterol levels rose rapidly as Americans consumed diets rich in meat and other sources of saturated fat. Scientists were misled into believing that the elevated cholesterol levels observed in the population were normal. However, we now know that such high levels are not healthy.

Current guidelines recommend that in adults without known heart disease or risk factors for heart disease, total cholesterol should be less than 200, HDL greater than 40 for men and greater than 45 for women, LDL less than 130, and triglycerides less than 150.

We need to emphasize a couple of important points here. The first relates to the relative importance of these different measurements. Although early attention centered on total cholesterol, remember that today we focus mostly on LDL cholesterol. The LDL level is the best predictor of the risk of heart attack and stroke, and the basic concept is simple:

lower is better. For example, an individual with an LDL of 125 has a higher risk of developing heart disease than someone of similar age and gender with an LDL of 90, even though both levels may fall in the normal range. In fact, this continuous relationship even extends to individuals with very low levels of LDL. Similar relationships hold true for HDL, where higher is better, although the strength of the relationship is somewhat less robust.

WHEN DO WE TREAT LDL CHOLESTEROL LEVELS?

Every time we bring a group of doctors together to determine when to treat LDL levels, we come away with new answers and recommendations. Today, most doctors rely on guidelines first developed in 1985 by the National Institutes of Health in collaboration with several professional medical societies known as the National Cholesterol Education Program (NCEP) Adult Treatment Panel (ATP). The most recent update to the guidelines (ATP III) was released in 2004, and an entirely new version (ATP IV) is due soon. The targets of cholesterol levels and their treatment continue to move.

The basic idea behind treatment guidelines is to treat elevated LDL cholesterol levels in people who already have coronary heart disease or who face a high likelihood of developing it. We use simple calculations to identify people who have a high risk of developing coronary heart disease and who therefore require cholesterol treatment. To determine who should be treated, we use a method known as the Framingham Risk Score, which incorporates seven risk factors to estimate a person's risk of developing coronary heart disease (CHD) over the next ten years.

FACTORS IN THE FRAMINGHAM RISK SCORE

Age

Gender

Total cholesterol

HDL

Tobacco use

Systolic blood pressure (the first number in the blood pressure reading)

Use of blood pressure medications

Knowing your risk, doctors choose a particular target for your LDL level and adjust the intensity of your therapy to reach that goal. (You can calculate your own risk of developing coronary heart disease over the next decade. Type the phrase "Framingham Risk Score" into an Internet search engine and you will find several online versions that allow you to enter your own data and compute your ten-year risk.)

In patients with preexisting coronary heart disease, the ten-year risk of a second heart attack or other serious heart problem usually exceeds 20 percent. For such patients, the guidelines recommend an LDL level of less than 100 mg/dL and suggest an optional goal of under 70 mg/dL in certain very high-risk patients—those with additional risk factors, including diabetes and a recent hospital admission for a heart attack. It is particularly important to achieve an LDL under 70 during the first two years following a heart attack. In our practice, we tend to be more aggressive than the guidelines: we want *most* of our patients with known CHD to aim for an LDL less than 70.

We also tend to be more aggressive in treating certain patients who have never had a heart-related problem but who have characteristics that cause them to have a risk equivalent to that of patients with established coronary heart disease. These risk-equivalent patients include individuals with blockages in arteries other than the coronaries, such as the arteries in the legs or the carotid arteries in the neck. Diabetes confers such a high risk of heart disease that traditional thinking considers people with diabetes to be risk-equivalent to those with known coronary heart disease. However, this principle has been challenged by some experts in recent years. A final category of risk-equivalent patients includes individuals with a Framingham Risk Score calculation that predicts a ten-year risk of CHD of more than 20 percent. In these patients, the guidelines target an LDL level of less than 100, but once again, we often aim for a level less than 70 if it can be achieved without causing unacceptable side effects from treatment.

We use the term *secondary prevention* to describe patients with established CHD or very high risk for its development; our goal with these patients is generally prevention of a second cardiac event. Everybody agrees with aggressive management of LDL as part of a program to try to prevent a second heart attack. The role of lowering LDL in primary prevention, where our goal is to prevent a first cardiac event, generates considerably more controversy. How should we treat the person with elevated LDL and risk factors who has not yet experienced a coronary event?

When it comes to primary prevention, current national guidelines are somewhat too conservative for our tastes. For primary prevention patients with two or more risk factors, such as smoking or high blood pressure, the Framingham Risk Score typically indicates a 10–20 percent probability of developing CHD during the next ten years. In these patients, the guidelines recommend achieving an LDL level under 130. For patients with two or more risk factors and a calculated ten-year risk under 10 percent, the goal is also for levels less than 130, but the guidelines recommend a conservative approach, relying primarily upon lifestyle changes rather than drugs. Finally, for individuals with zero or one risk factor, the guidelines suggest a target LDL less than 160 and recommend drug therapy only if LDL exceeds 190.

We take issue with these guidelines on two points. First of all, we don't think that anybody should be walking around with an LDL of 160. Second, we are more liberal in our use of statin medications to lower LDL cholesterol levels. If you are otherwise healthy and have an LDL greater than 130, we want you to achieve a lower value. Begin with lifestyle changes (see below), but don't be surprised or disappointed if you require a statin to further reduce your LDL.

Targeting Your LDL Cholesterol

CHD RISK	LDL TARGET
Known CHD	< 70 mg/dL
Diabetes	
Arterial blockages	
Framingham risk greater than 20 percent	
Aggressive target	< 70 mg/dL
Conservative target	< 100 mg/dL
No CHD, diabetes, or arterial disease	< 130 mg/dL
Framingham risk less than 20 percent	

MANAGING CHOLESTEROL WITH DIET AND EXERCISE

You may be surprised to find that a cholesterol-lowering diet is NOT the same thing as a low-fat diet. The NCEP's Therapeutic Lifestyle Changes (TLC) diet is rich in monounsaturated fats such as canola and olive oil, which tend to improve the ratio between LDL and HDL cholesterol. Saturated fats (typically found in meat and full-fat dairy products), which promote the production of cholesterol by the liver, are strictly limited. In addition, avoid trans fats, which adversely affect the balance of production between LDL and HDL. The message here: eat the right fats to control your cholesterol.

ATP III Guideline Recommendations for TLC Diet

NUTRIENT	RECOMMENDED INTAKE
Saturated fat	Less than 7 percent of total calories
Polyunsaturated fat	Up to 10 percent of total calories
Monounsaturated fat	Up to 20 percent of total calories
Total fat	25–35 percent of total calories
Carbohydrate	50–60 percent of total calories
Fiber	20–30 grams/day
Protein	Approx. 15 percent of total calories
Cholesterol	Less than 200 mg/day
Total calories	Sufficient to maintain ideal body weight

How does the cholesterol you eat affect your body's own cholesterol levels? Surprisingly, when it comes to influencing your cholesterol levels, your intake of saturated and trans fats plays a greater role than dietary cholesterol does. Foods rich in cholesterol, such as eggs, produce only modest changes in blood cholesterol levels. Your diet *can* include eggs, but no more than one to three per week if you need to lower your LDL cholesterol.

Certain foods have a beneficial impact on your LDL cholesterol levels. Soluble fiber, found in foods such as oatmeal, beans, and legumes, slightly decreases LDL levels in many people. National guidelines recommend eating foods (often margarines) fortified with certain plant stanols/sterols that slightly lower LDL. While many doctors support this recommendation, it is important to know that there is no strong scientific evidence documenting a clinical benefit (e.g., fewer heart attacks). While it is probably okay to purchase these fortified spreads, don't expect miracles.

There are no magic foods or supplements that can dramatically lower

LDL. Your dietary habits should be sensible rather than extreme. We do not recommend highly restrictive diets such as the Ornish, Esselstyn, or Pritikin diets: following these diets is challenging, and ultra-low-fat diets tend to have the unfavorable side effect of lowering levels of HDL, the "good" cholesterol.

Securing a favorable lipid profile also requires consistent exercise, maintaining an ideal body weight, and avoiding tobacco. Fortunately, each of these three factors helps to raise your HDL levels as well.

Lifestyle to Improve Your Cholesterol Profile

Diet

Avoid saturated fats	Limit red meats, processed meats, full fat dairy products, lard
Favor monounsaturated fats	Olive oil, canola oil
Favor dietary fiber	Whole grains, oats and oatmeal, beans, barley
Exercise	Aerobic exercise at least 30 minutes per day
Ideal body weight	Achieved by decreasing calories and increasing exercise
Quit smoking	Enough said!

What should you expect from the TLC program of diet, weight loss, and exercise? The program's effects on LDL levels are measurable but often quite modest. Because most of your cholesterol is manufactured in your liver, a reduction of more than 10–15 percent in LDL through changes in diet alone is unusual. If your LDL level is 140, you can probably get it down to 115–125 by adopting a healthy lifestyle. On the other hand, if your LDL is more than 20–25 percent above the target goal, you are unlikely to reach an optimal level through lifestyle changes alone.

This doesn't mean that you should abandon the TLC approach. Rather, embrace it as part of a broader program to bring down your LDL cholesterol levels. Understanding the limits of lifestyle modification in controlling LDL is important because many patients have an inordinate fear of taking cholesterol-lowering drugs. Our patients constantly tell us, "I know I can lower my cholesterol with diet. I'll cut out the french fries! Please don't put me on drugs!" For high-risk patients with very elevated LDL levels, this perspective can be lethal. As you work to control your LDL, begin with the TLC plan, but be prepared to take the next step to ensure your heart health.

THE STATINS ARRIVE

What Are Statins?

Because lowering LDL cholesterol is the primary goal of cholesterol management, drugs that reduce LDL levels are the big guns in our armamentarium. Statins, the most important class of LDL lowering drugs, have revolutionized modern cardiology. The first statin, lovastatin (Mevacor), reached the market in 1987, signaling a major breakthrough in the battle against CHD. Statins work by blocking a critical enzyme involved in the liver's production of cholesterol, reducing the amount of cholesterol the liver makes. Statins also increase the activity of receptors on the surface of liver cells, literally pulling cholesterol from circulating blood. As a consequence, blood levels of LDL and total cholesterol drop.

Lovastatin wasn't particularly potent by today's standards, but it was much more effective than anything previously available. Within a few years after the introduction of lovastatin, the FDA approved two more statins, pravastatin (Pravachol) and simvastatin (Zocor). Surprisingly, initial acceptance of statins by the medical community was relatively slow. Although these drugs were very effective at lowering LDL, there were not yet randomized clinical trials demonstrating that reducing LDL in patients with CHD would result in a reduced risk of future heart problems. The concept made sense, but a change in practice of this magnitude required solid evidence.

The proof came in 1994 with the publication of the landmark Scandinavian Simvastatin Survival Study, also known as the 4S Trial. A total of 4,444 patients with very high LDL levels who had suffered a heart attack were randomly assigned to receive either simvastatin or a placebo. After five years, simvastatin-treated patients had a 30 percent reduction in the risk of death due to all causes and a 42 percent reduction in the risk of death due to CHD. The risk of a second heart attack was also dramatically reduced, by 34 percent.

These results were stunning, and the medical community was positively giddy as a result of the 4S trial. Caught up in the enthusiasm, the two Nobel Prize winners who discovered the biologic mechanisms underlying the effects of statins wrote an editorial in the prestigious journal

Science predicting that by the turn of the twenty-first century heart attacks would be gone. Obviously, that prediction has not come to pass, but irrational exuberance notwithstanding, these drugs are incredibly useful. Today eight statins are marketed in the United States. Although all of these drugs substantially lower LDL cholesterol, they vary considerably in efficacy. The following table shows the most commonly used statins and the typical LDL-lowering effects that can be expected at various dosages.

HOW MUCH WILL A STATIN LOWER LDL CHOLESTEROL?

Drug	10 mg	20 mg	40 mg	80 mg
Pravastatin (Pravachol)	22 percent	28 percent	34 percent	40 percent
Simvastatin (Zocor)	28 percent	34 percent	40 percent	Not recommended
Atorvastatin (Lipitor)	34 percent	40 percent	46 percent	52 percent
Rosuvastatin (Crestor)	42 percent	48 percent	54 percent	Not available

Using this information, you can predict a particular statin's effect on your LDL level.

Does this mean that once you begin to take a statin, you can eat anything that you want? Don't make this mistake! By adhering to a heart-healthy, cholesterol-lowering diet, you can ensure that you can take a relatively low dose of your statin. Because statin side effects are dosage-related, this can represent a big advantage for you.

Diet is especially important in high-risk patients who may need to lower their cholesterol by 100 points or more. In these cases, no statin is likely to work on its own, but a combination of one of the most potent statins at the highest dosage and a heart-healthy diet will probably get you to your goal.

Patients often worry about the cost of statins. Statins need not be expensive. For many years statins were available only as brand-name drugs, and costs often reached $200 per month. In 2001, the first statin became generically available, but because lovastatin was not the most effective statin, branded drugs continued to dominate. In 2006, a medium-potency statin, simvastatin, became available as a generic, resulting in a gradual shift away from the more expensive brand-name drugs. An even more potent statin, atorvastatin, became generically available in November 2011, thus enabling even more patients to reach their LDL goals at lower cost.

If your doctor tells you that you need a statin, get involved with the decision making in order to maximize the effect on your heart and minimize the impact on your wallet. With your LDL level in hand, look at the table on the previous page. If you can achieve your LDL goal using a generic statin, we think such an approach makes the most sense. If the table predicts that you can't achieve optimal results generically, you may need to take the last remaining branded drug, rosuvastatin, or an additional drug (combination therapy) to further lower your LDL cholesterol.

WOULD YOU LIKE FRIES AND A STATIN WITH THAT?

Recognizing our infatuation with fast-food meals, British cardiologists proposed a novel concept to mitigate the risks associated with our dangerous eating behaviors. Their solution? Take a statin tablet with your Quarter Pounder! They calculated that most statins are sufficiently powerful to offset the cardiovascular risk associated with eating a meal such as a Quarter Pounder with cheese and a small milk shake. So why not put them together? After all, if you are going to put yourself at risk by driving ninety miles per hour, you might as well wear your seatbelt to ensure some protection from your dangerous behavior.

Of course, the British doctors offered this proposal with tongue in cheek. We do not really know whether or not statins, or any medicine for that matter, can reduce the deleterious effects of dangerous behaviors that are repeated over years or decades. It is unlikely that the condiment station at McDonald's will any day soon include salt, pepper, ketchup, and a statin. The British authors suggest that "no tablet can completely neutralize the harm to your individual health from eating unhealthy. Better ways to reduce your risk of death from heart attack include: eating healthily, exercising, maintaining a healthy weight, and not smoking." We could not agree more.

Statin Side Effects

Few drugs have been studied as carefully as statins. Scientists have examined statins in clinical trials involving hundreds of thousands of patients. These drugs are among the safest drugs in all of medicine, but they do have side effects. Because statins affect metabolic pathways in the liver, doctors initially worried about liver damage. Statin drugs can cause elevations in blood levels of liver enzymes that are commonly used as markers for liver injury, so the FDA has consistently recommended that physicians monitor liver enzymes in patients taking statins. Most doctors follow this advice, ordering blood tests every six to twelve months. We feel this is unnecessary.

Over the last twenty-five years of statin use, there have been *no* documented cases of serious liver damage in statin-treated patients that could not be attributed to another cause. While blood liver enzymes do sometimes increase, these levels usually eventually return to normal even if the drug is continued. The real risk to patients comes from the possibility that a physician will overreact to a small rise in liver enzymes and stop the drug, exposing you to the risk of a future heart attack. Therefore, we do not recommend routine monitoring of liver enzymes in statin-treated patients.

While statins do not harm the liver, there *is* a very small link between statins and the development of diabetes. The finding that treatment with statins increases the risk of diabetes generated a media frenzy, creating huge concerns for our patients. News reports were correct: statin use is associated with a slight increase in risk of developing diabetes. But this risk is extremely small and is more than offset by the medicines' benefits. The message is simple: whether or not you have diabetes, if you require a statin to lower your LDL cholesterol, the benefits far outweigh the risk.

The most serious adverse effect of statins is the breakdown of muscle tissue, a disorder known as rhabdomyolysis. Fortunately, this side effect is rare, occurring in about 1 of every 10,000 patients treated with the drugs. When it does occur, however, the consequences can be severe. Chemicals released by muscle destruction enter the blood and can damage the kidneys, causing acute kidney failure. If not recognized and treated promptly, the muscle damage of rhabdomyolysis can be fatal. Patients on statins should immediately report serious muscle pain or weakness, particularly if associated with dark, tea-colored urine. Rapid treatment with intravenous fluids protects the kidneys and aids recovery. Patients with an untreated underactive thyroid appear to have an increased risk of rhabdomyolysis with statins. If you have thyroid problems, make sure that your cardiologist knows about them before you take a statin.

Although rhabdomyolysis is rare, less severe muscle symptoms caused by statin administration are fairly common, ranging from vague, low-level muscle aches during exercise to severe and continuous pain. Blood tests used to diagnose rhabdomyolysis are often completely normal. Some patients are so bothered by these symptoms that they refuse to take statins. Don't give up so quickly.

If you suffer from muscle symptoms while taking a statin, you have options. Ask your doctor about switching to a different statin, particularly if you are taking simvastatin, which has the highest incidence of muscle problems. Inquire about a different dosing schedule. We often need to devise creative approaches to statin administration in patients with muscle symptoms, frequently relying on smaller dosages of a more potent statin three days per week. The most important advice is this: don't abandon statins because you develop muscle aches after taking just one drug in the class.

Statins and Other Drugs: Interactions You Should Know About

Many cases of statin-induced muscle toxicity can be traced to their interactions with other drugs. Most statins are metabolized by the same enzymes in the liver that break down other drugs. This means that other drugs "compete" with statins to be removed from circulation by the liver. This competition slows the removal of statins from the blood, thereby increasing their levels and in turn increasing the risk of statin-induced side effects. These drug interactions are most common with simvastatin but can occur with atorvastatin as well.

Certain drugs used to treat HIV infections are also capable of provoking statin toxicity. And finally, yes, it's true: if you are on a statin, you need to avoid consuming large quantities of grapefruit and grapefruit juice. Grapefruit juice increases blood levels of some statins by blocking the enzymes that normally break them down. This interaction seems the strongest with certain statins (atorvastatin, lovastatin, and simvastatin). An occasional glass of grapefruit juice or half a grapefruit won't cause a problem, but you should avoid large amounts.

OTHER ANTI-CHOLESTEROL MEDICINES

Ezetimibe (Zetia) and Vytorin

What if you follow a good diet, exercise, take your statin, and your LDL cholesterol is *still* too high? What's your next step? This question comes up for doctors, their patients, and, of course, the big pharmaceutical companies that are searching for the next blockbuster heart drug.

The answer to the question is controversial. While statins work at the level of the liver, ezetimibe reduces absorption of cholesterol from the intestine, lowering LDL by an additional 15–20 percent. Ezetimibe is available in two forms, as a stand-alone drug (Zetia) and as a combination product packaged with simvastatin (Vytorin). Both Zetia and Vytorin are not available in generic form yet and are relatively expensive.

Although ezetimibe seems like a logical choice for lowering cholesterol,

STATINS, INFLAMMATION, AND C-REACTIVE PROTEIN

While many people consider coronary heart disease a straightforward problem of arterial blockages caused by cholesterol, it is far more complicated. A variety of other factors contribute to its development, including inflammation. Boston researcher Paul Ridker confirmed the link between coronary heart disease and inflammation when he demonstrated that high blood levels of C-reactive protein (CRP), a substance related to inflammation, are associated with an increased likelihood of suffering a heart attack.

The higher your blood CRP level, the greater your risk of cardiovascular disease. We consider a value of 1 ideal, values of 1 to 2 intermediate, and values greater than 2 indicative of high cardiovascular risk. Fortunately, we can treat high CRP levels, and it turns out that the best treatment is the same as the treatment for high LDL cholesterol levels: statins. In addition to decreasing LDL cholesterol levels, statins lower CRP levels, and many scientists believe that this anti-inflammatory effect of statins contributes to their effects on cardiovascular health.

Do you need to know your CRP level? Maybe. Based upon the landmark findings of a study called the Jupiter Trial, we measure CRP levels in patients whose LDL and other risk factors put them on the borderline for requiring statins—for example, a fifty-five-year-old man with an LDL of 120, high blood pressure, and a low HDL. Some doctors would prescribe a statin and some wouldn't. We use the CRP to help us decide. If his CRP is low (less than 1), we defer statin treatment and concentrate on lifestyle factors. If the CRP is clearly elevated (greater than 2), we prescribe a statin in addition to lifestyle modification.

this drug has generated considerable controversy. In clinical trials, ezetimibe reduces LDL levels but has not been shown to reduce the risk of heart attack or stroke and failed to slow the progression of plaques in the carotid arteries in the neck. This raised questions about the ultimate effectiveness of the drug in improving heart health.

Today we use Zetia as a first-line agent rarely and only in patients who cannot tolerate any of the statins due to side effects, and as a second-line drug in those who cannot reach their LDL goals despite maximum doses of a powerful statin. We never use the combination drug Vytorin: there is simply no rationale for combining a medium-potency statin such as simvastatin with Zetia when there are more potent statins available. Why take an expensive combination product of uncertain benefit when a well-studied generic drug is readily available?

HOW TO INCREASE YOUR HDL CHOLESTEROL

Although current national guidelines focus on reducing LDL cholesterol, we have known for decades that low levels of HDL or "good" cholesterol are strongly associated with an increased risk of coronary heart disease. We generally want men to have HDL levels over 40 or 45, while women should aim for levels above 45 or 50. National guidelines do not make strong recommendations for treating low levels of HDL, citing the lack of high-quality trials confirming a benefit to raising them and noting that we have few drugs to do so. Some physicians also point to recent controversial studies suggesting that if your LDL level is low enough, your HDL level may be less important. We disagree with the concept of ignoring HDL.

Lifestyle Changes to Increase Your HDL

So how can you increase your HDL? We begin with lifestyle, and exercise is a key feature. Aerobic exercise can raise HDL levels by 10 percent, with the degree of HDL increase proportional to the amount of exercise. If you are currently sedentary, walking thirty minutes a day will cause a measurable increase in your HDL levels; walking further or engaging in more strenuous exercise, such as running, biking, and swimming, will increase your HDL levels even more. Resistance exercise such as weight lifting does not help with HDL levels.

If you are overweight, weight loss can also boost HDL levels. A loss of just six or seven pounds can increase your HDL by 1 mg/dL. If you are extremely overweight and lose twenty to thirty pounds, you will see a substantial increase in your HDL level. However, don't be discouraged if the effects are not immediate; the HDL levels may actually decrease during active weight loss, but they will eventually increase when your weight restabilizes at a lower level.

As with LDL, your diet influences your HDL levels. Dietary fat increases HDL levels, but you need the right fats. This means focusing on polyunsaturated and monounsaturated fats from vegetable sources such as olive oil and canola oil. Avoid trans fats and limit the saturated fats found in meats and full-fat dairy products. If your HDL is low, you should also shy away from trendy ultra-low-fat, high-carbohydrate diets, as these will actually decrease your HDL levels.

Stop smoking! Quitting smoking can increase your HDL by up to 10 percent. But you *can* have a drink. Moderate alcohol consumption (one drink per day in women, one to two per day in men) has been shown to increase levels of HDL cholesterol. This means that if you already drink alcohol, you can continue (in moderation), but we don't write prescriptions for people to start drinking just to treat a low HDL level.

Medicines to Raise HDL?

When diet, exercise, and smoking cessation are not enough to raise a patient's HDL to acceptable levels, physicians often turn to drug therapy. The problems here are a relative lack of options and no proven medical benefit for the few HDL-raising drugs that are available. Unlike statins, which can dramatically increase LDL cholesterol, medicines designed to raise HDL have limited effectiveness, and some have important side effects. Statins can increase HDL by 5–10 percent. There are small but potentially important differences in the effects of various statins on HDL. For patients close to their HDL target, switching from one statin to another may help to reach that goal.

One of the B vitamins, niacin, raises HDL levels up to 25 percent (and also lowers triglyceride levels) when taken at high doses. Therefore, until recently, we often prescribed Niaspan, a prescription form of niacin, to increase HDL in patients with very low levels. A recent study raised questions about this practice. The National Institutes of Health released results of a randomized controlled clinical trial investigating the impact of niacin in patients with low HDL levels. More than 3,000 patients with cardiovascular disease, low HDL levels, and high triglyceride levels were randomly assigned to either niacin or a placebo in addition to the statin that they were already taking. Niacin *did* raise HDL, as expected, but it did not reduce heart attacks and may have even slightly increased the risk of stroke. Based upon this finding, the Data Safety and Monitoring Board stopped the study eighteen months ahead of schedule. We have reduced our practice of prescribing niacin supplements to increase HDL levels pending review of this study when it is published.

Occasionally physicians employ another class of drugs to raise HDL, the fibric acid derivatives (fibrates). These include gemfibrozil (Lopid), fenofibrate (Tricor and other brands), and fenofibric acid (Trilipix). Fibrates raise HDL by 10–15 percent, which sounds appealing. Unfortunately, clinical trials have failed to demonstrate compelling evidence for a reduction in heart problems with fenofibrate, the most commonly used drug in the class. Gemfibrozil, another fibrate, has been associated with muscle damage when used with statins. For these reasons, we do not use fibrates to raise HDL in our patients.

NEW DRUGS TO INCREASE HDL CHOLESTEROL

We have progressed about as far as we can in lowering LDL cholesterol using statins. There are powerful new therapies under development to further lower LDL, but these will be useful only in the modest number of patients who can't get to goal using current drugs. However, many scientists remain cautiously enthusiastic about developing new medicines to raise levels of HDL cholesterol.

So far, the search for drugs to increase HDL has been an emotional and scientific roller coaster. After fifteen years of research costing more than $1 billion, Pfizer thought it had the answer with a medicine called torcetrapib. In animal experiments and preliminary studies, the drug worked as expected. It raised HDL 60 to 80 percent. But in a clinical trial involving 15,000 people, the medicine actually *increased* the risk of death and heart problems—a dead end for that medicine.

While Pfizer's experience left us disappointed and scratching our heads, we have not given up. Several drugs in the medical pipeline look promising. In a recent study of more than 1,600 patients, one of these new drugs more than doubled HDL levels while cutting LDL levels by 40 percent. If the next step, a larger study to assess the drug's impact on heart health, is successful, we may see the next blockbuster therapy for heart patients.

HIGH TRIGLYCERIDES AND METABOLIC SYNDROME

After LDL and HDL, the triglyceride level is the third most important value on your lipid blood test. What are triglycerides? Simply put, they are fat. Fat in your body and fat in food exist primarily as triglycerides. When we consume excess calories in any form, our body produces triglycerides, which are then stored in fat cells. Although we include blood triglyceride levels with every lipid panel, doctors argue about their relevance.

Of course, we have guidelines for normal values. We consider levels greater than 150 to be elevated and levels greater than 500 to be particularly concerning. What do high triglyceride levels mean for heart health? In comparison to our understanding of the relationship between LDL and heart disease, the evidence for an association between high triglycerides and coronary heart disease is relatively weak. Nonetheless, based on circumstantial evidence, we recommend treating high triglyceride levels in some patients with established coronary heart disease and in patients at high risk for heart disease.

Why do we assess and treat triglycerides for heart health? The issue relates to the strong association between high triglycerides, obesity, diabetes, and low HDL levels. Some authorities consider the combination of low HDL and high triglycerides levels to be a major cause of the development of heart disease in many patients without high levels of LDL cholesterol. These lipid abnormalities are components of a cluster of risk factors that has been dubbed metabolic syndrome.

The Metabolic Syndrome: High Triglycerides Keep Dangerous Company

FEATURE	MEASUREMENT
Abdominal obesity	
Men	Waist circumference > 40 inches
Women	Waist circumference > 35 inches
Triglyceride level	> 150 mg/dL
HDL cholesterol	
Men	< 40 mg/dL
Women	< 50 mg/dL
Blood pressure	≥ 130/85 mm Hg
Fasting glucose	>110 mg/dL

Because metabolic syndrome is tied to the development of heart disease and diabetes, the national cholesterol guidelines include it as a secondary target for ensuring heart health. This means that in addition to controlling your LDL cholesterol, you will need to manage these other risk factors as well.

The next time you go to your doctor, make sure that you leave with values for each of these factors; of course, you can measure your waist circumference on your own. Compare your values to those in the chart above. If three or more apply to you, you have metabolic syndrome.

Abdominal fat has long been thought to be the key driver of metabolic syndrome. Weight management and other lifestyle changes, not drugs, should be the primary focus for patients with metabolic syndrome and high triglycerides. Diet and exercise lower triglyceride levels and improve the other metabolic syndrome risk factors. The Mediterranean diet, with its wide array of healthful fats, is the best dietary choice. Low-fat diets such as the Pritikin diet actually elevate triglyceride levels, because excess carbohydrates are converted to triglycerides.

If elevated triglycerides persist after dietary changes, some authorities recommend fish oil supplements, which contain the two omega-3 fatty acids eicosapentaenoic acid (EPA) and docosahexaenoic acid (DHA). To lower triglycerides by 20 percent or more, you must take enough fish oil supplements to get 2 to 4 grams of these omega-3 fatty acids each day. A more potent prescription fish oil product, Lovaza, can lower triglycerides even more, up to 50 percent. Fibrates and niacin also reduce triglyceride levels. However, there is no evidence that this biochemical benefit, the lowering of triglycerides, actually improves cardiovascular outcomes. Our use of these agents may represent wishful thinking.

YOU AND YOUR CHOLESTEROL

The science of cholesterol is complicated. As researchers increase our understanding of the mechanisms by which lipids influence heart disease, our therapies will evolve, becoming better and more focused. But we have enough information right now to help you protect your heart. Make sure that you know your lipid numbers—your LDL, HDL, and triglyceride levels. Then use the information we have provided to determine your optimal target levels. Finally, work with your physicians to tailor the best strategy to reach your goals. Don't be afraid to take a statin. You will benefit from one of the greatest medical advances of the last one hundred years.

RX: CHOLESTEROL

Your liver makes most of the cholesterol in your body—only 20 percent comes from food

LDL cholesterol is the primary target

Know your target LDL:

- If you have coronary heart disease, your LDL cholesterol should be 70 mg/dL or less. If you have major risk factors for coronary heart disease, your LDL cholesterol should be 100 mg/dL or less
- LDL greater than 130 mg/dL is unhealthy even if you don't have heart disease

Lower your LDL level:

- Choose poly- or monounsaturated fats and high-fiber offerings
- Avoid saturated and trans fats
- Exercise
- Statins—make certain you get the right drug in the right dosage

HDL cholesterol: keep it up

Higher is better: over 40 mg/dL for men and over 45 mg/dL for women

Raise your HDL level:

- Exercise
- Weight loss
- Quit smoking

CHAPTER 4

YOUR WEIGHT AND YOUR HEART: HOW EXTRA POUNDS CREATE EXCESS RISK

THE BIG PICTURE

Right now, 55 percent of Americans are trying to lose weight. But in many cases they are dieting for the wrong reason. Their goal is to look better in that new bathing suit or fit into that favorite pair of jeans that seemed to be the perfect size last year but now feels just a little snug. These dieters are missing the point of weight loss efforts.

Being overweight threatens more than your appearance—it threatens your life. Today, two-thirds of Americans are overweight or obese (overweight is defined as a body mass index, or BMI, greater than 25, and obesity is defined as a BMI greater than 30). The heaviest among us will lose between five and fifteen years of life as a consequence of their extra pounds. The costs of the obesity epidemic ripple through society, from the impact on productivity to billions of dollars in health care expenditures, and there are no easy solutions.

Even those who are mildly obese face an increased risk of early death. The main health threat caused by obesity? You guessed it—heart disease. Obesity has become one of the most important reversible causes of heart disease. When a person loses weight, his or her risk factors for heart disease nearly always improve. Obesity is both preventable and treatable, but few patients are successful over the long run.

JIM FINNEGAN: "BIG MAN"

When Jim Finnegan played college football, his teammates christened him "Big Man" because he made big plays as a wide receiver, even though at a paltry five foot eleven and only 190 pounds he was dwarfed by the huge linemen.

A little too small for the NFL, Jim settled into a career as a stockbroker after his illustrious college experience. Jovial and well liked, he regaled clients with stories from his football days. His workweeks were filled with client meetings, often taking place over 18-ounce rib eye steaks or on the golf course, where Jim managed to play two or three times per week.

We met Jim when he was fifty-two years old, his football days three decades in the past. Jim came to us seeking cardiac clearance before undergoing knee replacement surgery. This type of examination is used to determine whether his heart would be able to tolerate the strain of the procedure.

Jim no longer looked like a college football star. He now carried 245 pounds on his five-eleven frame, having gained two to three pounds a year since college graduation. The year-to-year change in Jim's physique was not that great, but over the years the cumulative impact was huge. And so was Jim's waistline.

Jim told us that he had not seen a doctor in ten years. We did a few basic tests and were not surprised by the results. Jim's blood pressure was 160 over 90—high blood pressure. His blood glucose was 130 mg/dL—diabetes. His LDL cholesterol was 160 mg/dL—high cholesterol. His wife reported that he had started to snore loudly, and a simple test confirmed that he had sleep apnea. When we presented Jim with his test results and new diagnoses, he responded, "I was healthy until I met you guys. Now I have all of these diseases. What happened?"

We explained that "what happened" was a 55-pound weight gain. His diabetes, hypertension, high cholesterol, and sleep apnea were all direct results of his bulging waistline. In addition, the extra weight probably stressed his joints and contributed to the arthritis in his knee. Because he also had some chest pain when walking briskly on the golf course, we performed a nuclear medicine stress test, which demonstrated strikingly inadequate blood flow to portions of the left ventricle, the heart's primary pumping chamber. At cardiac catheterization, we found coronary heart disease with severe blockages in all three of the heart's arteries—yet another new diagnosis for Jim.

We explained the results in the recovery room. Jim did not take this news well. "Now I've got heart disease, too? Unbelievable!" He liked our next recommendation even less: he needed bypass surgery. Jim bellowed, "You mean open heart surgery?" His wife managed to calm him down, and we arranged to discuss the details the following day.

The next morning, Jim appeared at our office with a legal pad filled with neat, careful writing. He put it on our desk and said, "This is the plan." He had outlined the next year of his life, beginning with coronary artery bypass surgery, proceeding through knee replacement, and ending with Jim in fighting shape. He was going to change his diet immediately, moving his business meetings to a Mediterranean-style restaurant that offered salads, fish, and chicken dishes. Once his knee was fixed (three months after the heart surgery) he planned on beginning an exercise program, starting with walking and gradually adding swimming and bicycling. There was no need to give up golf, but he needed to add some more vigorous exercise.

Jim had his heart surgery and his knee replacement. Both procedures went well. He stuck to his plan, asking us to repeat all of our tests at his one-year appointment. When he came to the office to go over the results, he was trim and bristling with energy. His numbers were good: weight 205 pounds, blood pressure 130/80, blood sugar 70 mg/dL, LDL cholesterol 65 mg/dL. And his wife even reported that his snoring was gone, the sleep apnea having subsided.

Gaining just a couple of pounds per year after college had contributed to a smorgasbord of diseases, including coronary heart disease and diabetes. But Jim turned things around. By improving his lifestyle, he achieved gradual and sustained weight loss, and improved his health across the board. You can do the same. The time to start is now.

OBESITY: THE SIZE—AND COST—OF THE PROBLEM

Today, obesity is a grave health threat. About 200 million Americans—two-thirds of us—are either overweight or obese, a figure that has increased dramatically over the last four decades. The prevalence of obesity was relatively low and constant for a long time, increasing from 13.4 percent to 14.4 percent of the population between 1960 and 1980. But from 1980 to 2000, obesity doubled. Experts predict that 44 percent of Americans will be obese by 2020.

This epidemic spans all strata of society, but some groups face greater risk than others. Blacks are 50 percent more likely to be obese than are whites, with black women facing a particularly high risk. Obesity is 20 percent more common among Hispanics than among whites. Economic status is also linked to obesity. Before the dawn of the twentieth century, increased weight was associated with prosperity, a bulging belly serving as a declaration that a person had enough money to afford large quantities of food and did not need to perform manual labor. Today, the poor and un-educated have higher rates of obesity than do the wealthy.

Southerners and midwesterners tend to have bigger waistlines than those in the Northeast and West. For five years running, Mississippi has had the heaviest people in the nation, while only Colorado and the District of Columbia have obesity rates of less than 20 percent. The District of Columbia is the only region in the country with declining obesity rates.

TOO FAT TO FIGHT

The rise of obesity actually represents a threat to our national security. That is the conclusion of Mission: Readiness, a group of retired military leaders who analyzed the impact of obesity on our armed forces. They found that over the last fifteen years, the proportion of potential recruits who failed their physical exam because of their weight increased by 70 percent. Among those who do pass the physical exam and enlist, obesity is a critical and expensive problem—the military spends $60 million per year to recruit and train replacements for enlistees who are discharged due to weight problems.

In order to combat this problem, the army has revamped its menu and its fitness program. Mess halls now feature more green leafy vegetables, less fried food, and milk and water instead of soda. Drill sergeants monitor soldiers' food choices and provide important tips on nutritional needs in combat, explaining that a cup of coffee and a Snickers bar do not constitute the best preparation for battle. The army takes the obesity epidemic seriously. According to retired Navy rear admiral James Barnett Jr., "When over a quarter of young adults are too fat to fight, we need to take notice."

Beyond the health risks, it is the staggering financial cost of America's collective weight gain that has captured the attention of our policy makers. It costs an extra $1,429 per year to cover the health care of an obese person. This year we will spend 10 percent of our health care dollars, between $150 billion and $200 billion, to treat obesity-related health problems, a dramatic increase from 6.5 percent of the health care budget in 1998. Employers are also acutely aware of the cost of obesity, paying a $73 billion price tag for their obese workers, who miss more work and are less productive on the job.

OBESITY: RISKY BUSINESS

Obesity accounts for 300,000 American deaths per year, and this number is increasing. A recent study in the *New England Journal of Medicine* quantified the increase in the risk of death with increasing BMI. Although previous studies suggested that being mildly overweight was neutral or even beneficial when it came to health, this new study of nearly 1.5 million people laid that incorrect assertion to rest. The safest BMI is 20 to 25. Once a person exceeds this range and becomes overweight, the risk of death increases with every pound that is gained. Scientists predict that if left unchecked, the worldwide obesity epidemic will cause life expectancy in the United States to level off or even decline by 2050, reversing a 150-year upward trend.

Excess body weight means that the heart has to do more work. A normal heart in an obese person is like a Volkswagen engine in a Mack truck. Responding to the excess work requirement, the heart undergoes structural changes, including a thickening of its walls, an increase in the size of the its chambers, and unfavorable alterations in heart function. Some very obese people even develop fatty infiltration of the heart muscle, causing damage to the heart's conduction system and a reduction in the heart's pumping power. Obesity also makes it harder to diagnose heart problems, as many standard diagnostic tests are more difficult to perform and interpret in obese people.

While people may not notice thickening of their heart muscle, they will certainly take note of the chest pain associated with coronary heart disease. Obesity increases the risk of developing coronary heart disease. Today, obesity represents a major modifiable risk factor, approaching the importance of smoking, because it affects so many of the other known risk factors for heart disease.

HOW OVERWEIGHT AFFECTS RISK FACTORS
FOR CORONARY HEART DISEASE

LDL cholesterol increases

HDL cholesterol decreases

Triglycerides increase

Blood pressure increases

Diabetes/glucose intolerance increases

Blood vessels become dysfunctional

Inflammation increases

Increased blood clotting

A small but vocal cadre of doctors believes that obesity and heart health are not mutually exclusive. They use the term "metabolically healthy obese" to refer to people who are obese but who do not have changes in lipids, blood pressure, or other standard cardiac risk factors, suggesting that these people have nothing to worry about. However, recent, careful studies in this group demonstrate that they face an increased risk of developing heart disease when compared to metabolically healthy people of normal weight. The message here is clear: excess weight is a real and independent risk factor for heart disease even when other standard risk factors are absent. Don't be lulled into a false sense of security if your weight is high but your cholesterol is normal.

In addition to increasing the risk of coronary heart disease, obesity is associated with a broad range of other cardiovascular problems, including heart failure, abnormal heart rhythms (most notably atrial fibrillation), and increased risk of stroke. Well-recognized non-cardiovascular problems include osteoarthritis and increased risk of certain cancers. With all of these negative consequences, it is no surprise that obesity reduces both the quality and the duration of life.

While all excess fat is unhealthy, the location of excess fat appears to influence a person's risk of developing diabetes and heart disease. As we discussed in Chapter 2, people who are "pear-shaped" have excess fat around the thighs, hips, and buttocks. Other people are "apple-shaped," carrying extra fat in the belly. In terms of heart health, pears are better than apples.

The apple-shaped person has fat in and around the organs of the abdomen. These intra-abdominal fat cells (also called adipocytes) are metabolically active, releasing at least eighty different chemicals and hormones that lead to insulin resistance (a precursor to diabetes), inflammation, and lipid changes, including elevated triglyceride levels and reduced HDL cholesterol. In fact, even if overall weight is normal, extra fat around the midsection is associated with these risk factors for coronary heart disease (CHD). So getting rid of a big belly is a special imperative for weight loss.

ARE YOU OVERWEIGHT OR OBESE?

How do you know if you are overweight or obese? Most of us can answer this question with a mirror and an honest appraisal. But in our data-driven society, we like to add measurements and numbers. While no single number tells you for sure that you are overweight or obese, measurements can help track your progress toward a normal weight.

Let's start with your waist circumference. Take a simple tape measure and wrap it around your midsection, halfway between the bottom of your rib cage and the top of your pelvis. If you are a man, you want the number to be less than 40 inches. For women, it should be less than 35 inches. Higher numbers generally indicate abdominal obesity. If your waist circumference is high, losing enough weight to reduce your waist size by 2 inches may reduce your risk of developing coronary heart disease by 10 to 15 percent.

Your doctor may talk about a different number—your BMI. This is the measurement that doctors and scientists generally use to classify people as overweight or obese. Body mass index is calculated by taking your weight in kilograms and dividing it by the square of your height in meters. You don't have to do the math yourself—you can go to the government website www.nhlbisupport.com/bmi and calculate your BMI. A normal BMI is between 20 and 25. A BMI between 25 and 30 puts a person in the overweight category. A BMI 30 or greater is in the obese category.

If you are a woman of average height, five feet four inches, and you weigh 174 pounds or more, your BMI is 30, and you are probably obese. Similarly, a man who is five foot ten and weighs more than 208 pounds is likely to be obese.

Notice that in these examples we said "probably obese" and "likely to be obese." We hedged here because BMI is not 100 percent accurate in determining whether or not a person is obese. Many factors can limit the usefulness of BMI as a screening tool for obesity. For example, muscle weighs more than fat, so a very muscular person will have a high BMI without being overweight or obese. At six foot eight and 250 pounds, basketball star LeBron James has a BMI of 27.5. This puts him in the overweight category; obviously, he is not overweight.

So to figure out if you are overweight, combine a measurement (waist circumference or BMI) with a look in the mirror. There are no tricks. Your answer should come easily.

THE OBESITY EPIDEMIC: WHY NOW?

In order to develop the most effective weapons to combat obesity, we must ask two important questions: What caused the obesity epidemic? And why is it occurring now?

Can We Blame Genes or Infections?

The obesity epidemic dates back to the 1980s, when we started to witness a steady, relentless increase in the proportion of individuals who are overweight or obese. While the National Institutes of Health has classified obesity as a disease since 1985, we can't blame its rise on either infectious agents or genes, two of the most common causes of other diseases. Rather, the explosion of obesity was caused by changes in our environment and our behaviors.

Let's lay the "obesity is in your genes" argument to rest. Obesity is rarely an inevitable, direct consequence of a person's genetic makeup. More than forty sites in the human genome affect susceptibility to obesity, including genes that regulate body fat distribution, metabolic rate, and responses to exercise and diet. Together, these genes can influence body weight, but they do not cause obesity. After all, over the last three decades, our gene pool has not changed, but the percentage of overweight and obese Americans has doubled. Genes play only a minor role in the development of obesity.

IS OBESITY "SOCIALLY CONTAGIOUS"?

We all know that friends, family, and peers influence our behaviors. For example, teens who fall into a "bad" crowd of smokers and drinkers tend to take up these damaging habits as well. Could the same peer influence hold for eating and obesity? Researchers from Harvard Medical School addressed this question, examining the spread of obesity in a large social network over a thirty-two-year period. They found that obesity tended to occur in clusters, and examination of these clusters of obese people confirmed that obesity is socially contagious. A person's risk of becoming obese increased by nearly 60 percent if he or she had a friend who became obese over the course of the study. Similarly, a sibling or spouse becoming obese resulted in a 40 percent chance that other siblings or the other spouse would also become obese. This obesity effect was transmitted over long distances—friends separated by thousands of miles had the same influence as those who lived next door.

Study authors speculate that having obese friends and relatives changes our perception of what's normal in terms of body size. As a result, one person's obesity can ripple through a social network. The converse may also be true: normal weight, good dietary habits, and a heart healthy lifestyle may improve the health of those around you. Test this hypothesis with your own friends and family. Maintain a healthy weight and spread good health through your own social network.

Bad Habits: Too Many Calories, Too Little Exercise

We all recognize the behaviors that lead to obesity: too many calories and too little exercise, supported by the death of the home-cooked meal and the rise of fast-food meals that simply contain too many calories. We frequently make token efforts toward healthy eating. but do we really believe that we can create a healthy meal by adding low-calorie Apple Dippers to a Big Mac, large fries, and large Coke (a total of 1,350 calories, according to the McDonald's website)? For those of us not training for a triathlon, frequent meals like this can lead to only one outcome.

Like family dinners, regular exercise—even just a simple evening walk through the neighborhood—conjures up thoughts of times long gone. These days, we don't run into our friends when we are out for a walk or riding bicycles with our kids. Instead, social interactions occur when we drive over for a visit—even when we live only a short distance away.

Huge portions, calorie-dense foods, and limited exercise . . . what did we think was going to happen to our waistlines?

Soda, Sugar-Sweetened Beverages, and High-Fructose Corn Syrup

Fueling the obesity epidemic is what we drink—specifically, our love affair with high-calorie beverages, many of which contain high-fructose corn syrup. High-calorie drinks are everywhere, from Coke to sugar-sweetened sports drinks to kids' boxes of fruit juice. Sugar-sweetened beverages are the number one source of added sugars in the American diet, and the largest source of dietary carbohydrate in the United States.

We have evidence supporting an association between sugary drinks and obesity. The obesity epidemic and the increase in consumption of these beverages have occurred over the same time frame. In the last two decades, consumption of sugar-sweetened beverages has increased 61 percent. Today, 9 percent of total calories come from such drinks, and the average American consumes twenty-eight ounces of them each day, taking in more than 250 empty calories per day with the drinks. Drinking just one can of regular soda per day could lead to an annual weight gain of fifteen pounds.

Large observational studies find that high-calorie soft drinks are associated with obesity, increased blood pressure, diabetes, and unfavorable lipid profiles, including elevated LDL cholesterol and triglycerides. Of course, each of these factors increases the risk of developing heart disease. Just two sugar-sweetened beverages per day may measurably increase the risk of coronary heart disease. Researchers from the University of California at San Francisco estimated that in the decade from 1990 to 2000, consumption of sugary drinks contributed to 130,000 new cases of diabetes and 14,000 new cases of coronary heart disease in the United States.

Many experts argue that the high-fructose corn syrup found in sodas is the real villain when it comes to sugary drinks and obesity. High-fructose corn syrup is the primary sweetener in most U.S. sodas today and is also used extensively in baked goods. It is actually sweeter than glucose or sucrose (common table sugar), but the real reason that food manufacturers use it is that it's cheap, thanks to government quotas on domestic sugar

THE DANGER OF DRINKING YOUR CALORIES

Our bodies respond differently to calories in liquids than to calories in solid food. These differences help explain why sugar-sweetened beverages are so dangerous for our waistlines. Scientists conducted a study in which half of their subjects took in 450 calories per day in sugar-sweetened beverages while the other half consumed the same number of daily calories by eating jelly beans. Subjects assigned to the jelly bean group naturally adjusted their intake of other foods so that their total daily calorie intake was maintained or even slightly reduced. In contrast, those assigned to sugary drinks actually *increased* their consumption of other foods. As a consequence, subjects in the sugar-sweetened beverages group gained weight, while those eating jelly beans did not. Along similar lines, researchers at Penn State University studied the impact of different types and sizes of drinks on food intake in thirty-three volunteers. All subjects were offered the same foods for lunch, but beverage type (cola, diet cola, or water) and portion size (12 fl oz or 18 fl oz) were varied. The question was, do people decrease their intake of calories from solid food if they consume liquid calories at a meal? The answer is no. Study subjects ate the same amount of food, whether their drink was a large, sugar-filled soda or a smaller glass of water. Drinking sugar-sweetened beverages with meals increases total calorie intake. And we know where that leads—obesity, diabetes, and coronary heart disease.

production, import tariffs on foreign sugar, and subsidies to United States corn farmers. In contrast, it is used less in Europe, where it is more expensive.

Over the last four decades, our consumption of high-fructose corn syrup has increased by more than 1,000 percent. Although the media focus has been on high-fructose corn syrup, scientific evidence suggests that if there is any special problem with this sweetener, it actually stems from the fructose it contains. Whether derived from high-fructose corn syrup or regular table sugar (sucrose, which is a combination of glucose and fructose), fructose is more likely than glucose to stimulate fat production, particularly dangerous visceral fat. In laboratory studies, fructose causes increases in blood pressure, inflammation, triglycerides, and other heart-disease-causing lipids.

Some evidence suggests that fructose is less effective than glucose at inducing satiety. In other words, fructose doesn't quell your hunger pangs.

HIGH-FRUCTOSE CORN SYRUP:
A SUGAR BY ANY OTHER NAME IS STILL A SUGAR

There has been such a backlash against high-fructose corn syrup that many food manu-facturers have removed it from their products. Hunt's and Heinz ketchups, Gatorade, and Pepsi Throwback are just a few of the foods that no longer contain this substance. Hop-ing to increase sales, manufacturers are publicizing this change to "healthier" sweeteners. Meanwhile, the Corn Refiners Association is formulating strategies to try to convince the public that high-fructose corn syrup is safe and natural—after all, it's made from corn. With polls showing that 53 percent of Americans are concerned about health effects of high-fructose corn syrup, a name change is a key component of this strategy. The leading candidate? *Corn sugar.* The FDA has approved this name change, but the Corn Refiners Association now faces a challenge from the competing Sugar Association, which does not want to see high-fructose corn syrup benefit from the word *sugar* in its new name.

Only a minority of experts favor the term *corn sugar.* When asked his opinion by the *New York Times,* Michael Pollan suggested "enzymatically altered corn glucose." We don't think that one will do much to dispel fears or increase sales.

Glucose ingestion releases insulin and other hormones into the body, send-ing satiety signals that tell the brain it is time to stop eating. In contrast, because fructose does not have the same effect on insulin and other satiety hormones, it does not induce satiety. People continue to eat and drink.

While the damage associated with the extra calories in sugar-sweet-ened beverages may be increased by the presence of fructose, we feel it's most important to change the type of drink, not just the type of sugar. Cutting back on sugary beverages facilitates weight loss and maintenance and reduces both blood pressure and glucose intolerance—changes that are likely to reduce the risk of heart disease. Pause for a moment the next time a soda machine swallows your dollar bill, and choose water over soda. You will quench your thirst and improve your health just by pushing the right button.

A SODA TAX: TIME FOR GOVERNMENT ACTION?

The negative health consequences of sugar-sweetened beverages are clear. Decreasing consumption is a key imperative and is supported by many experts. But some authorities believe that the government should do more than simply educate—it should tax. Currently, forty states impose modest sales taxes on soft drinks. These taxes (generally about 5 percent) raise some money, but they are too small to discourage consumption. In contrast, experts predict that a 1-cent-per-ounce excise tax—which would increase the cost of a 20 ounce soda by 15 percent to 20 percent—would reduce soda consumption by 10 percent or more, as well as generate $15 billion in the first year. Polls show that consumers favor such a tax, particularly if the proceeds are targeted toward programs to reduce obesity and improve health. Predictably, major corporations oppose this concept. When New York State proposed an 18 percent tax on sugar-sweetened beverages, PepsiCo threatened to move its corporate headquarters from New York City. The measure died. However, there is important historical precedence for this sort of government action. In 1776, Adam Smith wrote in *The Wealth of Nations,* "Sugar, rum, and tobacco are commodities which are nowhere necessaries of life, which are become objects of almost universal consumption, and which are therefore extremely proper subjects of taxation." Today we tax rum and tobacco. Maybe sugar, in the form of sugar-sweetened beverages, should be next on our agenda.

STRATEGIES TO COMBAT OBESITY

Therapies to combat obesity fall into three broad categories: diet and behavior, medicines, and surgery. Lifestyle therapies (diet, exercise, behavioral changes) should always be the first line of defense. Remarkably, fewer than half of overweight and obese people are ever advised by their doctors to lose weight or provided with a program to help them. After looking in a mirror and performing a measurement or two, you have an idea of where you stand. If you are overweight, let us help you improve your cardiovascular and overall health by lowering your body weight.

Diets and Behaviors: The "Secret" of Calories

Seeking a magic bullet, Americans spend $59 billion per year on diet books, diet plans, and weight loss products. While we wholeheartedly support this focus on achieving a healthy weight, we don't want you to be duped into exhausting your money and time chasing impossible results promised by diets that make no sense. The best diet choice is to go "low fad," and we'll help you by dispelling the myths and revealing the truths about dieting to lose weight.

For years, diet enthusiasts, government agencies, and medical societies have incorrectly linked weight loss to the proportions of macronutrients in the diet. The three macronutrients, or basic energy sources, are carbohydrate, fat, and protein. The standard, government-approved food plate (previously a pyramid) emphasizes fruits, vegetables, and grains, indicating that a healthful diet includes about 55–60 percent of calories from carbohydrate, 10–15 percent from protein, and less than 30 percent from fat. Many popular diet programs promise to deliver a slimmer body by emphasizing one or two macronutrients while virtually eliminating the others. As a result, controversy and confusion abound. Atkins demonizes carbohydrates. Pritikin, Esselstyn, and Ornish rail against fat. Who is right?

To answer these questions, you need to understand the basic principle of dieting to lose weight. Recent studies comparing a variety of different diets, from low-carbohydrate to low-fat and everything in between, prove that the proportion of carbohydrates, proteins, and fats in your diet *does not influence weight loss*. Period. You can lose weight with any diet, as long as you burn more calories than you take in. This is the "secret" of calories.

So the first thing you need to know before you begin to diet is how many calories you should consume. Although half of Americans are actively dieting at any given time, only 12 percent know how many calories they require each day. You don't begin a five-hundred-mile trip in your car without a good idea of your route, whether obtained from a road map, MapQuest, or your GPS unit. The same is true for your diet. You need a plan, beginning with pinpointing the number of calories you need for weight maintenance (or loss). That number depends primarily upon your age, gender, and activity level.

			Calorie Requirements for Weight Maintenance by Age, Gender, and Activity Level	
GENDER	AGE	NO EXERCISE	PHYSICAL ACTIVITY EQUIVALENT TO WALKING 1½–3 MILES PER DAY	PHYSICAL ACTIVITY EQUIVALENT TO WALKING MORE THAN 3 MILES PER DAY
Female	19–30	2,000	2,000–2,200	2,400
	31–50	1,800	2,000	2,200
	51+	1,600	1,800	2,000–2,200
Male	19–30	2,400	2,600–2,800	3,000
	31–50	2,200	2,400–2,600	2,800–3,000
	51+	2,000	2,200–2,400	2,400–2,800

If your goal is weight loss, you need to consume fewer calories than you burn—that is, aim for numbers lower than those displayed in the table.

Weight loss hinges on the simple equation of calories taken in minus calories burned. Don't be fooled by fad diets that make unrealistic promises or promise quick weight loss. Any weight loss of more than one to two pounds per week generally represents loss of water weight, and many studies suggest that the quicker the weight comes off, the faster it goes back on. Therefore, we recommend targeting weight loss of one to two pounds per week, which will usually mean cutting your daily intake by 500 to 1,000 calories.

This clarifies the picture and simplifies your task. Weight maintenance and weight loss require that you manage calories, and no particular diet is better than any other. In carefully monitored clinical trials, dieters tend to lose five to ten pounds over the course of a year, no matter what the diet plan. The challenge is to choose a diet that works for you and that you can stick to. In most studies, half of people assigned to a diet regain all of the weight that they lost within two years. If you have tried a diet and it did not work, choose a different diet for your next attempt.

A successful weight loss program—combining an effective diet with appropriate exercise (see Chapter 7 for the exercise part of the equation)—has impressive health benefits. Important changes begin after a loss of just 5 percent to 10 percent of initial body weight. Diabetes often improves.

Blood pressure decreases. Cholesterol profiles become more favorable. The risk of coronary heart disease declines. Heart structure and function return toward normal. Meanwhile, cancer risks are lower, arthritis is reduced, and your energy level is restored.

THE DIET WAR:
LOW CARBOHYDRATE VERSUS LOW FAT

We would be remiss if we did not talk a little about the diet war—the fight for supremacy between those who advocate low-carbohydrate diets and those who favor low-fat plans. Zealots on both sides raise important questions about the competing diets. Won't a high-fat diet hurt the heart? Can fat-free, carbohydrate-rich foods make you lose fat? Recent studies address these questions, as well as the big question for scientists: is it possible that both diet programs could work equally well for weight loss?

The medical establishment has traditionally favored a low-fat diet for weight loss and heart health. Intense media campaigns and educational efforts have touted the heart-healthiness of this type of diet. The truth is that this sort of diet, like any diet, can help you lose weight as long as calories are controlled. But the public went too far with the low-fat concept, embracing *all* low-fat and fat-free foods, including those that are high in sugar and calories. We call this the "SnackWell phenomenon," and it has contributed significantly to the obesity epidemic.

A healthful-appearing green package of SnackWell cookies promises that the contents are "reduced fat" and have "no cholesterol." But the nutrition label on the back of the box tells a different story, reminding us that a single serving (only two cookies) has 110 calories. If you eat half a box of cookies—pretty easy to do while watching television or surfing the Web—you take in 500 excess calories. Repeat this regularly, and the resulting weight gain a few months down the road should come as no surprise. This gorging on low-fat, high-carbohydrate, high-calorie foods is the primary danger of low-fat diets.

While many doctors endorse limiting fat intake, today there is increasing public enthusiasm for low-carbohydrate diets. The Atkins diet is the best-known of these programs, but the low-carbohydrate foundation of the Atkins diet is not a new idea. In 1863, William Banting alerted the medical profession to the weight loss potential of a low-carbohydrate diet. More than a hundred years later, cardiologist Robert Atkins reintroduced the concept.

The principle of these diets is to restrict carbohydrate intake while consuming unlimited quantities of fat and protein. Early, rapid weight loss is impressive, but it results primarily from fluid shifts and water loss. Some claim that subsequent, sustained weight loss on low-carb diets is caused by selective burning of fats, with chemicals called ketones created as a by-product of fat metabolism. But ketosis—an increase in blood concentration of ketones from burning fat—usually does not occur, and if it does, the ketosis itself does not cause weight loss. People who achieve sustained weight loss on low-carbohydrate diets do so the old-fashioned way: they take in fewer calories than they burn.

So, how do low-carb and low-fat diets stack up? Large, randomized controlled clinical trials demonstrate that early weight loss is slightly greater with low-carbohydrate diets than with low-fat diets. Over time, however, the gap closes. By one to two years, weight loss is similar between low-carbohydrate, low-fat, and even the centuries-old Mediterranean diet. Any diet that controls calories creates weight loss.

Do these two distinctly different paths to weight loss (low-fat versus low-carbohydrate) have disparate effects on heart health? The truth is that we don't know yet. There are no long-term studies examining the impacts of low-fat and low-carbohydrate diets on development or progression of heart disease. We do, however, have insight into the effects of these diets on risk factors for heart disease.

These two diets differ in their effects on blood lipids. Low-carbohydrate diets cause greater increases in HDL cholesterol and larger decreases in triglyceride levels. These are favorable changes. On the other hand, low-fat diets are associated with greater decreases in LDL cholesterol, the lipid that is most closely associated with development of coronary heart disease. These findings have been borne out by several clinical studies.

The most recent diet study to make headlines was a two-year trial comparing low-fat and low-carbohydrate diets in 307 obese subjects. The media summarized the study's findings with the claim "Atkins diet best for heart health." If you had stopped reading there, you would have thought that the final answer was available.

As is often the case, however, the headlines did not tell the entire story. The real finding of this study was that *both* diets caused weight loss and improved cardiac risk factors. Both diets caused reductions in LDL cholesterol, triglyceride levels, and blood pressure. Both diets were associated with increases in HDL cholesterol. But the increase in HDL cholesterol was greater among those who followed a low-carbohydrate diet. This is where the headlines came from. A more accurate summary would have read, "Low-carbohydrate and low-fat diets both cause weight loss and improve cardiac risk factors."

If you feel that you must choose either a low-fat or a low-carbohydrate diet, go with the diet that fits you best. First, determine which you are most likely to follow. Sticking to a diet—any diet—is key. Also consider your personal cardiac risk factors. If you have a high LDL cholesterol, a diet low in saturated fats is best. If you have high triglycerides or low HDL cholesterol, a low-carbohydrate diet is most likely to help your lipid profile.

The bottom line is this: you can shed pounds with a wide variety of diets. When it comes to the relationship between diet and obesity, calories are king. But we do have our favorite diet. Check out Chapter 5 to find out why the Mediterranean diet is best for the heart.

Regardless of the diet you choose, burning more calories via exercise is absolutely essential. Studies have shown that individuals who lose weight without increasing exercise nearly always regain the lost weight within two years.

THE SAD SAGA OF DIET PILLS

If obesity is a disease, why don't we have medicines to treat it? We have antibiotics to cure infections, drugs to lower cholesterol, and a host of medical options for chronic diseases ranging from hypertension to gout. A drug that causes weight loss would have a dramatic impact on obesity and all of its accompanying illnesses, including heart disease.

We're working on it. Currently, there are more than eighty anti-obesity drugs in development. Scientists are developing agents that influence eating behavior, food intake, nutrient absorption, and energy expenditure. Pharmaceutical companies, salivating over a multibillion-dollar market that is growing by the day, are happy to fund these efforts. But so far, the story of medicines for obesity is a collection of disappointing and occasionally tragic vignettes. The fen-phen debacle is our most spectacular failure in this arena.

Fen-phen was a combination of two different drugs, each one individually approved by the FDA as an appetite suppressant for the treatment of obesity. The "phen" part was phentermine, an amphetamine-like agent that was approved in 1959. It both suppresses appetite and increases the rate at which calories are burned. It was combined with fenfluramine (or the related drug dexfenfluramine), the "fen" in fen-phen. Fenfluramine increases levels of a hormone called serotonin. Increased serotonin in the brain decreases appetite, resulting in weight loss.

While fen-phen did cause weight loss, it had a much more dramatic effect in many patients—heart valve damage. After Mayo Clinic researchers recognized this deadly side effect, the drug was withdrawn from the market, its legacy a new form of heart disease and thousands of lawsuits against the manufacturer.

The fen-phen disaster temporarily dampened enthusiasm for diet pills, but neither the public nor pharmaceutical companies were permanently dissuaded. Today, the demand for a "real" diet pill is stronger than ever.

Ironically, phentermine (alone, this time) is now the most widely prescribed anti-obesity medication in the world, with more than 1 million patients taking it. It is FDA-approved for short-term use, generally for about three months. In this time frame, it is associated with modest weight loss, usually in the range of 5 to 10 pounds. Although possibly safe, it is far from ideal for long-term treatment of obesity.

In spite of intense scientific effort and billions of dollars in funding, at the beginning of 2010 there were only two drugs on the U.S. market approved for long-term weight loss—sibutramine (Meridia) and orlistat (Alli, Xenical). Amid newspaper headlines that recalled the fen-phen experience, Meridia was withdrawn from the market on October 8, 2010.

There were two problems with Meridia. Over a three-year period, Meridia was responsible for an average weight loss of only five to ten pounds. The cost of losing these few pounds was high—a 16 percent increase in the risk of heart attack or stroke among those who took Meridia. As FDA panel member Dr. Lamont Weide commented, "This is a unique drug; you can lose weight without getting any of the benefits of doing so." Modest weight loss with *increased* cardiovascular risk? Not a good deal.

Today orlistat stands alone as the only FDA-approved agent for long-term treatment of obesity. It acts by reducing absorption of dietary fat from the GI tract. By taking this medicine, patients generally lose five to ten pounds in a year. The good news is that there are no apparent cardiovascular side effects. But other side effects abound. The unabsorbed fat in the GI tract causes predictable issues that many find socially challenging, including excessive flatulence and incontinence of stool. The medicine won't cause you to die of a heart attack, but you may die of embarrassment.

Although success has been elusive, we may see an increase in our pharmaceutical options for weight loss over the next few years. To achieve FDA approval to treat obesity, a drug must demonstrate only modest effectiveness—the FDA is looking for agents that sustain a 5 percent or more loss of body weight for at least two years. While the bar is set low for weight loss, it is high for safety. Weight loss should prevent, rather than cause, heart attacks, strokes, and the need for heart surgery.

A SURGICAL SOLUTION

Although headway with medicines has been slow, bariatric surgery—surgery to treat obesity—is on the rise. In 2008, 344,000 patients worldwide had an operation for the express purpose of losing weight. Although the idea of weight loss surgery may seem drastic, bariatric surgery is currently the most effective and durable means to achieve weight loss in the severely obese patient.

While lifestyle changes—diet with calorie control and exercise—are always the first line of anti-obesity therapy, in most people they produce a weight loss of only five to ten pounds after one year. This modest weight loss does have a modest cardioprotective effect. But if your heart and overall health depend upon your shedding fifty or a hundred pounds, success with conventional approaches is unlikely, so it is worth considering bariatric surgery.

Bariatric surgery is usually reserved for people with a BMI of at least 35. Before a visit to the operating room, severely obese patients must make a good effort at standard lifestyle therapies for weight loss. If these attempts fail, it is reasonable to think about surgery. But bariatric surgery is not a quick fix, and it does have risks, most notably a small (about 1 in 500) risk of dying as a result of the procedure. Some doctors are concerned about the use of bariatric surgery in adolescent girls and young women who may later become pregnant, because the operation may cause nutritional deficiencies that may result in birth defects.

The two most popular bariatric procedures are gastric banding and gastric bypass. In gastric banding, an adjustable, circular band is tightened around the top part of the stomach, limiting the transfer of food from the esophagus to the stomach and requiring that people eat small amounts of food slowly. In most cases, after a gastric banding procedure, meal size is reduced to about ½ cup of food, which must be thoroughly and carefully chewed. In addition to restricting the intake and passage of food, new research suggests that gastric banding actually decreases appetite as well, since the band compresses the nerves associated with feelings of satiety.

Gastric banding is an attractive option because it can be done minimally invasively via very small incisions. In addition, the band is adjustable, meaning that it can be tightened or loosened at a subsequent procedure in order to optimize control of appetite. Approximately 10 percent of patients undergo such a second procedure to maximize the band's effect.

The second common bariatric surgery, gastric bypass, involves reducing the size of the stomach. The surgeon creates a very small pouch by separating a small section of the upper stomach from the body of the stomach. This small pouch is attached to the intestine downstream, allowing food to bypass the rest of the stomach. While a normal stomach may stretch to hold about 4 cups, the pouch—which serves as the entire stomach after surgery—generally holds less than ½ cup, and it empties slowly. The new, smaller stomach causes patients to restrict their food intake. Weight loss is further enhanced as the operation decreases downstream absorption of food. Like gastric banding, this operation can be performed minimally invasively.

Gastric banding and gastric bypass create impressive results. Weight loss tends to plateau at about a year, with the average person shedding sixty to eighty pounds. This usually represents about 50 percent of the individual's excess weight. Over time, there is often some weight regain, but after ten years most people have maintained weight reduction of at least 25 percent. This degree of weight loss has a substantial impact on measures of cardiovascular health.

IMPROVED CARDIOVASCULAR HEALTH WITH BARIATRIC SURGERY

Diabetes improvement or remission

Decreased blood pressure

Decreased total and LDL cholesterol

Decreased triglycerides

Increased HDL cholesterol

Heart size and thickness decrease toward normal

Other health benefits associated with bariatric surgery include improvements in sleep apnea, gastroesophageal reflux, asthma, and depression. Combined with the cardiovascular impacts, these translate to longer life. In a Swedish study of more than 4,000 obese individuals, those who had bariatric surgery saw their risk of dying over an eleven-year period reduced by nearly 30 percent. An American study demonstrated that this improved survival was attributable to reduced risks of death from coronary heart disease, diabetes, and cancer. These two studies of the impressive health impact of bariatric surgery represent our best evidence to date that weight loss prolongs life.

RX: YOUR WEIGHT AND YOUR HEART

Know your numbers:
  Waist circumference and BMI: are you overweight?
  Calories: how many you need, and how many you are consuming

If you are overweight or obese, take charge and make a plan for weight loss

Choose a diet that works for you:
  Go "low fad"
  Think Mediterranean diet (Chapter 5)
  Control calories
  Watch portion sizes
  Never finish an entire restaurant meal
  Use smaller bowls and plates at home
  Avoid sugar-sweetened beverages

Burn calories—exercise

When diet and exercise fail, consider bariatric surgery if you are severely overweight and have major health issues related to obesity

A PLAN FOR PREVENTION

FOOD FOR THE HEART

THE BIG PICTURE

In the last chapter, we explained the risks of obesity and the "secret" of calories. But in addition to taking stock of calories, you need to understand the specific foods that are good (and bad) for your heart. Bad food choices can land you in the coronary care unit or the cardiac operating room. A good diet can have the opposite effect, preventing the development and progression of coronary heart disease. So where do we find the best diet for your heart? (Hint: think seaside villas and olive groves.)

Hundreds of diet books and thousands of websites promise to deliver *the* diet that will secure your heart's health. Don't believe everything that you read. Few of the recommendations are supported by reliable, evidence-based research. The data on diets and heart protection are out there, but you need to know where to look and how to interpret the information once you find it.

We can point you to the best heart diet with one word: Mediterranean. We recommend the Mediterranean diet—rich in fresh fruits and vegetables, whole-grain products, fish, and olive oil—to our patients. This is the only diet whose long-term impact has been studied in randomized, controlled trials. Compared to other diets, it comes out the clear winner.

Within the Mediterranean diet you have a wide variety of food choices. These choices sometimes confuse people, particularly when it comes to determining which fats and carbohydrates they should eat. The truth is that you need both types of nutrients, but you need the "best in class" for each.

A heart-healthy diet can—and should—be interesting and varied. You don't have to give up everything that tastes good to ensure your heart's health. For example, dark chocolate won't make you live forever, but it can be part of a good diet. A glass of wine is probably a good thing for your heart. And coffee, though much maligned, has no established cardiovascular risks. On the other hand, the message is clear on salt, particularly if you have hypertension: most American eat too much of it.

BOB VENTURI AND THE TWELVE-INCH MEATBALL SUB

At six foot three and 240 pounds, Bob Venturi fit in perfectly with his crew of five burly men who had been moving furniture into our new house all morning. These guys were working very hard, but they looked like they needed some fuel, so we offered to get them lunch. Bob asked which fast-food restaurants were nearby. We responded with a roundup of the usual suspects—McDonald's, Burger King, Wendy's, and Subway.

Bob made a quick choice: "Let's go with Subway. It's healthier." A frequent visitor to Subway, Bob rattled off his usual order: foot-long meatball sub with provolone on Italian bread, Sun Chips ("healthier" than regular chips), and a 20-ounce bottle of Coca-Cola. That sounded like a good plan to the other guys, so they all had the same thing, except for Jim, who was allergic to cheese and asked for extra marinara sauce instead of the provolone.

The next day, Bob and his team returned to finish the job. Partway through, while the rest of the guys were taking a break, Bob came into the living room and said, "Your wife mentioned that you are a heart doctor. What is the best diet for my heart?"

Bob explained that his worries stemmed from a family history of heart disease. His father had had a heart attack at age fifty-eight. One of his brothers had a stent placed in a coronary artery when he was forty-seven years old. His other brother was overweight and had diabetes. Bob was forty-three and had high blood pressure. He wanted to avoid the family tradition that included heart disease, diabetes, and obesity.

Bob knew that good dietary habits can help prevent coronary heart disease, but his doctor had never discussed diet with him, beyond the general advice to "lose a few pounds." Bob was frustrated by confusing and contradictory information on the Internet. Fats, sugars, fiber, olive oil, coffee, fish oil, dark chocolate—what should he eat? His Subway order of the previous day illustrated his challenge: his lunch had contained nearly enough calories for an entire day, with more than a day's allotment of saturated fats, trans fats, sugar, and sodium.

There was absolutely nothing wrong with choosing Subway for lunch. The restaurant has plenty of healthy offerings. But Bob ordered a meal high in saturated fats (meatballs), salt (chips, marinara sauce), and added sugar (regular Coke). Enough meals like this and Bob would become our patient rather than our mover.

After a few minutes' discussion—the other guys came over to listen, too—Bob had the simple training that he needed to make the right choices. Now it is your turn to learn the facts of food for the heart.

THE MEDITERRANEAN DIET

We told Bob that of all the diets that have been studied, the Mediterranean diet has the strongest claims to promote heart health.

In the 1950s, University of Minnesota researcher Ancel Keys recognized that there was something special going on in the Mediterranean. In his landmark Seven Countries Study, Keys reported a twenty-year analysis of heart disease and dietary habits among 12,000 men from communities in Italy, the Greek islands, Yugoslavia, the Netherlands, Finland, Japan, and the United States. He found that despite a high fat intake, people from the Greek islands had very low rates of coronary heart disease and long life expectancies. He linked this to their diet, and the term *Mediterranean diet* was coined.

While particular foods vary somewhat from region to region—more than fifteen countries border the Mediterranean Sea—clear patterns emerged as scientists extended Keys's work and examined the cardioprotective elements of diets in these countries.

COMPONENTS OF THE MEDITERRANEAN DIET

Plant foods: fresh fruits and vegetables, beans, nuts, seeds, legumes, whole grains

Olive oil

Poultry: moderate amounts

Fish: moderate amounts

Eggs: fewer than 4 per week

Dairy: low-fat offerings, moderate consumption of cheese and yogurt

Wine: moderate consumption with meals, usually red

Very little red meat

The Mediterranean diet arose because poverty in the region forced people to eat fresh, unprocessed, locally produced foods. Plant-based foods are the most important, so the diet is high in fiber. Poultry and fish serve as additional sources of protein, while red meat is virtually absent. Low-fat dairy products and modest egg consumption are included. The diet contains very low levels of saturated fats and refined carbohydrates. Red wine frequently accompanies meals. And, of course, there is olive oil—lots of olive oil.

The Mediterranean diet is relatively high in fat, with olive oil as the primary source of fat. Olive oil is rich in "good" fats, particularly the monounsaturated fat oleic acid, and contains less saturated fat. While olive oil was initially favored because of its easy availability and good taste, it turns out to have cardiac benefits, too. Olive oil is associated with decreases in triglyceride levels, inflammation, and blood clotting and better blood vessel function.

Which type of olive oil should you use? The terminology can be confusing and misleading. "Light" olive oil refers to color and flavor, rather than calories; like all olive oil, the light variety contains about 115 calories per tablespoon. Compared to refined olive oil, extra-virgin olive oil may increase HDL cholesterol. We recommend using the cold-pressed, extra-virgin variety as a dressing for salads and vegetables and as a dip for your whole-grain breads. Enjoy the taste and improve your heart health.

THE MAGIC OF OLIVE OIL

Much of the mystique of the Mediterranean diet centers on the "magical" properties of olive oil. Olive oil was used to anoint the ancient Israelite priests and kings; in 1988, Vendyl Jones (the real-life model for Steven Spielberg's Indiana Jones) found a flask in a Jerusalem cave with the royal crest engraved on the outside and the residue of olive oil inside. In ancient Greece, Homer called olive oil "liquid gold" and Hippocrates extolled its medicinal properties, referring to it as "the great therapeutic." The ancient Greeks and Romans believed that olive oil conferred strength and youth, and it was used to produce both medicines and cosmetics. The Romans planted olive trees along the entire Mediterranean, profiting from commerce in this special commodity. Today, that commerce continues, and 99 percent of the world's olive oil is produced by countries bordering the Mediterranean Sea. Building on Hippocrates' conjecture, we now recognize that olive oil contains a wide variety of substances that can affect cardiovascular health. These range from its monounsaturated fatty acids to components that reduce inflammation and may act as antioxidants. For scientists, olive oil remains an object of fascination, as we work to improve our understanding of the mechanisms by which it may influence the heart. For the rest of us, olive oil offers a combination of good taste and good health.

Carefully designed randomized controlled trials and observational studies suggest that the fruit-, vegetable-, and olive-oil-based Mediterranean diet has favorable effects on cardiac risk factors.

MEDITERRANEAN DIET IMPROVES CARDIOVASCULAR RISK FACTORS

Decreases total cholesterol

Decreases LDL cholesterol

Decreases triglycerides

Reduces blood pressure

Increases HDL cholesterol

Improves insulin sensitivity

Improves blood vessel function

Improves heart rate regulation

Reduces inflammation

Although many of these benefits have been ascribed specifically to olive oil, it is difficult to separate out the effects of individual components of the diet. You should think of the Mediterranean diet as a package deal, filled with many tasty, healthy choices. Olive oil is best in the context of this diet, rather than as an add-on to a typical Western diet. Put another way, dressing a dinner salad with extra-virgin olive oil does not "erase" a main course that includes an 18-ounce rib eye steak smothered in blue cheese.

Moving beyond our examination of risk factors, observational studies suggest that the Mediterranean diet may offer protection from clinical heart problems. In a study of more than 22,000 Greek adults, those adhering to a Mediterranean diet had a reduced risk of dying from heart disease. In keeping with our thinking, no single component of the diet emerged as the key factor responsible for this benefit. The same findings hold in the United States, where a 400,000-person study sponsored by the National Institutes of Health and AARP recorded similar cardiac benefits in those following a Mediterranean diet.

To date, we have more data supporting the Mediterranean diet than we have for any other diet when it comes to heart health, although critics are correct in their claim that we do not yet have iron-clad proof that this diet reduces the risks of "hard" clinical endpoints such as heart attack and stroke. None of the dietary studies meets our contemporary gold standard for medical evidence: a large randomized clinical trial. Nonetheless, we think that the Mediterranean diet is the best choice for heart health, in large part because it incorporates the right fats and the right carbohydrates. Let's start with the fats.

FAT IS NOT A BAD WORD

When it comes to diets, the bad word is *fad,* not *fat*. In fact, your body needs fats. The idea that fat is bad for your heart is simply incorrect. Just because a food is low in fat does not mean that it is heart-healthy. Total fat intake does not correlate with development of coronary heart disease.

But the type of fat is important. As we discussed on page 82, the Atkins diet has created too permissive an approach to dietary fat, empowering people to eat large quantities of all sorts of fat. This is a mistake. The fat from bacon is not the same as the fat in salmon or olive oil. Some fats are good for your heart. Others are associated with coronary heart disease.

The Mediterranean diet is the best diet for your heart, but it's not just *what* you eat that matters: *how* you eat counts as well. Think of Fellini's classic movie *La Dolce Vita,* with its leisurely lunches at sidewalk cafés, enjoyed over the course of two hours and uninterrupted by work and emails. Experiencing lunch in this fashion remains the norm in many Mediterranean countries, and it turns out that reasonable science supports this approach.

Studies show that people who eat more slowly consume significantly fewer calories than do people who gobble down their meals. It takes our brains twenty minutes to register satiety, so by rushing our meals we tend to eat more food than we actually need. In contrast, eating leisurely often means eating less. While few of us can set aside two hours a day for lunch, trying to carve out at least thirty minutes for our meals will pay off.

Many of us eat our meals while seated in front of the television, surfing the Web, checking emails, or even talking on the telephone. (It's still impolite to talk with your mouth full, even if the other person cannot see you.) Like rushing through a meal, this sort of distracted eating causes people to overeat. Mindful eating—focusing on your food and noticing and enjoying the tastes and the experience of eating—is associated with reduced calorie intake.

Try an experiment. Choose the right foods, and eat them in the right way: sitting down at a table with the television screen dark and your computer and cell phone out of reach. Find a half hour for the event. Use attractive dishes. You may enjoy the meal more, eat less, and do your heart a favor.

There are four basic kinds of dietary fat. From worst to best: trans fats, saturated fats, polyunsaturated fats, and monounsaturated fats. The names refer to their chemical structures, but the key for us is to understand that each type of fat has different effects upon cardiac risk factors and development of heart disease.

Dietary Fats, Common Food Sources, and Heart Disease

	FOOD SOURCES	EFFECT
Trans fats (partially hydrogenated vegetable oils)	Deep-fried foods Fast foods Commercial bakery products Shortening Stick margarines	Increases heart disease the most
Saturated fats	Red meats Dairy products Coconut oil Palm oil Eggs	Increases heart disease
Polyunsaturated fats (PUSFs)	*Omega-3s* Fish Walnuts Flaxseed Canola oil *Omega-6s** Soybean oil Safflower oil Corn oil	Decreases heart disease
Monounsaturated fats (MUSFs)	Olive oil Canola oil Sesame oil Avocado Nuts	Decreases heart disease the most

* The evidence supporting the cardiac benefits of omega-6 fatty acids is not as strong as that for the omega-3s.

Trans Fats

There is no safe quantity of trans fats—our recommended intake is as close to zero as you can get. While they do exist in milk and meat from cows and sheep, most of the trans fats we consume are man-made. They are produced by bubbling hydrogen through heated vegetable oil, producing a semi-solid fat. The addition of trans fats to crackers, cookies, and baked goods became common because trans fats increase shelf life and enhance taste, giving some foods that melts-in-your-mouth sensation. Trans fats have also been widely used in commercial cooking and in the production of stick margarine (although some, but not all, stick margarines now contain reduced amounts of trans fats).

By the 1980s, the cardiac dangers of trans fats were becoming clear. They increase triglycerides, total cholesterol, and LDL cholesterol; promote inflammation, blood vessel dysfunction, and blood clotting; and decrease HDL cholesterol. With such wide-ranging effects on cardiac risk factors, the evidence began building for a direct relationship between dietary trans fat intake and coronary heart disease. Observational studies suggest that every 2 percent of energy derived from trans fats increases your risk of coronary heart disease by as much as 25 percent. For this reason, many scientists would like to see trans fats eliminated from the food supply.

Governments, food producers, and consumers have responded to the medical profession's warnings. Denmark and Switzerland have banned trans fats. Restaurants in Boston, Philadelphia, New York City, and California are prohibited from using trans fats in food preparation. Large food producers have reduced or eliminated trans fats in many products. The Girl Scouts eliminated trans fats from their cookies in 2006 (and they still taste good). Fast-food chains such as Wendy's, Burger King, KFC, Arby's, Taco Bell, and Chick-fil-A have all removed trans fats. And, after years of secret experiments to ensure that their signature taste was preserved, McDonald's recently cut trans fats from its french fries.

Even Crisco, the original trans fat product, was reformulated. In 2007, Procter and Gamble released a new version of Crisco that met the FDA standard for zero trans fats per serving. However, this FDA standard merits discussion. Although FDA has mandated that all nutrition labels include trans fat content, they left a giant loophole. Foods may be listed as "zero trans fats" if they contain less than 500 milligrams of trans fat per serving. Five hundred milligrams is not the same as zero. Even that small quantity might be bad for your heart health.

Be vigilant. When buying baked or packaged snacks, check the label for trans fat content. Then examine the list of ingredients. If the ingredients include "partially hydrogenated vegetable oils" (another name for trans fats), try to choose a different product.

Fig Newtons: Nutrition Label and Ingredients

Nutrition Facts

Serving Size: 1 (2 cookies, 31 grams)

Amount Per Serving

Calories 110	Calories from Fat 18

	% Daily Value*
Total Fat 2g	3%
Saturated Fat 0g	0%
Trans Fat 0g	
Cholesterol 0mg	0%
Sodium 120mg	5%
Total Carbohydrate 22g	7%
Dietary Fiber 1g	4%
Sugars 12g	
Protein 1g	2%
Calcium	

* Percent Daily Values are based on a 2,000 Calorie diet. Your daily values may be higher or lower depending on your Caloric needs.

	Calories	2,000	2,500
Total Fat	Less than	65g	80g
Sat Fat	Less than	20g	25g
Cholesterol	Less than	300mg	300mg
Sodium	Less than	2,400mg	2,400mg
Total Carbohydrate		300g	375g
Dietary Fiber		25g	30g

*Calories per gram:
Fat 9 • Carbohydrate 4 • Protein 4

Ingredients: Enriched Flour (Wheat Flour, Niacin, Reduced Iron, Thiamine Mononitrate {Vitamin B1}, Riboflavin {Vitamin B2}, Folic Acid, Figs Preserved with Sulfur Dioxide, Corn Syrup, High Fructose Corn Syrup, Sugar, Soybean Oil, Whey (from Milk), **Partially Hydrogenated Cottonseed Oil,** Salt, Baking Soda, Calcium Lactate, Malic Acid, Soy Lecithin (Emulsifier), Potassium Sorbate Added to Preserve Freshness, Natural and Artificial Flavor.

Unfortunately, a second loophole exists when it comes to trans fats. Restaurants, bakeries, and bulk food producers are not required to report trans fat content. As a result, we don't know the trans fat content of the food that schools serve our children or, ironically, that hospitals provide their patients. While there is no doubt that trans fat use has been reduced, it's still widely available. Concerted government action and continued consumer awareness are necessary to limit and eventually eliminate trans fats.

Saturated Fats

Red meats and full-fat dairy products are the primary sources of saturated fat. Saturated fats are not as bad as trans fats, but in excess they pose a threat to heart health. For sixty years the medical profession has recommended that these fats be restricted, particularly in heart disease patients. High saturated fat intake increases total and LDL cholesterol levels, well-known risk factors for coronary heart disease. Therefore, the American Heart Association recommends limiting saturated fats to 7 percent or less of calories, which results in daily saturated fat intakes of 11–14 grams for women and 14–17 grams for men. We agree with this recommendation. Today most Americans eat nearly twice this amount. We need to cut back on red meats and full-fat dairy foods. But we have to do this strategically, choosing healthier replacements for dietary saturated fats.

FOOD	SATURATED FAT (GRAMS)
American or cheddar cheese (4 oz)	24
T-bone steak	18
Butter (2 tablespoons)	14.5
Quarter Pounder with cheese	12
Ice cream (1 cup, standard ice cream)	10
Ice cream (1 cup, Häagen-Dazs butter pecan)	22
Hershey's chocolate bar	8
Eggs (2)	4
Most fruits and vegetables	0

RED MEAT: IS IT REALLY THAT BAD FOR YOUR HEART?

Red meat is relatively high in saturated fat, and as a result, it gets a bad rap. But how much are your heart and arteries really going to pay if you succumb to temptation and grill a steak on your backyard barbecue? This question has generated a great deal of controversy. In evaluating the cardiac impact of red meat, the most important point is to distinguish between processed and unprocessed products. Processed red meat is meat that has been smoked, cured, salted, or subjected to chemical preservatives such as nitrates: think hot dogs, pepperoni, and bologna. A recent observational study of more than 1 million people found that those who ate large quantities of processed red meat seemed to face increased risks of coronary heart disease and diabetes.

What is the issue with processed meats? It goes beyond the fat. Compared to unprocessed meats, processed meats have similar contents of saturated fat and cholesterol. The key difference is that they have four times as much sodium (600 versus 150 mg per serving) and 50 percent more nitrates and nitrites. The sodium can increase blood pressure, while the nitrates may promote atherosclerosis and diabetes.

In general, you should limit all red meats because of their high saturated fat content and try to avoid processed red meats. An occasional meal that contains a reasonable quantity of unprocessed red meat (a 6- to 8-ounce steak, *not* a 22-ounce rib eye) is unlikely to cause harm. However, try to choose healthier sources of protein such as fish, poultry, soy, nuts, and beans.

Recently, several large controversial studies suggested that high saturated fat intake does not increase the risk of coronary heart disease. One doubting editorialist commented that this message is akin to telling people that it is a good idea to ride a motorcycle without a helmet. The problem with many of these studies is that they compare two different unfavorable dietary strategies: diets with high saturated fat content versus diets with an excess of refined carbohydrates. Replacing saturated fats with high-calorie, refined carbohydrates does not reduce the risk of heart disease. Stop and read that last sentence again; it's important. *When you cut your saturated fats, you must replace them with better choices.*

When saturated fats are replaced by refined carbohydrates—particularly those that are high in calories and low in fiber—LDL and total cholesterol fall (good news), but HDL cholesterol also decreases while triglyceride levels increase (bad news). In contrast, replacing saturated fats with mono-unsaturated fats (MUSFs) or polyunsaturated fats (PUSFs) is associated with reduced inflammation, triglycerides, and LDL and total cholesterol. A meta-analysis of randomized controlled trials including more than 13,000 people revealed that coupling a 5 percent decrease in intake of saturated fats with a 5 percent increase in PUSFs reduced the risk of coronary heart disease by 10 percent. Our recommendation is this: get your dietary fat by replacing saturated fat with PUSFs and MUSFs.

Polyunsaturated Fats

Most experts believe that PUSFs are good for your heart. The best PUSFs are probably those that come from fish, in particular fatty fish such as salmon, mackerel, herring, and trout. The story of fish and heart disease began with Greenland Eskimos, Alaskan natives, and Japanese fishermen, groups that consume diets high in both fish and fat. Scientists confirmed that their very low risk of developing coronary heart disease was a consequence of high fish consumption coupled with low intake of saturated fats. Subsequent observational studies in the continental United States and Europe suggested that the more fish people ate, the less heart disease they developed.

This evidence led researchers to investigate the cardiovascular effects of omega-3 fatty acids found in oily fish. The two important fish-derived omega-3 fatty acids are eicosapentaenoic acid (EPA) and docosahexaenoic acid (DHA). Ironically, these fats are not produced by the fish themselves. Fish obtain omega-3 fatty acids by ingesting plankton, the real producers of these beneficial fats.

EPA and DHA have a wide variety of potential benefits for the heart and vascular system. These include reductions in the tendency of blood to clot and in blood triglyceride levels. In addition, studies suggest that fish oil may improve blood vessel function, stabilize atherosclerotic plaques, and decrease heart rate, blood pressure, and inflammation.

As a consequence of these cardiovascular effects, many scientists believe that fish oil both prevents the development of coronary heart disease and reduces the risk of death in people who already have coronary heart disease. The potential benefit to oily fish and fish oil supplements has been studied most frequently in those who have already suffered a heart attack.

One of the most important of these studies comes from Italy, where

11,234 heart attack survivors were randomly assigned to receive either 1 gram of fish oil per day or placebo, beginning within 3 months of their heart attacks. After three and a half years, those receiving fish oil supplements had a 20 percent reduction in the risks of dying from heart disease or having another heart attack. However, this study result has not been replicated in subsequent clinical trials, and many experts doubt whether the reported benefit is real.

At this time, the benefit of supplemental omega-3 fatty acids in heart patients is controversial. In a recent report from the Netherlands, omega-3 supplements appeared to help only female heart patients and those with diabetes. The authors postulated that because all of the heart attack survivors in their study received state-of-the-art medical therapy (aspirin, statins, anti-hypertensive medicines), it may have been more difficult to show further benefit by the addition of omega-3 fatty acids. In addition, the Dutch study participants already consumed large quantities of fish—three times as much as the average American—so they may have been already experiencing benefits from fish before receiving any supplements. Finally, the study used a low dose of omega-3 fatty acids and started the therapy late, generally years after the heart attack.

This study and others like it raise questions concerning the value of fish oil supplements in people with coronary heart disease. While the American Heart Association recommends daily fish oil supplements (1 gram per day of combined EPA and DHA), we do not yet have conclusive proof of a benefit from supplements. But we do think that oily fish should be part of your diet, particularly as a replacement for red meats. If you have suffered a heart attack, when you stop at the supermarket on your way home from the hospital to stock up for your Mediterranean diet, make sure that you visit the fish counter and choose a nice piece of fresh salmon.

Let's expand that recommendation. Bypass red meats and go to the seafood counter *every* time you are at the supermarket, whether you have had a heart attack or not. Every person should include fish in his or her diet. The benefit is double: reduced intake of unhealthy saturated fats and ingestion of (potentially) heart-healthy fish oils.

Omega-3 Fatty Acids (EPA/DHA) in Fish

FISH	OMEGA-3 FATTY ACIDS (GRAMS PER 3-OZ SERVING OF FISH)
Herring	1.7–1.8
Salmon	1.0–1.8
Sardines	1.0–1.7
Mackerel	0.3–1.6
Halibut	0.6–1.2
Tuna (fresh or frozen)	0.2–1.1
Rainbow trout	0.8–1.0
Swordfish	1.0
Albacore tuna (canned in water)	0.7
Flounder/sole	0.4
Red snapper	0.3

DOES MERCURY IN FISH POSE A DANGER?

There is some concern that increasing fish intake might expose people to the damaging effects of mercury, polychlorinated biphenyls (PCBs), and dioxin. These toxic chemicals are most commonly found in large, predatory fish. While exposure to PCBs can be lessened by removing the skin before cooking fish, this does not affect mercury exposure, as mercury is distributed throughout the muscle. For most of us, the small amount of mercury in fish is not dangerous. But the FDA has advised that pregnant or nursing women, women who are likely to become pregnant, and children avoid eating the four species of fish that are most likely to be contaminated—shark, swordfish, king mackerel, and tilefish (also called golden bass or golden snapper). People in these categories should also limit albacore (white) tuna to one 6-ounce serving per week; they may consume up to 12 ounces per week of other fish. In contrast, for middle-aged and older men and women, the tiny risk of contamination associated with fish consumption is outweighed by the potential health benefits. Among these groups, including oily fish in just two meals per week (particularly when replacing red meat) may reduce the risk of developing heart disease.

If you don't like fish, you can get plant-based omega-3 fatty acids (called alpha-linolenic acid, or ALA) from flaxseed, walnuts, green vegetables, and some vegetable oils, including canola oil. Incorporating these foods in your diet is relatively easy: sprinkle ground flaxseed on your cereal or yogurt, eat a handful of walnuts as a snack instead of a candy bar, or make a salad dressing with flaxseed oil. But the evidence that plant-based omega-3 fatty acids are heart-healthy is substantially weaker than the evidence in favor of fish-based omega-3s. We prefer fish, both for taste and for heart health.

Monounsaturated Fatty Acids

MUSFs are found in olive oil, canola oil, avocados, and nuts. Like PUSFs, MUSFs are "good" fats. They do not increase the risk of developing heart disease. MUSFs have favorable effects on the lipid profile, and replacing dietary saturated fats with MUSFs helps to lower total and LDL cholesterol levels and may increase HDL cholesterol. As such, olive oil and canola oil are excellent choices for cooking and baking, and as we discussed on page 94, olive oil has other, potentially beneficial effects on cardiovascular risk factors.

Most versions of the Mediterranean diet include both MUSFs from olive oil and PUSFs from fish. This is ideal, and likely explains some of the benefits of that diet. While some argue that MUSFs are superior to PUSFs, none of the evidence comes from high-quality randomized trials measuring heart outcomes. But we can confidently recommend including *both* MUSFs and PUSFs—instead of trans and saturated fats—to provide a varied and interesting diet that ensures an adequate intake of heart-healthy fats. Including fish as a source for omega-3 fats also makes solid sense.

GOOD CARBS, BAD CARBS

A Carb by Any Other Name: Deciphering the Terminology

We have reviewed the science on fats and determined that some fats are good, while others are bad. What about carbohydrates? Television commercials and Internet advertisements talk about good carbs and bad carbs, added sugars, the glycemic index, fiber, and whole grains. Don't be taken

NUTS: GOOD FAT

Frequently maligned because they are high in fat and calories, nuts are often one of the first foods that people eliminate when they diet. But there are observational studies (albeit our weakest category of medical evidence) suggesting that you can enjoy nuts and maintain a healthy diet. The FDA recently permitted a health claim stating that eating 1½ ounces of most kinds of nuts per day may reduce the risk of coronary heart disease. Studies find that people who eat nuts five times per week have a decreased risk of developing heart disease compared to those who do not eat nuts at all. This benefit has been linked primarily to the specific fat composition of nuts. While nuts are typically 50–75 percent fat, they are low in saturated fats and high in MUSFs and PUSFs. Nuts also contain dietary fiber and plant sterols, which may help to lower total and LDL cholesterol and triglyceride levels in people with abnormal lipid profiles. Other suggested beneficial cardiovascular effects of nuts include improved blood vessel function and reduced inflammation. Our prescription for nuts is to include them in your diet, favoring walnuts and almonds. Avoid cashews, Brazil nuts, and macadamia nuts; these have a greater content of saturated fats than most other nuts. And, of course, steer clear of those tempting salted and sugar-coated nuts. Peanuts are okay and are superior to peanut butter, which often contains added sugar and salt.

But don't go nuts over nuts. Remember that nuts are high in calories. A typical serving of nuts is 1 ounce, about a handful. A *single* handful of nuts per day is a good snack, but it generally contains about 180 calories. Therefore, you shouldn't merely add them to everything else you eat; the best strategy is to use nuts to replace less healthful foods, such as those rich in saturated fats, processed meats, or high-calorie, refined carbohydrates.

in by misinformation and hype. Let us fill you in on the true identities of the good and bad members of the carbohydrate family as we craft a heart-healthy prescription for carbohydrates, centered on whole grains and an increased intake of fiber.

First, let's clarify the confusing terminology and dispel the myths. All carbohydrates share a single basic property: in the body they can be converted to sugar—specifically, glucose. Many people don't understand this, and split carbohydrates into "simple" and "complex," alleging that simple carbohydrates are bad and complex carbohydrates are good.

Simple carbohydrates are those that are digested and absorbed quickly, best represented by sugars themselves. Complex carbohydrates include starches. While many believe that dietary starches cause a slower rise in

EGGS AND DIETARY CHOLESTEROL

Everybody knows that eggs contain cholesterol, and it is widely believed that eating foods rich in cholesterol leads to heart disease. Ergo, we should not eat eggs, right? Not exactly. Today we understand that most people can have one to three eggs per week. Eighty percent of your body's cholesterol is made by your liver, with diet contributing only about 20 percent. Among dietary factors, saturated fats and trans fats have a greater impact on blood cholesterol levels than does dietary cholesterol. So in most cases, the cholesterol that you eat does not play too large a role in determining your blood cholesterol levels. This is not a reason to fill your meals with cholesterol, but it does mean that you can keep eggs in your diet.

On average, a single egg contains 213 mg of cholesterol, bringing you close to the daily limit of 300 mg of cholesterol. Eggs are also good sources of protein, unsaturated fats, and vitamins. Large observational studies in healthy people demonstrate that eating up to five eggs per week does not increase the risk of developing coronary heart disease. However, these findings may not hold true for people who already have coronary heart disease or who have elevated cholesterol levels or diabetes; such individuals should restrict intake of eggs to no more than once or twice per week. A good strategy is to substitute eggs for red or processed meats, or for high-calorie, refined carbohydrates. Whether you are allowed three eggs per week or only one, be honest about portion sizes. A large omelet from Denny's contains enough eggs for an entire week's allotment. If you simply must have more eggs, try making your omelet with egg whites, egg substitutes, or one whole egg mixed with several egg whites.

blood glucose levels than do simple sugars, this is incorrect. Many starchy foods—white bread and baked potatoes, for example—cause rapid and large increases in blood sugar, just like simple sugars.

Sugar is not entirely bad for you. Your body requires 200 grams of sugar per day, and sugar is the primary fuel for your brain. But sugar has been vilified of late, particularly in the discussion of added sugars. Added sugar is any caloric sweetener that is added to a food as it is prepared or processed. So if pineapple, which contains natural sugars, is sold in a can that contains syrup, the syrup includes added sugars. Primarily because of our love affair with sugar-sweetened beverages (see page 76), Americans consume an average of 21 teaspoons of added sugar each day, amounting to an astounding 16 percent of our total calories. Added sugars are everywhere; they hide out in ketchup, barbecue sauce, cream substitutes, many reduced-fat salad dressings, and granola bars.

Although added sugars are chemically the same as naturally occurring sugars, they are not an innocent part of our diets. They provide empty calories—those with no nutritional value. Excess added sugar in the diet is associated with obesity, diabetes, hypertension, and an unfavorable lipid profile that includes reduced HDL cholesterol and increased triglycerides.

The American Heart Association recommends that women consume no more than 100 calories per day of added sugars (6 teaspoons) and men 150 calories per day (9 teaspoons), amounting to about 5 percent of total energy. For reference, a 12-ounce can of regular soda has 8 to 10 teaspoons of added sugar and a serving of a standard breakfast cereal has about 4 teaspoons.

How do you know if there are added sugars in a product? The American Heart Association has petitioned the FDA to require manufacturers to include added sugar content on food labels. This may be part of our future. For now, when the ingredient list includes the word *syrup* or has words that end in *-ose* (such as *sucrose, glucose, fructose,* and *dextrose*), these are added sugars. People are often misled by other terms that indicate sugar, including *agave sugar* or *nectar, corn syrup, honey,* and *molasses.* Some of these are touted as being healthier than others. But basically, sugar is sugar! To limit added sugars, check labels and know the vocabulary. The simplest way for you to cut down is to eliminate full-calorie sodas and sports drinks from your diet and to minimize your reliance on processed foods.

In 1981, a researcher named David Jenkins added to the confusing lexicon of carbohydrate terminology with his development of the glycemic index. His goal was to add science and measurement to carbohydrate classification, focusing on sugar. The glycemic index ranks carbohydrates according to the rise in blood glucose that occurs after a food is eaten. Foods with a high glycemic index cause large and rapid increases in blood glucose. Refined carbohydrates—such as sugar-sweetened beverages, candy, cakes, white bread, white rice, and potatoes—generally fall into this category. Foods with a low glycemic index cause smaller increases in blood glucose. Low-glycemic-index foods include those made from whole grains and most fruits and vegetables. The key question is this: does the glycemic index influence heart health?

We have some data to suggest that high-glycemic-index carbs might be "bad carbs." Heavy consumption of foods with a high glycemic index is associated with adverse changes in the lipid profile, including elevated tri-

ARTIFICIAL SWEETENERS AND *INCREASED* WEIGHT

While our consumption of added sugars has skyrocketed, there has also been a concurrent proliferation of non-caloric sweeteners. We have blue packets, yellow packets, pink packets, and a variety of other products in this category. Once reserved for sweetening coffee, these compounds are now widespread in our food supply; over the last decade, food companies have added non-caloric sweeteners to more than 6,000 new food products. Are these sweeteners safe? And do they help you lose weight?

The safety question is easy. Although there were early concerns of cancer risks, these sweeteners do not cause cancer and have not been linked to other illnesses. The question about weight loss is a little tougher. When used alone—rather than as part of a comprehensive weight loss plan that includes caloric restriction and exercise—these sweeteners do not cause weight loss and are even associated with weight *gain* in some studies. Yale University biologist Qing Yang notes that one reason for this paradox is that sweet tastes, whether from sugar or artificial sweeteners, tend to increase appetite. In addition, neurologists have hypothesized that the coupling of sweet taste with no calories "confuses" satiety centers in the brain and stimulates overeating.

The take-home message: artificial sweeteners are safe, but alone they do not result in weight loss.

glyceride levels and reduced HDL cholesterol. There is also some evidence (from observational studies only) that a diet rich in high-glycemic-index carbohydrates increases the risk of developing diabetes. So it is possible that carbohydrates with a low glycemic index are preferable.

But at this point there is no clear evidence that the glycemic index of foods has an impact on the development of heart disease. As a result, the 2010 United States dietary guidelines recommend that we not focus on the glycemic index of foods. Rather, when considering carbohydrates, the guidelines suggest that we keep it simple: focus on total calories and fiber content while limiting added sugars. We agree.

Whole Grains and Fiber

When it comes to carbohydrates and heart health, the key distinction is between whole grains, which tend to be high in fiber, and refined grains, which are generally low in fiber. This leads to our definition of "good carbs" versus "bad carbs." Good carbs include whole-grain foods with high fiber content. Choose relatively low-calorie, high-fiber carbohydrates. Avoid bad carbs—those that are highly refined, high in added sugar, and low in fiber.

Whole grains include all parts of the plant—germ, bran, and endosperm. The germ and bran contain the majority of the plant's beneficial components, including fiber and a variety of bioactive chemicals. In contrast, the endosperm is the starch-filled, carbohydrate-rich part of the grain; the endosperm is the principal component of refined grains. When grain is refined, the milling process removes much of the fiber and other healthy components, leaving nutrient-poor flour or meal. The flour is used to make white bread, pastries, and a variety of other foods that have had the good stuff stripped from them.

How can you tell if something contains significant amounts of whole grain? Check the ingredient list on the label. The first ingredient should be "whole grain," such as whole-grain oats, whole-grain wheat, whole-grain rice, whole-grain corn, or whole wheat.

Large, population-based studies have suggested cardiovascular benefits for diets rich in whole grains and fiber. Increased intake of whole grains is associated with decreases in BMI, total cholesterol, LDL cholesterol, and fasting insulin levels. The effect of fiber intake is modest; three servings of oatmeal per day reduce total cholesterol by about 2 percent. The cholesterol-lowering feature of fiber is limited to soluble fiber, which is present in beans, peas, oats, barley, citrus fruits, strawberries, and apples. Although small, this effect of fiber on cholesterol is real, especially when the high-fiber offering replaces less favorable foods.

There appears to be a relationship between whole-grain, high-fiber diets and health outcomes. High intake of fiber and whole grains is associated with reduced incidence of hypertension and a decrease in the risks of developing type 2 diabetes and cardiovascular disease. Aim for at least three servings of whole grains per day. Do this by making virtually all of your grains whole grains. Don't be fooled by the color of breads—just because bread is brown does not mean that it is high in fiber. The addition of molasses or brown sugar to bread makes it brown but does nothing to enhance its fiber content.

Recommended Daily Fiber Intake (Institute of Medicine)		
	AGE 50 OR YOUNGER	OVER AGE 50
Male	38 grams	30 grams
Female	25 grams	21 grams

The decision to enrich your diet with whole-grain, high-fiber foods does not mean that you have to limit yourself. The wide variety of available high-fiber, whole-grain foods ensures a satisfying and variety-filled carbohydrate presence in your diet.

SOURCES OF WHOLE GRAINS

Toasted oat cereals

Shredded wheat

Barley

Buckwheat

Bran flakes

Low-fat granola

Oatmeal

Brown and wild rice

Popcorn

100 percent whole-grain bread and crackers

Rye bread

Whole-wheat pasta

Fruits and Vegetables

Like whole grains, fruits and vegetables contain fiber, so they are included in our list of "good carbs." A high intake of fruits and vegetables has been associated with a decreased risk of cardiovascular disease. Aim for five or more daily servings of fruits and vegetables. Green leafy vegetables (spinach, broccoli) and citrus fruits (oranges) are best. Fruit juices don't count toward your daily goal, and fruits packed in high-calorie, sugar-filled syrups may do more harm than good.

The mechanisms by which fruits and vegetables help heart health remain controversial. Plant-based diets rich in fruits and vegetables are associated with decreased total and LDL cholesterol and reduced risk of high blood pressure. The effect on blood pressure may be related in part to the low sodium and high potassium content of many fruits. Some scientists tout the theoretical benefits of antioxidants in fruits such as blueberries, but there are no convincing clinical data linking antioxidants in fruit to reduced heart disease. Blueberries taste good, but they are not a "superfood," as suggested by zealots. However, they can be part of a heart-healthy diet that substitutes fresh fruits and vegetables and whole grains for refined, low-fiber carbohydrates and unhealthy saturated fats.

SALT AND HIGH BLOOD PRESSURE

Diet and, in particular, salt intake strongly influence blood pressure. Blood pressure, in turn, is a key factor in determining your risk of heart attack, stroke, and other cardiovascular disease. Just as you need to know your daily calorie requirement, you should know your blood pressure; both of these numbers should influence your dietary choices.

Blood Pressure Values		
	SYSTOLIC PRESSURE (MM HG)	DIASTOLIC PRESSURE (MM HG)
Hypertension	140	90
Prehypertension	120–139	80–89

Blood pressure is expressed by two numbers: the larger number is the systolic blood pressure, while the smaller number is the diastolic blood pressure. (See Chapter 10 for a more detailed discussion of blood pressure.) Elevation of either is bad, but the top number is the most important. While we call 120 over 80 a normal blood pressure, the risk of developing cardiovascular disease actually begins to increase once blood pressure exceeds 115 over 75.

Salt intake is the most important dietary factor influencing blood pressure. Stick with a typical high-salt American diet and you will likely develop hypertension as you age; it is almost a guarantee. In fact, hypertension is so common that many believe that it is an inevitable consequence of aging, almost like gray hair (or, for some of us, no hair). This is not true.

Societies with plant-based, low-salt diets have no age-related increase in blood pressure. By contrast, in most Western countries, hypertension develops with age as a result of decades of poor health habits, including excess salt intake. But this is not inevitable. A low-salt diet can prevent hypertension in people who don't have it and help reduce blood pressure in those with high blood pressure. Decreased salt consumption has the greatest impact in those who are already hypertensive, African American, or elderly. But no matter what your blood pressure, ethnicity, or age, don't wait until you have hypertension to reduce sodium intake.

When we measure salt intake, we usually focus on sodium (a component of sodium chloride, the entire salt molecule). Current recommendations state that adults should consume no more than 2,300 mg of sodium per day (the amount in 1 teaspoon of table salt); however, African Americans, people older than forty, and those with hypertension or prehypertension are advised to limit daily sodium consumption to 1,500 mg per day (⅔ teaspoon). In fact, new dietary guidelines may soon recommend that all adults target a sodium intake of 1,500 mg/day. At first that does not sound too difficult—just avoid the saltshaker and you will be fine, right?

Wrong. The challenge with cutting sodium intake is that sodium is everywhere. Seventy-five percent of dietary sodium comes from processed, prepared, and restaurant foods. As a consequence, the average sodium content in the American diet is 3,900 mg per day, more than double the recommended allowance. Only a small percentage of that comes from home cooking or excessive use of the salt shaker at the table.

Today, it is difficult for most people to reduce their daily sodium load to 1,500 mg. But even cutting back by one-third (from 3,900 mg per day to 2,600 mg per day), a realistic goal, might prevent 50,000 to 100,000 heart attacks, 30,000 to 60,000 strokes, and 40,000 to 90,000 deaths annually. The annual savings in health care dollars has been estimated at $10 billion to $24 billion. Some authorities claim that reducing salt intake may produce as many benefits as quitting smoking, although this hypothesis has not yet been tested.

WHY WE PUT SALT IN OUR FOOD

For the first few million years of our evolution, humans ate a diet very low in salt. This all changed about 5,000 years ago, when the Chinese discovered that salt could be used to preserve food. This revelation dramatically changed patterns of food preparation and distribution, injecting large quantities of salt into the diet. Salt became so valuable that in ancient Rome soldiers were paid with a handful of salt each day. When soldiers were later paid with coin, their wages were termed their "salt money"—our word *salary* derives from the Latin for "salt." By 1870, salt was the most heavily traded commodity in the world and was present throughout the food supply. Then technology stepped in. Development of refrigeration reduced the need for salt-based preservation, and salt consumption declined precipitously. However, over the last three decades, food manufacturers have increased production of highly processed and salted foods. As a result, we are now back to the level of salt consumption in 1870. The difference is that in 1870 there were reasons to add salt to food. In 2012 there are more compelling reasons to remove it.

So the question is, how can you cut sodium from your diet? The first step is to make educated food choices. This requires knowing where sodium hides. One deli sandwich can have 2,000 mg or more of sodium. Salt also hides in pizza, pasta, and condiments. And you probably recognize the high salt content of Chinese food served in American restaurants—that sodium is the reason that you wake up thirsty at two in the morning. And while they taste good, a single salt bagel or salted soft pretzel has two to three days' worth of sodium.

You don't need to memorize lists of foods' sodium content—the information is right there in the labels. If you just take a moment to look, you will often find salt lurking in unexpected places. For example, many breads and cookies have high sodium contents, even though they do not taste salty. Limit condiments—ketchup is a major source of salt (and sugar). Choose fresh fruits and vegetables over processed or canned foods whenever possible, as fresh produce has very little sodium. Frozen vegetables without salt are a good alternative. If you do buy canned vegetables, make sure that they are the low-salt variety. Finally, don't be fooled into thinking that sea salt won't negatively influence your blood pressure; it has just as much sodium as the kind that comes out of the saltshaker.

By following these measures, you can make a difference in your dietary sodium intake and in your blood pressure.

THE DASH DIET

Salt is the major focus when discussing diet and blood pressure. But, as we keep emphasizing, you need to consider your whole dietary program, not just one component. The DASH (Dietary Approaches to Stop Hypertension) diet is the most closely studied food prescription for blood pressure reduction. This diet is low in sodium, as you would expect. But it also emphasizes fresh fruits and vegetables, low-fat dairy products, whole grains, poultry, fish, and nuts. Fruits and vegetables are high in potassium, which is associated with reduced blood pressure. Saturated fats, red meat, sweets, and sugar-sweetened beverages are discouraged. This diet echoes the Mediterranean diet.

Sticking to the DASH diet for just thirty days can lower blood pressure by 10 mm Hg; this is similar to the effect many people achieve with blood pressure medicines. This diet is particularly effective in hypertensive African Americans. If your doctor recommends a medicine for high blood pressure, ask whether dietary changes such as switching to a Mediterranean-style or DASH diet can save you from having to add another drug to your list of medicines.

The next step toward reining in salt consumption involves society-wide initiatives to reduce salt in the food supply. This requires interaction between government and food manufacturers. Such efforts require time and negotiation, but several countries have achieved success. Finland took aim at salt in the 1970s, and since then the Finns have cut salt intake by 40 percent. This has been associated with a population-wide drop in average blood pressure (10 mm Hg on average), a 75 percent decrease in the death toll from heart disease and stroke, and a five-year increase in average life expectancy. In the United Kingdom, coordination between government and the food industry has produced a 20 to 30 percent reduction in salt content of processed foods, and salt intake among the population there is down by 10 percent. Similar efforts to reduce salt intake are under way in Australia, France, New Zealand, and Japan.

What about the United States? In 2007, the American Medical Association petitioned the FDA to remove sodium from the list of ingredients that are "generally recognized as safe," which would have gone a long way toward controlling the salt in our food supply. But the FDA did not respond. Fortunately, several major food companies have developed plans to lower sodium content in their products. Kraft, the largest North American food maker, plans to cut sodium 10 percent by 2013. Campbell has reduced sodium content in its soups and V8 drinks. And Pepperidge Farm and Conagra (makers of Chef Boyardee meals, Orville Redenbacher's popcorn, Hunt's brands, and others) are planning major salt reductions, too. The New York City Health Department is coordinating the National Salt Reduction Initiative, with the ambitious goal of cutting salt intake by 20 percent in five years.

Some people worry that if we decrease the salt content of foods, the taste will suffer. The truth is, when salt is slowly removed from foods—over the course of months—it takes less salt to give us that salty taste. And food manufacturers need not worry about sales—food sales in the United Kingdom were unaffected by reductions in salt content.

IS CHOCOLATE A HEALTH FOOD?

Red heart-shaped boxes of chocolate are ubiquitous on Valentine's Day. The intriguing question, debated by scientists for decades, is whether the chocolate inside those boxes actually helps your heart and cardiovascular system. If chocolate turned out to be an effective heart medicine, we would foresee no problem with getting people to comply with the prescription. In fact, the average American is already ahead of the game, consuming 14 pounds of chocolate per year.

When it comes to chocolate and the heart, the focus is on dark chocolate. Studies of dark chocolate have suggested potentially beneficial cardiovascular effects, including decreased blood pressure and blood clotting, improved blood vessel function and insulin sensitivity, and decreased oxidation of LDL cholesterol.

Of these, chocolate's effect on blood pressure has been examined most carefully. In most studies, short-term administration of dark chocolate causes blood vessels to dilate (expand), which in turn causes a modest reduction in blood pressure (2 to 5 mm Hg). A study of heart transplant recipients showed that coronary artery blood flow increased after eating dark chocolate.

We accept the evidence that dark chocolate can reduce blood pressure

READING FOOD LABELS

Knowing what you *should* eat and knowing what you *are* eating are two different but essential components of a heart-healthy diet. The FDA has mandated that all packaged foods contain a Nutrition Facts panel, and by now we are all familiar with the displays on the backs of food containers. Read them! First, note the serving size. One package does not always equal one serving. For example, the common 20-ounce soda bottle contains 2.5 servings. Then check the composition, and choose foods with the following characteristics: 0 grams trans fats, low in calories, low in sodium, low in saturated fat, and, if the food contains carbohydrate, high in fiber and whole grains. Look for foods containing polyunsaturated or monounsaturated fats.

Don't be swayed by flashy health claims on the fronts of packages. Health claims on the front are frequently misleading, and sometimes flat-out lies. "Made with whole grains" might mean that whole grains actually make up only a tiny fraction of the product. "Includes natural antioxidants that promote heart health" may not have any relevance. Consumers tend to assume that front-of-package labels imply some sort of government approval. Not so.

The FDA is cracking down on misleading front-of-box health claims. If a pharmaceutical company wants to claim that a drug reduces cholesterol, it must complete a large, randomized controlled study and gather real data on cholesterol levels in thousands of people before obtaining FDA approval to market the drug for this purpose. Until recently, food companies could get away with these claims without the supporting data. For example, General Mills used to advertise that Cheerios could reduce cholesterol, and by implication the risk of coronary heart disease. In 2009, the FDA warned the company that these claims violated federal law. General Mills changed the wording to comply with the law, but the package still touts the "toasted whole grain oat cereal" inside and notes that "three grams of soluble fiber daily from whole grain oat foods, like Cheerios cereal, in a diet low in saturated fat and cholesterol, may reduce the risk of heart disease." And, of course the Cheerios box displays the cereal in a red, heart-shaped bowl. Cheerios are fine, but we don't want you to think that a bowl a day will protect you from heart disease.

Our goal here is not to beat up General Mills or Cheerios. Rather, we want to illustrate the way manufacturers manipulate the fronts of packages to convey the notion that a food is healthy. Until the United States goes the way of the United Kingdom, which places a stoplight-like red, yellow, or green dot on the front of foods to indicate their fat, saturated fat, sugar, and salt content, read the back-of-package Nutrition Facts panel first. Don't judge a food by its front cover. Use the data on the back and your own knowledge to determine whether a food meets the standard for heart-healthiness.

in the short term. But there are very few data to determine whether this translates into clinically meaningful long-term reductions in blood pressure and reduced risk of heart disease. At this point, the effect of chocolate on long-term cardiovascular outcomes is unknown—some studies suggest that those who eat chocolate live longer and have a reduced risk of cardiovascular disease, while other studies find no such effect.

Why does dark chocolate dominate the discussion of chocolate's cardiovascular effects? Dark chocolate has a higher cocoa content than milk chocolate, and cocoa is rich in a group of antioxidants called flavonols—believed to be the ingredient in chocolate that might confer cardiovascular benefit. Experimental studies demonstrate several potential benefits of flavonols, including dilatation of blood vessels (lowering blood pressure) and inhibition of platelet function (reducing blood clotting). Thus, we give the nod to dark chocolate over milk chocolate for its potential cardiovascular benefits.

But there is a catch: neither the color of the chocolate that you buy nor the cocoa content (frequently displayed prominently on the packaging) necessarily correlates with its flavonol content. Flavonols impart a bitter taste, so manufacturers often remove them when processing the cocoa. Because flavonols may be the most important component of the chocolate—after taste, of course—we would like to see them listed on the package. But methods for processing cocoa are trade secrets, so we consumers are not privy to this information.

Our conclusion on the chocolate question is this: in small amounts, chocolate can be part of a heart-healthy lifestyle. But don't forget about the calories. A standard Hershey's chocolate bar has 210 calories. Dark chocolate is probably more reasonable, in general, than milk chocolate. So if you return to your hotel room at night and find two chocolates on your pillow, one milk and one dark, choose the dark chocolate and have a good night's sleep.

COFFEE AND TEA

Coffee has a bad reputation when it comes to heart health, while tea is generally accorded special healing properties. We have good news for both coffee and tea drinkers: neither is bad for the heart.

Interest in the links between coffee and health is not new. In seventeenth-century Europe, coffee was thought to aid digestion and gout but cause impotence and paralysis—not a favorable trade-off, and also not correct. Today the coffee-health question focuses on the heart.

While some scientists have suggested that coffee might be bad for the heart, others (probably coffee drinkers) have repeatedly rebutted their findings. Among people who are *not* habitual coffee drinkers, the caffeine from two cups of coffee increases blood pressure by 2 to 3 mm Hg. This effect is short-lived and is usually absent among those who drink coffee regularly. Coffee can cause a temporary increase in heart rate, but it is an uncommon cause of abnormal heart rhythms. Boiled or unfiltered coffee contains oils that may increase total and LDL cholesterol levels, but these chemicals are removed by the filtering process, so most coffee has no effect on cholesterol. Finally, some studies suggest that coffee contributes to arterial stiffness. However, other research suggests that two cups of coffee per day actually causes arteries to relax.

In studying the health effects of coffee, cardiologists have focused on hypertension. Coffee does not cause high blood pressure. If you have high blood pressure and you like coffee, you can continue to drink it.

Turning to the heart, large studies demonstrate no increased risk of coronary heart disease among coffee drinkers, whether they prefer regular coffee or decaf. While we have no prospective, randomized comparative studies examining cardiac outcomes over ten to twenty years among people assigned to drink coffee or another beverage, there is enough evidence for us to conclude that coffee does not cause heart disease and that it can be part of a heart-healthy diet.

Recently scientists have raised concerns that coffee might be harmful to people with preexisting coronary heart disease. The question raised by scientific studies and media reports is whether coffee can trigger a heart attack in people with coronary heart disease. The answer is yes, but the risk appears to be extremely small and does not apply to all coffee drinkers.

Among sedentary people who are not habitual coffee drinkers and who have risk factors for heart disease, a morning cup of coffee may cause a very, very small increase in the risk of a heart attack. People with these characteristics may have exaggerated changes in blood pressure and nervous system activity after a cup of coffee, and these factors could cause disruption of a vulnerable plaque in a coronary artery. Additional research suggests that the link between coffee and heart attacks might be mediated in part by a person's genes. A Costa Rican study determined that people who are genetically programmed to be slow caffeine metabolizers have an increased risk of suffering a heart attack as a result of coffee. However, the overall the risk of coffee triggering a heart attack is so small that it is not worth worrying about it or attempting to identify people who might have a genetic susceptibility.

What about tea? It is difficult to compare coffee and tea because tea drinkers tend to have healthier diets and lifestyles when compared to coffee drinkers. So we can't really tell you which one is better. But like coffee, both black tea and green tea have been associated with reduced risk of developing coronary heart disease in observational studies. However, the potential cardiac benefits of tea require drinking five to six cups per day.

What should you drink? The data suggest that neither coffee nor tea is bad for the heart and the possibility that both may confer cardiac benefits. Choose your drink based upon your taste preference. Avoid boiled or unfiltered coffee, which increases cholesterol. And if you must add a sweetener or cream, use low-calorie and low-fat varieties.

ORDERING AT SUBWAY: THE NEXT VISIT

With the principles of a heart-healthy diet in hand, let's return to the counter at Subway and choose Bob Venturi's next lunch. By selecting a 12-inch turkey sub on whole-grain bread with lettuce, tomatoes, peppers, and cucumbers, two packages of apple slices, and water to drink, Bob will make his heart a lot happier. His calorie intake will drop from 1,730 to 640, a major improvement given that Bob is currently overweight. His sodium content will still be high at 1,830 mg, but considerably better than 3,505 mg. Saturated fat intake will fall to 2 grams instead of 25.5 grams, and trans fats will be zero. He could even get adventurous and sprinkle a bit of oil (olive oil, of course) on the sandwich. Bob's educated choices will get him a tasty, filling, heart-healthy lunch and put him on track for weight control, blood pressure reduction, and a life free of heart disease.

RX: FOOD FOR YOUR HEART

Go Mediterranean:

Fresh fruits and vegetables

Whole-grain products

Lean meats: poultry and fish (fatty fish at least twice per week)

Low-fat or non-fat dairy

Olive oil

Replace saturated fats with polyunsaturated or monounsaturated fats

Avoid these:

Trans fats

High-sodium foods

Processed meats

Sugar-sweetened beverages

Read food labels (the back label first)

It's okay to reward yourself with a small piece of dark chocolate and perhaps an espresso as well

CHAPTER 6

RED WINE AND YOUR HEART: A DRINK A DAY MAY KEEP THE CARDIOLOGIST AWAY

THE BIG PICTURE

Is red wine good for your heart? Ask your doctor, and you are likely to get a lot of hemming and hawing. This question generates tremendous controversy, and frankly, many doctors don't want you to know the answer. Here is the truth: drinking a daily glass or two of red wine a day is probably good for your heart. Digging deeper, we find that white wine, beer, and spirits are also acceptable. However, we all know that there are downsides to consuming excessive amounts of alcohol, so the key is to determine the right "prescription" for you. If you do drink alcohol, a few simple facts will ensure that you get the health benefits and avoid the dangerous side effects. Consider the case of Gianni Toso, the Venetian glassblower and heart patient who ignited our interest in the controversy about red wine and the heart.

GIANNI TOSO: HIS WINE AND HIS CORONARY ARTERIES

Although almost everyone is familiar with the conventional wisdom that wine is good for your heart, we had never looked into the science behind this concept until we met Gianni Toso. A sixty-six-year-old Italian glass artist, Gianni came to us for surgery to fix a leaking heart valve. Before having open heart surgery, patients undergo intensive medical testing that provides us with a detailed "road map" of the heart and ensures the safety of the operation. We told Gianni that one of his preoperative tests would be a cardiac catheterization, a procedure in which dye is injected into the heart's arteries while X-ray pictures are taken. The resulting images allow us to visualize the blocked or narrowed arteries characteristic of coronary heart disease. Patients with blocked arteries require bypass surgery if they are having other kinds of heart surgery.

Bearing a striking resemblance to the famed opera singer Luciano Pavarotti, Gianni told us in his rich Italian accent that he did not need a cardiac catheterization. He asked, "Don't you know that wine is good for the heart?" For two decades he had been making his own red wine and drinking at least a glass (sometimes a bottle) a day. His conclusion was simple—years of drinking his homemade red wine had protected the arteries in his heart.

Some doctors don't like to be told their own business, but we always enjoy a spirited discussion with a patient. Being the data-driven, white-coat-wearing doctors that we are, we countered with statistics: based on his age and sex, he stood about a one-in-ten chance of having life-threatening coronary heart disease. We needed to know the state of his coronary arteries *before* subjecting his heart to the stress of a heart valve operation. We did not want to find out that he had coronary heart disease by watching him have a heart attack on the operating table. Besides, we explained (somewhat smugly), the condition of his heart's arteries was determined mainly by his family history, his diet, and his lifestyle, rather than by the amount of wine that he drank.

In the end, Gianni decided that it was not a good idea to upset his heart surgeon, and he submitted to an uneventful cardiac catheterization. When the results demonstrated pristine coronary arteries, similar to those of a healthy twenty-five-year-old, we both claimed victory. We told him that we now had the information we needed to proceed with his surgery; Gianni told us that we had demonstrated the heart-healthy benefit of his red wine. Gianni had successful mitral valve repair surgery and for the next few days passed out celebratory drinks from his hospital bedside to visitors and medical staff alike. Before returning home, he and his wife presented us with a bottle of his merlot and offered a toast to our health. The wine was quite good. In addition to generating an enduring friendship, the experience with Gianni and his wife piqued our curiosity about the relationship between red wine and coronary heart disease. As we began to sift through the evidence for a link between alcohol and heart health, we found that this story, like most stories involving wine, began in France.

DOCTORS AND WINE THROUGHOUT THE AGES

We doctors are interested in wine and have been for a long time. In fact, physicians' interest in wine predates even their love affair with golf. The belief that wine possesses medicinal properties has endured for centuries. In ancient Egypt, wine was used to treat ear infections. A pharmacopoeia from the year 2200 BCE lists wine as a medicine. Hippocrates (450–370 BCE), the "Father of Medicine," used wine as a key component in many of his remedies, and prescribed it as a treatment for fevers, a diuretic, an antiseptic, and a general aid for convalescence. Displaying his customary wisdom, Hippocrates wrote, "Wine is fit for man in a wonderful way provided that it is taken with good sense." Other ancient physicians used wine as a sedative, a treatment for anemia, and an appetite stimulant. Clearly, the medical profession has long been comfortable with the idea that wine may be used to promote health. Today we finally have the data to back up this belief.

THE FRENCH PARADOX

In 1979, an English researcher named St. Leger published an influential scientific paper suggesting a correlation between a lower rate of development of coronary heart disease and wine consumption. He discovered that France, a country renowned for making fine wine and drinking plenty of it, had the lowest coronary heart disease mortality of any developed country. This finding was surprising, if not counterintuitive. Despite a high-fat diet rich in heavy sauces, crepes, and croissants, French people died from coronary heart disease at a rate less than one-third that of Americans. St. Leger's analysis suggested that generous wine consumption was the key factor protecting the French from developing heart disease.

Other scientists and doctors soon jumped on the bandwagon, undertaking large-scale observational studies to examine St. Leger's findings. For the most part, these new studies bore out his results, and the media coined the term "French Paradox." Today the idea that alcohol is good for your heart receives a great deal of media attention, with some stories discussing alcohol consumption in general and others focusing specifically on wine. Although St. Leger did not distinguish between red and white wine, much subsequent research focused on red wine, in part because of early studies suggesting that red wine drinkers from the Bordeaux region in France live longer and have a significantly lower rate of heart-related mortality than do white wine drinkers from Alsace. But you need not choose between red and white wine quite yet. We will have more about this piece of the puzzle shortly.

ALCOHOL HELPS THE HEART: THE EVIDENCE

The beneficial effects on the heart of moderate alcohol consumption have gained the attention not just of the popular press but of public health experts and policy makers. Alcohol is even mentioned in the American Heart Association's guidelines. The bottom line: in observational studies, moderate alcohol consumption is associated with a reduction in the risk of dying from coronary heart disease.

Skeptics remain, however, and some scientists question whether or not alcohol consumption itself is the *cause* of this improved health. The data are based on hundreds of observational studies comparing drinkers with non-drinkers. But none of these studies meet the scientific gold standard of a randomized controlled clinical trial. In such a trial of alcohol as a protector of heart health, similar people would be randomly assigned either to receive alcohol or to abstain, and scientists would measure participants' rates of heart disease and survival over a specified time period. Although such a study would produce a definitive answer to an important health question, a clinical trial assigning people to drink alcohol would certainly push the bounds of medical ethics.

Because the available studies of alcohol and heart health are not randomized controlled trials, participants were not randomly assigned to either drink or abstain; they made that choice themselves. So it is possible that the drinkers and non-drinkers already differed at the outset of the study. For example, researchers have found that moderate drinkers tend to be younger, fitter, and more physically active than people who don't drink. They are also more likely to be married, and generally make more money. These are all factors that have been shown to influence the risk of developing coronary heart disease. Perhaps these factors, rather than the alcohol consumption, account for the improved health and survival among moderate drinkers?

Other scientists have asked whether the category of abstainers, who seem to fare worse in the studies, includes "sick quitters"—people who stopped drinking because they already suffered from heart disease or other serious ailments. If the abstainers include people who are, at the outset of the study, generally sicker than the population of moderate drinkers, then it stands to reason that, as a group, they would have significantly worse outcomes.

In response to these questions, doctors have investigated the possibility that these confounding factors, rather than the alcohol itself, are responsible for alcohol's perceived benefit. Although controversy remains—and most likely always will—most results support the theory that yes, it *is* the alcohol.

HOW DOES ALCOHOL PROTECT YOUR HEART?

The main health benefit of moderate alcohol consumption is a reduction in heart attacks. In this context, scientists believe that alcohol works via two mechanisms: by bringing about favorable changes in HDL cholesterol levels and by causing a reduction in blood clotting.

The best-documented mechanism for alcohol's protective effect is its impact on cholesterol, specifically the effect on HDL cholesterol. As we discussed in Chapter 2, your levels of the different types of cholesterol help determine your risk of heart disease. HDL or "good" cholesterol prevents the development of plaques in the arteries of the heart, so you want this number to be high. In contrast, LDL or "bad" cholesterol encourages heart-attack-causing plaques to form, and it is advantageous for this level to be low.

Alcohol affects both LDL and HDL cholesterol levels. Laboratory studies demonstrate that alcohol blocks the oxidation of LDL, which is favorable, because oxidation of LDL leads to the formation of fatty plaques in the arteries of the heart. However, the effect of alcohol on HDL is likely more important. Moderate alcohol consumption increases HDL by about 12 percent, which in turn may reduce the risk of developing heart disease. Proponents claim that 50 percent of alcohol's heart benefit can be attributed to this change in HDL cholesterol levels. By way of comparison, this extent of increase in "good" cholesterol is similar to the effects of an aerobic exercise program.

A second property of alcohol that may reduce the risk of heart attacks is its effect on blood clotting. We all know that cholesterol-filled plaques in the arteries of the heart put people at risk for heart attacks. But in order for a heart attack to occur, a blood clot must form at the site of a plaque in an artery.

Alcohol inhibits blood clotting by reducing the viscosity or thickness of the blood, as well as by reducing the actions of platelets and certain proteins that cause blood to clot. An important protein called fibrinogen is critical for clot formation, and a study recently demonstrated that by reducing the fibrinogen level in your blood, alcohol makes blood clotting less likely. It also makes platelets less "sticky," which makes it more difficult for blood clots to form. Together, these effects of alcohol may reduce the risk of clot formation in coronary arteries, which is the chief cause of heart attacks.

Several other effects of alcohol may be good for the heart, but none has been studied as extensively as the increase in HDL and the reduction in blood clotting. Alcohol improves glucose metabolism and significantly reduces inflammation. Inflammation recently made headlines for being a prime suspect in the development of heart disease and the occurrence of heart attacks. These effects may contribute to alcohol's cardiac benefits.

Taking all of the evidence together makes a good story for alcohol's role in heart health. Hundreds of observational studies supporting alcohol's cardiac benefits, combined with other scientific studies that explain the mechanisms of these benefits, lead us to conclude that moderate alcohol consumption can be part of a heart-healthy lifestyle.

RED WINE, WHITE WINE, BEER, OR SPIRITS?

When people talk about alcohol and the heart, the conversation almost always turns to red wine. Much of the earliest research studying the cardiac effects of moderate alcohol consumption focused on red wine. Many patients ask us whether white wine, beer, and spirits have the same effects. We cannot begin to tell you how many times patients have asked us this question—but we can tell you the answer. The evidence suggests that red wine may have benefits that are not found in other types of alcoholic beverages.

A short course on winemaking helps us understand why red wine is special. Red wine gets its color from fermenting the juice together with the grape skins for a longer period than when white wine is made. In addition to the rich color, the grape skins contribute certain chemicals to the fermenting wine, many of which may be good for your heart. Recently, chemicals called polyphenols, which are derived from grape skins, have received widespread attention for a variety of potential heart-healthy features. The polyphenol compounds in red wine have antioxidant properties, beneficial effects on arteries that may help prevent plaque formation, and anti-clotting characteristics.

Resveratrol, a polyphenol chemical found in grape skins, has been examined most closely. Experimental studies suggest that resveratrol improves the health of arteries by causing them to relax, and reduces the blood's ability to clot. Resveratrol has generated so much interest from both the public and the scientific community that it is now marketed as a pill, much like a vitamin. St. Leger, who first identified the French paradox, correctly predicted that scientists would try to isolate the chemicals in wine that promote heart health and put them in pill form. But he was against this idea, noting that "the medicine is already in a highly palatable form (as every connoisseur will confirm)."

To date, there is not sufficient evidence to support the notion that taking a resveratrol pill each day will ward off heart disease. We do know, however, that if you do not like or cannot drink red wine, you can get an equivalent dose of resveratrol by drinking a glass of dark grape juice every day.

RESVERATROL: THE FOUNTAIN OF YOUTH?

Resveratrol is present in peanuts, blueberries, and cranberries as well as grapes—and today it is also found in health food stores, where it is aggressively marketed as a nutritional supplement. Some scientists believe that resveratrol may become a useful medication. Preliminary studies suggest that resveratrol may help the heart recover after the damage of a heart attack, assist in managing diabetes, and prevent some cancers. But where resveratrol really captures public imagination is its purported effects on aging. In a recent *60 Minutes* story entitled "Fountain of Youth in a Wine Rx," scientists suggested that resveratrol activates a "longevity" gene called the sirtuin gene. When activated, the sirtuin gene extends life—at least in fruit flies and mice. But in order to duplicate the dose the mice received, a human would need to consume 10,000 bottles of wine! Based upon these findings, drug companies reignited the quest to find the fountain of youth, investing more than $1 billion in efforts to create resveratrol-based drugs.

So far, success has been elusive. Pharmaceutical giant GlaxoSmithKline terminated a clinical trial of a resveratrol-like compound after discovering associated kidney complications. Undaunted, a small cadre of zealous scientists continues to test resveratrol-like drugs, searching for an agent that protects the heart and slows aging without causing side effects. Meanwhile, your best source of resveratrol comes in a bottle of red wine. Choose your wine based upon your palate, but if you are looking for resveratrol, Australian pinot noirs contain the highest concentrations.

Short-term data from studies in humans support the concept that red wine is the most heart-healthy form of alcohol. In one study, ninety-two people were given a daily glass of red wine for a three-week period, then instructed to abstain from drinking alcohol for three more weeks. During the period of wine drinking, the subjects of the study had documented lower fibrinogen levels and lower blood viscosity, both features helpful in preventing heart attacks. In another study, people were given red grape extract—alas, they did not get to enjoy the wine itself—which was found to improve vascular health, as evidenced by increased blood flow. Other studies in humans demonstrate that de-alcoholized red wine decreases oxidation of LDL cholesterol, which has the potential to reduce arterial plaque formation.

What if you don't like red wine? Do other types of alcohol—in moderation, of course—help the heart? Probably. While red wine contains sub-

GRAPE JUICE AND YOUR HEART

Because they contain chemicals from the grape skins, red and purple grape juice offer many of the same benefits to your heart as red wine. Scientists have shown that dark grape juice has beneficial effects on cholesterol and on the heart's arteries. Juice made from Concord grapes is the best. White grape juice tastes good but does not have the same impact on your heart.

stances that may be particularly good for the heart, alcohol itself is the key ingredient. It is the alcohol that has the greatest effects on HDL cholesterol, blood clotting, and inflammation. At this point, we don't think that anybody is going to do a large study comparing the health effects of red wine to those of white wine, beer, or spirits, so you should let your palate determine your drink choice. Our bias is to choose a good cabernet or merlot, both for the potential extra heart benefits conferred by red wine and for its taste.

HOW MUCH SHOULD YOU DRINK?

In this chapter, we keep talking about moderate alcohol consumption. People who drink alcohol in moderation have a reduced risk of a heart attack and live longer than people who don't drink at all. They also enjoy better health than those who drink heavily. How much alcohol is a moderate amount? "Moderate" typically means one or two drinks per day. Many Americans like to supersize their food, and some of us might be tempted to be a little too generous in our definition of a drink. You don't get that kind of leeway when discussing alcohol and your heart. In scientific studies, a drink is precisely defined as 1½ ounces of liquor, 5 ounces of wine, or 12 ounces of beer. So when we tell you about the health benefits of moderate alcohol, we are talking about one or two normal-sized drinks per day.

The quantity of alcohol is the key factor affecting your health. Binge drinkers—those who have more than three drinks per hour—not only lose out on the heart benefits conferred by alcohol but actually put themselves at greater risk for other health problems.

WOULD YOU LIKE A GLASS OF MERLOT WITH YOUR CORONARY ARTERY STENT?

Despite the challenges associated with formulating a safe and effective resveratrol pill, researchers have not given up in their quest to develop novel medicines from red wine. Most recently, these efforts have focused on coronary artery stents. Before they are used to prop open patients' coronary arteries, most stents are designed to be "drug-eluting"— that is, they are coated with medicines to prevent restenosis, a condition in which the stent becomes clogged because of the body's natural inflammatory response to a foreign body. Manufacturers traditionally employ chemotherapy drugs for this purpose. Recently, scientists tested a new strategy: they coated stents with an extract that included resveratrol and other antioxidant chemicals found in red wine. To the delight of cardiologists (and perhaps wine connoisseurs), this special coating reduced inflammation and restenosis in an animal model. While the concept of resveratrol-coated stents is highly speculative and the benefits in humans are entirely untested, these preliminary results in animals might someday pave the way for testing in people.

We know the general rule that white wine goes best with fish and red wine with meat. Now we must extend the rules of wine etiquette and answer this question: which red wine goes best with a coronary artery stent?

No medicine works in everyone, and alcohol, though not generally considered a medicine, follows the same rule. Nearly all of the scientific studies of alcohol and the heart focus on people who are middle-aged. So, as far as we know, the heart-healthy benefits of alcohol apply only to people in this age group. This makes sense, because these are the people most at risk for coronary heart disease and heart attacks. We must include a note of caution for the older drinker, too. As we age, we metabolize alcohol less efficiently. Drinking two or three beers at age seventy has about the same impact that four or five have at age fifty, and the elderly are particularly vulnerable to the negative effects of alcohol, including insomnia and depression. Therefore, people in their seventies and eighties who drink should aim for the lower end of moderate, meaning no more than one drink per day.

ALCOHOL AND SEX

Don't get too excited by the title of this section. We know that alcohol and sex frequently go together, but that is the subject for a different kind of book. The point of this discussion is that alcohol has different health effects on men and women. The effects of alcohol, both beneficial and adverse, occur at lower levels of intake in women. Thus, a woman drinking the same amount of alcohol as a man will wind up with a higher blood alcohol concentration, a result of both her lower body weight and the fact that she metabolizes alcohol more slowly. While this may not seem fair, it is a medical fact. For men, the magic number for cardiovascular health is one to two drinks per day; for women, it is one. Of course, pregnant women should not drink at all.

The risk of cancer associated with alcohol consumption also differs in women. Although moderate alcohol consumption protects the heart, alcohol increases the overall risk of developing cancer. While alcohol decreases the risks of certain cancers (thyroid and kidney cancer), it increases the risks of other cancers (breast and rectal cancer). The increased risk of cancer caused by alcohol is greatest in women (see below). The bottom line here is that because alcohol's effects on both cardiovascular and general health differ in men and women, women should not exceed one drink a day.

We want to cover one additional gender-related issue, and this one spells good news for women who drink. It relates to the impact of alcohol on body weight. We all tend to gain weight as we move into middle age, but women who drink in moderation seem to put on fewer pounds than those who don't drink. In a large observational study that followed women with an average age of thirty-nine for more than a decade, scientists observed an average weight gain of only three pounds in moderate drinkers, compared to more than seven pounds in teetotalers. Although alcohol contains calories (100–200 calories in an average glass of wine or serving of beer), women who drink tend to compensate by reducing their food calories. In contrast, male drinkers simply add the calories from alcohol to their food calories, perhaps explaining the genesis of the "beer belly."

I HAVE HEART DISEASE. CAN I DRINK?

The answer is yes. But controversy abounds: the FDA warns that patients with heart disease should abstain from drinking, while the American Heart Association suggests that in patients with cardiovascular disease, moderate alcohol consumption can be part of a healthy lifestyle.

The data compel us to side with the American Heart Association on this one. We have consistent evidence supporting cardiovascular benefits in patients with coronary heart disease. In a 2010 meta-analysis examining people with cardiovascular disease, moderate drinking reduced the risk of dying from heart disease and the overall risk of death. Among heart attack survivors, a daily serving of alcohol was reported to decrease the risk of early death. In men who have undergone bypass surgery, two drinks per day appeared to reduce the need for repeat bypass surgery, and also reduced the risk of stroke and heart attack

Before you raise your glass to toast, remember that alcoholic beverages taste good but act like medicines. This means that they can interact with other medications, particularly the blood thinners and anti-platelet agents that we often prescribe in heart patients. If a person requires a blood thinner (warfarin) or anti-platelet agent (aspirin or clopidogrel), alcohol can increase the risk of gastrointestinal bleeding. Therefore, the heart patient who takes one of these medicines and who has a history of gastritis or ulcer disease should avoid drinking alcohol. Otherwise, if you take an anticoagulant or anti-platelet drug, limit alcohol to no more than two drinks per day.

CAN YOU HAVE TOO MUCH OF A GOOD THING?

One to two drinks per day can be part of a heart-healthy lifestyle, but we cannot ignore the risks of excessive alcohol. Moderate drinking with meals, as practiced in many Mediterranean countries, is the best strategy for optimizing the protective effects of alcohol. People who drink more than this increase their risks of a whole host of serious illnesses, some of which are even life-threatening.

The risks associated with heavy drinking and binge drinking are best illustrated in Russia. The stereotype involving Russians and their vodka is based upon a painful reality. In recent years, alcohol abuse has been responsible for more than half of all Russian deaths among people fifteen to fifty-four years old. We have not escaped this problem in America—each month, nearly one of every three American drinkers drinks to excess, contributing to 79,000 deaths each year.

BINGE DRINKING

In order to tease out the cardiac risks of binge drinking, French researchers compared Irish drinkers to French drinkers. The Irish were twenty times more likely than the French to be binge drinkers, often consuming five or more drinks in a single sitting; they tended to concentrate their alcohol intake on Saturdays (perhaps in association with soccer games). In contrast, the French spread their alcohol evenly throughout the week.

Over a ten-year period, in this observational study binge drinkers were twice as likely to suffer heart attacks or to die from heart disease when compared to more moderately paced drinkers. Scientists continue to investigate the mechanisms by which binge drinking might damage heart health. Leading candidates include binge-drinking-related changes in the heart's conduction system and a failure of binge drinking to increase HDL cholesterol levels (these levels appear to increase with more regular alcohol consumption).

It is okay to relax and have a drink or two on weekends, but stop there. Don't finish the entire bottle of wine or six-pack of beer: let your friends help you with that, and maybe you'll improve their heart health, too.

RISKS OF EXCESS ALCOHOL: BINGE DRINKING AND HAVING MORE THAN FOUR DRINKS PER DAY

Like any medicine, alcohol has side effects, which can be devastating. While it protects the heart, alcohol increases the risks of developing certain forms of cancer (including cancers of the liver, mouth, esophagus, larynx, and breast), cirrhosis of the liver, high blood pressure, pancreatitis, damage to the heart muscle (alcoholic cardiomyopathy), abnormal heart rhythms, and fetal alcohol syndrome. In addition, alcohol is the cause of many accidental deaths, especially those caused by car accidents. So, just as it would be irresponsible for a doctor to prescribe a one-size-fits-all medicine for every one of his patients, it would be similarly irresponsible for us to tell every one of our readers to open a bottle of wine with tonight's dinner. The "medicine" must be tailored to the individual patient.

The largest study to date that examines the relationship between alcohol and cancer was the Million Women Study, published in 2009, which enrolled almost 1.3 million middle-aged women in the United Kingdom and correlated their alcohol consumption with the development of cancer. In this study, drinking alcohol—whether in the form of wine, beer, or hard liquor—increased women's risk of developing breast cancer, liver cancer, and rectal cancer. The combination of alcohol and tobacco was even more concerning (it is thought that the alcohol acted as an accelerating agent), possibly increasing cancers of the mouth, throat, esophagus, and larynx in drinkers who also smoked. Interestingly, alcohol seemed to *decrease* the risk of developing thyroid cancer, kidney cancer, and non-Hodgkin lymphoma. Overall, however, alcohol increased cancer risk by 6 percent, and the more alcohol a person consumed, the greater the risk. The study's authors estimated that 30,000 American women develop breast cancer each year as a result of alcohol consumption.

So what do we do with the information that alcohol is a double-edged sword for your health? Joanne Silberner of National Public Radio posed this question on February 25, 2009, to Dr. JoAnn Manson, professor of medicine at Harvard Medical School and chief of preventive medicine at Brigham and Women's Hospital. Dr. Manson responded, "A woman with a high risk of breast cancer and an average risk of heart disease may want to avoid alcohol. But a woman with a high risk of heart disease and an average risk of breast cancer might find the trade-off acceptable."

Our take on this is similar. Young women (and men) have a low risk of developing coronary heart disease and therefore receive little cardiac benefit from alcohol consumption. In contrast, middle-aged and elderly people may lower their risk of heart disease substantially with a drink or two a day. Nonetheless, people in that age group with a strong family or personal history of the cancers listed above would do best to avoid alcohol altogether.

RX: ALCOHOL

The ever-increasing number of conflicting studies can be confusing and stressful. One day alcohol is good for you; the next day it is bad. As the old joke goes, it's enough to drive a person to drink. Our goal here is to help you make an informed and intelligent choice about alcohol. Ask yourself whether you want to drink, and then consider your answer in the context of your personal medical history. Involve your doctor—the American Heart Association recommends that every person discuss the risks versus benefits of alcohol with his or her physician. Remember that we have a great deal of information concerning the health impact of alcohol, but we have very few randomized controlled trials, our strongest source of medical evidence.

Our final thoughts on alcohol and the heart inevitably return to the old saying "Everything in moderation." In this case, the adage is supported by the majority of scientific studies.

RX: ALCOHOL

If you already drink:

Drink in moderation

- Men—no more than two drinks per day
- Women—no more than one drink per day; if there is family or personal history of breast, liver, or rectal cancer, or if pregnant, do not drink at all

Avoid overdosing and bingeing

Consider red wine as your drink of choice

If you don't or can't drink:

Maintain a heart-healthy lifestyle on other fronts

Drink dark grape juice on occasion, as it may confer some of the non-alcohol-related heart benefits of red wine

CHAPTER 7

EXERCISE AND YOUR HEART: WHICH TYPE AND HOW MUCH?

THE BIG PICTURE

You can fib to your friends that you are active and athletic, and wear baggy clothes to hide your physique, but you can't fool your heart. If you don't exercise regularly, you increase your risk of developing coronary heart disease, and you cut years from your life. Being a couch potato may be nearly as bad for your heart as smoking cigarettes. Everybody should exercise. Whether your workout includes a brisk walk through your neighborhood or training for the New York City Marathon, your heart appreciates the effort.

Today we have more health clubs, gyms, and space-age exercise machines than ever before. But overall, we devote less and less time to physical activity. Only one-third of Americans exercise regularly. We sit down for hours on end—driving, working at computers, and relaxing in front of flat-screen TVs. The average American takes about 5,000 steps per day (1 mile equals about 2,000 steps), while Swiss and Australians average nearly twice that. We consider somebody to be active if he takes at least 10,000 steps each day. Most of us are inactive, and it's time to change our ways.

Nobody denies that exercise is good for heart health. But like all broad statements, this one generates as many questions as it answers. How much exercise does a person need in order to reap health benefits? Is aerobic exercise better than resistance training (i.e., weight lifting)? Can exercise ever be dangerous? Why do Olympic athletes and world-class runners sometimes die suddenly from a heart problem? Should people see a cardiologist before beginning an exercise program?

Exercise is a big part of our prescription for heart health. But it is also fun. We are going to make sure that you get the right exercise prescription, including important tips to guarantee your safety. There is some truth to the notion that exercise can have risks for heart patients. With our prescription, you will stay out of trouble and avoid the fate of famed runner and author Jim Fixx.

EXERCISE AND THE FOUNDING FATHERS

The United States of America was founded on lofty ideals, including the rights to life, liberty, and the pursuit of happiness. But the Founding Fathers also highlighted the importance of exercise. Benjamin Franklin recommended stair climbing for at least fifteen minutes per day, advising the addition of swimming and weight lifting to enhance health. Thomas Jefferson was more aggressive in his prescription, writing, "Not less than 2 hours a day should be devoted to exercise, and the weather shall be little regarded. If the body is feeble, the mind will not be strong." While our nation follows many of the principles established by Franklin and Jefferson, today fewer than half of Americans exercise regularly. This is one of the key reasons that coronary heart disease is the leading cause of death in our country. We are going to tell you how to heed the advice of the Founding Fathers and begin a safe exercise program that will extend your life. Our recommendations fall somewhere between Franklin's fifteen minutes and Jefferson's two hours of daily exercise.

JIM FIXX: LESSONS OF A RUNNING GURU, BEST-SELLING AUTHOR, AND HEART ATTACK VICTIM

At the age of fifty-two, when he was in what appeared to be the best shape of his life, Jim Fixx died while running. Fixx was not always an athlete. In fact, before becoming a runner, he was a setup for heart disease. He was overweight, smoked two packs a day, and spent most of his time at a desk. In addition, he had a family history of premature coronary heart disease. As a boy, Fixx had watched a heart attack cripple his thirty-five-year-old father. Years later, he resolved not to suffer the same fate.

His solution—and, he thought, his salvation—was long-distance running. Fixx began running when he was thirty-five years old, and it became the center of his life. He logged thousands of miles, quit smoking, and shed thirty-five pounds. Outwardly, he was the picture of athletic good health.

Compelled to share his love of running, Fixx put his passion on paper. In 1978, *The Complete Book of Running* reached number one on the *New York Times* best-seller list. Fixx's well-toned legs, featured on the cover of the book, became famous, and his name was known throughout America.

Fixx enjoyed the celebrity. He gave talks across the country, always taking his running shoes with him when he traveled. Even when he experienced chest pain and tightness during his runs, Fixx would not consider the possibility that he might have a heart problem. He ignored his wife's pleas and refused to see a cardiologist.

On July 21, 1984, Fixx collapsed and died of a heart attack while running in Vermont. His autopsy showed severe coronary heart disease, with blockage of all three major arteries of the heart.

Runners and exercise enthusiasts were shocked. Some suggested that long-distance running and excessive exercise were harmful. Others felt that if Jim Fixx could suffer a heart attack, nobody was safe. The truth is that Fixx's heart disease was predictable and his death preventable. He had risk factors—a family history of premature heart disease and a personal history of smoking and obesity—that should have triggered a doctor's visit *before* he started running. More important, he had warning signs. Chest pain and tightness during exercise were his body's way of telling him that something was seriously wrong.

In his pursuit of fitness and running, Fixx was both right and wrong: right to think that exercise could improve his health and wrong to ignore the warning signs of heart disease. We are going to help you steer clear of the problem Fixx encountered as we plot your course to cardiovascular fitness. There is no question that exercise is good for you and for your heart. But we think of exercise as a medicine, and like any medicine, you need the right type and the right dose. Different people get different prescriptions. The key to a healthy heart is to get the prescription that is right for you.

IS EXERCISE DANGEROUS?

Five to 10 percent of all heart attacks follow vigorous physical activity. So it is reasonable to ask whether exercise is dangerous.

Vigorous exercise—the kind of exertion that makes you sweat—causes acute increases in heart rate and blood pressure, and these factors can precipitate a heart attack or an abnormal heart rhythm. During and immediately after strenuous exercise, the risk of heart attack is increased. However, the size of this risk depends upon the person's level of fitness. If a person is fit and exercises frequently, the exertion is associated with only a very small risk. In contrast, for the person who rarely exercises, strenuous activity—such as shoveling snow—increases the risk of a heart attack substantially.

So, returning to the question of whether exercise is good for you, the overall answer is unequivocally yes. The long-term benefits of exercise far outweigh the risk associated with exertion. People who exercise regularly live longer. If you are just beginning an exercise program, the key is to start slowly and proceed gradually. This enables you to increase your fitness bit by bit, reducing your risk and maximizing your benefit. The more fit you become, the safer your exercise program and the greater your long-term protection from heart disease.

WHY YOU SHOULD EXERCISE

Exercise Prevents Coronary Heart Disease

Here is the first take-home message: *exercise reduces the risk of developing coronary heart disease.* In your quest to avoid heart disease, regular exercise is every bit as important as a heart-healthy diet and quitting smoking. Large observational studies suggest that middle-aged people who exercise regularly reduce their risk of dying from heart disease by as much as 40 to 50 percent. Medically speaking, that is a huge effect.

You'll notice that we keep saying "regular exercise." "Regular exercise" means exercising just about every day. You can take a day off every now and then, but you need to find a minimum of thirty minutes per day to exercise As far as your heart is concerned, any exercise is better than no exercise. The biggest health benefit comes when those who don't exercise at all begin. Walking just thirty minutes per day confers major benefits. However, the more you exercise, the better.

One study compared men who walked one mile per day to those who walked at least two miles per day. Over a twelve-year period, the men who walked two or more miles per day were more likely to remain alive and well. Extending this concept, we find that world-class aerobic athletes (such as competitive runners), for whom exercise is a way of life, live, on average, five years longer than the rest of us.

Many people in their twenties and thirties think this discussion does not apply to them, but they're wrong. You don't get a free pass if you are young and apparently healthy. The seeds of heart disease are planted early. Young adults (and even kids) must exercise for heart health. The Coronary Artery Risk Development in Young Adults (CARDIA) study assessed the impact of physical fitness on risk factors for heart disease in nearly 2,500 young adults ages eighteen to thirty. The least fit people were more than twice as likely to develop diabetes, hypertension, cholesterol abnormalities, and obesity over a fifteen-year period—all important risk factors for heart disease. So even if you are eighteen years old, newly arrived at college, and having the time of your life, take a break from the library (or the parties) and visit the gym.

What if you are sixty-five years old and have never exercised? The answer is the same as for the college student—get started. A recent study of sedentary seniors demonstrated that exercise training improved physical fitness, blood vessel function, and heart muscle efficiency. No matter what your age, if you start to exercise today, you will improve your fitness within just three months. Note that we said *today,* not tomorrow. Don't procrastinate. We are thrilled that you are reading this. But if you have not exercised yet today, stop and take a thirty-minute break right now and go for a walk, or get on the elliptical trainer or treadmill. Then return to the book.

The mission here goes beyond looking good in a bathing suit for summer. We want to get you in shape for life. Exercise needs to become a part of your daily routine. Exercise is like sleep; you can't store it up. You have to develop a program—we will help with that. And you have to stick with it— that part is up to you. The cardiovascular benefits of exercise set in quickly, but if you stop exercising, the conditioning disappears just as rapidly.

IS SEX EXERCISE?

The answer depends on what you do and for how long. Because this book is rated PG, we won't go into the details of this topic, but we can give you some general guidelines. On average (and of course none of us wants to lay claim to being average), sex lasts for five to fifteen minutes and consumes about as much energy as walking one mile in twenty minutes. The younger and more vigorous among us may double or even triple this figure, reaching the threshold of vigorous exercise. Alas, these people are the exception. So can we make an argument for sex, heart-wise? The answer is probably yes. A healthy sex life correlates with a healthy heart. A recent observational study made headlines with the finding that men who had sex at least twice per week were less likely to develop cardiovascular disease compared with those who had sex once a month or less. While this observation does not necessarily mean that sexual activity prevents heart disease, it suggests that sex can be part of a heart-healthy lifestyle.

One note about sex for those with diagnosed coronary heart disease: sex is safe and has an extremely low risk of precipitating a heart attack. But men with coronary heart disease do need to follow the rules. When heart attacks occur during or after sex, they almost always involve older men in extramarital affairs with younger women. For those men, it would have been safer to stay at home and burn off excess energy on a treadmill in the basement.

Exercise to Treat Coronary Heart Disease

So far, we have presented a strong case for exercise in the prevention of heart disease. What about people who already have coronary heart disease? Should they exercise, too? The answer, of course, is a resounding yes. It is a myth that people should not exercise if they have a heart condition. The truth is that nearly all people with heart problems should exercise.

People who have coronary heart disease *must* see a doctor before beginning an exercise program. Those with symptoms such as chest pain and shortness of breath will usually undergo an exercise stress test to ensure the safety of exercise and determine the appropriate type and intensity of exercise. Once heart patients get the green light, they should make exercise a key part of their heart program.

When people talk about exercise for heart patients, they often use the

SLEEP IS IMPORTANT, TOO

We know that a good night's sleep makes us feel better. But is it important for heart health? Former president Bill Clinton thinks so. After a recent hospitalization to treat a blocked artery on his heart, Clinton commented, "I didn't sleep much for a month. That probably accelerated what was already going on." Our evidence suggests that Clinton was probably right.

The benefits of sleep go well beyond the resting of muscles made sore by exertion. Sleeping a solid seven or eight hours per night is a marker of good heart health. A recent study showed that inadequate sleep is associated with increased calcium buildup in the heart's arteries. This calcium is a component of the plaques that cause heart attacks. One hour less sleep each night increased the risk of arterial calcification by 33 percent. People who slept less than six hours per night had the greatest risk of developing changes in the arteries of the heart.

Exactly how sleep influences the coronary arteries is unknown. But we do know that not getting enough sleep is associated with risk factors for heart disease. Those who sleep less than six hours per night tend to have higher blood pressure, higher blood sugar, greater inflammation, and more obesity than those who sleep longer. In a recent study from Columbia University, sleep-deprived subjects consumed an average of 300 additional calories compared to those who enjoyed a full night's sleep: ice cream was the preferred food among those who were tired. People with chronic sleep disturbances such as insomnia (30 percent of us) have an increased risk of high blood pressure and a shorter life expectancy compared to those who sleep well. (We hope we haven't just added another worry to keep you up at night.)

Our advice is to respect your body's need for sleep, aiming for seven to eight hours per night. Turn off your BlackBerry and cell phone before you go to bed, and leave them off while you are driving to work after a good night's rest. This is the best strategy for you, your heart, and everybody else on the road.

term "cardiac rehab." Cardiac rehab is a comprehensive program to improve heart health in people with heart disease, and includes exercise, diet, weight management, smoking cessation, psychosocial support, and management of conditions that lead to heart disease, such as diabetes and high blood pressure. Cardiac rehab is safe and effective: it improves heart health and prevents death. Each year in the United States, cardiac rehab *should* be offered to more than 2 million people, but doctors prescribe it for only 10 to 20 percent of those who need it. Women and the elderly are least likely to get the referral that could save their lives. If you or a family member has heart disease, ask your doctor for a referral to cardiac rehab. It works.

As with any exercise program, the habits taught in a twelve-week cardiac rehab program are meant to last a lifetime. But most people don't understand the need for persistence. One year after completing cardiac rehab, only 37 percent of heart patients continue to exercise regularly.

Some patients stop exercising because they are afraid to do it on their own, especially if they have had a serious heart problem. Instead, they should be scared of the consequences of *failing* to exercise. With a doctor's okay, exercise is definitely safe after a heart attack, angioplasty, stenting, or bypass surgery. In people with coronary heart disease, an exercise program substantially reduces the risk of death from a subsequent heart attack. In addition, exercise improves the efficiency of the heart and increases blood flow, thereby raising the threshold for development of chest pain (angina). This means that people with coronary heart disease who exercise regularly can perform a wider variety of activities without pain.

If you have had an angioplasty and placement of a stent or if you have had bypass surgery, *you need to understand that you are not cured.* Coronary heart disease is not like appendicitis, which goes away once the appendix is removed. After angioplasty or bypass surgery, your plumbing is better, but you still have coronary artery disease. Your mission is to prevent the coronary heart disease from progressing. That is where exercise and cardiac rehab are critical.

Along with medicines and diet, exercise has scientifically proven benefits in people with coronary heart disease. In one study, 118 patients who had coronary angioplasty or stenting were randomly assigned to either a program of exercise three times per week or to usual medical care without exercise. After six months, those who exercised had fewer heart problems, less progression of heart disease, fewer hospital readmissions, and better heart function. In a more recent study of nearly 19,000 heart attack survivors, sticking with cardiac rehab for six months—exercise, good diet, quitting smoking, taking their medicines—substantially reduced the risk of suffering another heart attack. People who stayed in the program felt better, too.

For heart patients, exercise and cardiac rehab should begin under medical supervision, preferably in a formal cardiac rehab program. If you have just had a heart attack, angioplasty, or bypass surgery, you will need to recover for two weeks before beginning regular trips to the rehab facility. Once you begin going, you need to go at least three times a week. Yes, we know it is hard to get there that often—but it is not nearly as inconvenient as another heart attack or encounter with the heart surgeon. Actually, we recommend that you go five times a week. After a few weeks, though, you can do the exercises on your own if you choose. Supervision during the first few weeks is key to get your exercise prescription in order and to ensure your safety.

HOW DOES EXERCISE HELP THE HEART?

Coronary heart disease looks fairly simple on an angiogram or X-ray. The arteries on the heart are like pipes that carry blood to the heart muscle. In people with coronary heart disease, the pipes become partially or completely blocked. The heart muscle does not receive enough blood flow, and heart cells are starved for oxygen and nutrients. When a blood clot forms in the artery, the patient often has a heart attack.

The concept is simple, but the causes are complex. A wide variety of conditions contribute to the development of coronary heart disease, including elevated LDL cholesterol, low HDL cholesterol, inflammation, high blood pressure, increased blood clotting, diabetes, and malfunction of the inner lining of the arteries. No single medicine addresses all of these dangerous risk factors for heart disease. Remarkably, exercise—simple and inexpensive—affects every single one.

EXERCISE MAKES A HEALTHY HEART

Many people believe that exercise's only impact on heart disease is due to its ability to increase HDL cholesterol levels, But this is only one of many benefits. Moderate exercise increases HDL cholesterol levels by 2 or 3 mg/dL (about 5 percent), while more vigorous exercise, such as running, results in larger increases. These increases in HDL cholesterol may be small, but they count; an increase of just 1 mg/dL appears to decrease the risk of coronary heart disease by approximately 3 percent. Exercise also decreases LDL cholesterol, total cholesterol, and triglyceride levels. Overall, exercise remains an important component of a program to manage cholesterol levels, particularly when combined with diet and, often, statin medications.

Inflammation works in concert with LDL cholesterol to cause the plaques of coronary heart disease. Because many people with coronary heart disease are in a constant state of low-grade inflammation, some scientists wonder if anti-inflammatory strategies might retard or prevent heart disease. While researchers have not yet fully answered this question, we do know that regular exercise reduces inflammation in the body. Studies demonstrate that people who exercise have lower blood levels of C-reactive protein, or CRP, an important marker of inflammation and heart disease risk.

Although diet is important for weight loss, exercise training greatly helps sustain weight loss. Exercise in young adults helps to stave off the typical weight gain of middle age. In a recent study of 3,000 young adults who were followed for more than twenty years, men who exercised at least thirty minutes per day gained six fewer pounds than those who were inactive; the benefit was even greater in women, with exercise trimming an average of thirteen pounds off middle-aged weight.

As exercise prevents weight gain, it leads to a more favorable body composition, with increased lean body mass. This is associated with lower risk of both heart disease and diabetes. The impact of exercise on diabetes is particularly important, as diabetics face an increased risk of developing coronary heart disease.

Focusing directly on the heart and blood vessels, we see that in people who exercise regularly, the heart does not have to work as hard to pump the blood. This increased efficiency contributes to a drop in resting heart rate. In most cases, a low heart rate (60 beats per minute) is a sign of good heart health. Many long-distance runners have heart rates of 40 to 50 beats per minute, and Lance Armstrong's resting heart rate is said to be in the thirties.

Exercise also directly affects the heart's arteries. A healthy endothelium—the inner lining of the artery—enables the coronary arteries to dilate and increase blood flow when the heart needs more nutrients and oxygen, such as during exercise. If the endothelium is damaged, blood flow becomes abnormal, setting the stage for development of the plaques of coronary heart disease. Exercise helps keep the endothelium healthy by stimulating production of chemicals such as nitric oxide and proteins that maintain the function of the endothelium.

Through its impact on arteries in the rest of the body, regular exercise causes a decrease in blood pressure and can even prevent development of hypertension. In people with high blood pressure, exercise can lower blood pressure by as much as 10 mm Hg, often reducing the need for expensive medications. Even a 3 mm Hg drop in blood pressure substantially reduces the risk of developing heart disease or stroke. So people with high blood pressure need not fear exercise; they should embrace it.

In addition to all of these preventive features, exercise sets in motion a number of events that benefit people who already have coronary heart disease. In heart patients who exercise, the endothelium's health is improved and blood flow to the heart increases, helping to compensate for arteries that are blocked. Increased blood flow can also reduce anginal chest pain. Unfortunately, exercise does not cause regression of coronary heart disease, nor does exercise cause growth of new arteries (called collaterals); these often-discussed attributes of exercise are myths. But exercise *does* increase blood flow to the heart in people with diseased arteries.

FLEXIBILITY, YOUR ARTERIES, AND YOUR HEALTH

Normal arteries are elastic, which helps keep blood pressure normal. Stiffening of the arteries is associated with high blood pressure and heart disease. How can you know if your arteries are flexible? Researchers recently discovered that flexible muscles and joints are signs of flexible arteries. Scientists had volunteers sit down with their backs against a wall and their legs stretched in front of them. Subjects then reached forward as far as they could and tried to touch their toes. In people who were middle-aged or older, flexibility on this test directly correlated with arterial flexibility. Give this a try and test your own flexibility. Other studies have determined that people who stretch regularly have decreased arterial stiffness. The cause-and-effect relationship between arterial and physical flexibility is not confirmed. But for a variety of reasons, including avoidance of orthopedic injury, it is a good idea to include stretching in your exercise program.

Exercise provides one other crucial benefit to people with coronary heart disease. Through at least three mechanisms, regular exercise helps to prevent formation of blood clots that cause heart attacks. Exercise makes platelets in the blood less sticky, which reduces their ability to initiate blood clotting. Exercise also promotes the production of proteins that travel in the blood and help to break down clots. Finally, the healthy endothelial lining of exercise-trained arteries resists blood clot formation.

EXERCISE MAKES YOU HEALTHIER . . . AND SMARTER

In addition to advancing cardiovascular health, exercise has a wide range of other major benefits, including reducing the risks of developing colon or breast cancer. Many scientists are particularly intrigued by the large number of observational studies suggesting that exercise improves cognitive ability. Yes, it appears plausible that exercise makes you smarter. In a study of 1.2 million Swedish men, cardiovascular fitness, but not muscle strength, was associated with increased intelligence. In that study, superior cardiovascular fitness at age eighteen was associated with higher educational attainment and better jobs down the road. Delving more deeply into the relationship between cognitive function and exercise, a meta-analysis of twenty-nine randomized controlled trials found that aerobic exercise was associated with improvements in attention, processing speed, and memory, with the addition of resistance training enhancing these benefits. The impact of exercise on both physical and mental health knows no age limits. Among older adults, increased physical activity is associated with reduced risk of dementia.

Recent studies in animals suggest that exercise increases blood flow to the brain and can even cause an increase in the size of the hippocampus, a part of the brain associated with memory. Is higher intelligence a consequence of fitness, or do people who are more intelligent choose to exercise? We don't know the answer. Although the scientific evidence explaining the association is limited, we generally agree with Thomas Jefferson's assertion that a strong mind lives in a healthy body. Exercise helps to achieve both.

THE EXERCISE PRESCRIPTION

Exercise is good for your heart. It both prevents heart disease and helps treat heart disease if you already have it. We understand the biology of how this works—exercise attacks a wide variety of the factors that hurt your heart. Now it is time to give you the prescription. How do you start? How much should you exercise? Do you go with Jillian Michaels, the P90X program, or something entirely different? To answer these questions, we return to our medicine analogy. For you, exercise should be fun. But for your heart, exercise is a medicine—it comes in different strengths. We are going to help you figure out the dose that is right for you, crafting a prescription that includes both aerobic and resistance training.

TAKE THE STAIRS

Are you one of those people who gets in the elevator and takes it up (or down) one floor? Take the stairs—doctor's orders! You will avoid disapproving stares from other people in the elevator, and you will help your heart. In the Geneva Stair Study, nurses and doctors at the University Hospital of Geneva were encouraged to use stairs instead of elevators for a period of twelve weeks. Climbing 100 to 150 floors per week corresponded to eight to twelve minutes of daily exercise. That does not sound like much, but the payoff was real and measurable. People who took the stairs lost weight, had decreases in blood pressure and LDL cholesterol, and saw a 10 percent improvement in exercise capacity. This increase in fitness was achieved in only twelve weeks. Take the stairs!

Aerobic Exercise

The ultimate goal is to reach thirty minutes of aerobic exercise at least five days per week. If you currently do not exercise at all, we will get you to this goal in four weeks. Start today. Walking is the easiest way to fill this prescription. Begin by walking twenty minutes per day, three days per week. Walk briskly—faster than your normal pace, but slowly enough that you can speak comfortably while walking. This will generally mean a pace of approximately 3 or 4 miles per hour. If this level of exercise causes chest pain or shortness of breath, stop; these are signs that you need to see your doctor before resuming the program.

After two weeks, increase your walking time to thirty minutes per day three times per week. Do this for two weeks. The next step is to exercise every day, but we'll be a bit lenient and suggest that you walk *at least* five days per week. Really, though, walking every day is optimal.

You can make this fun. Walk with a friend or family member. You can break up the walking into ten-minute intervals or mix it with other enjoyable activities. Play basketball in your driveway or throw a Frisbee back and forth. Set up a badminton net in the backyard. Join an aerobics class. Play golf, walking part of the course. The options are nearly endless. The goal is to choose an activity that you like enough to make it part of your daily routine.

VIDEO GAMES AS EXERCISE

One creative way to get your daily dose of exercise is to play games on the Wii. One-third of the activities in the Wii sports video and fitness packages require enough energy expenditure to qualify them as moderate-intensity exercise. Golf and bowling involve only low-level exertion, but you can work up a real sweat on the Wii with boxing and tennis. Although we recommend real sports over virtual sports, these video games can help you exercise if you can't get to a gym or a park.

We tested the "sports" ourselves. After an hour of Wii boxing, we woke up the next day with muscle soreness. We're all familiar with sports-related injuries, and it turns out that Wii sports are no exception. An article in the *New England Journal of Medicine* coined the new term "Wiiitis" to describe joint or muscle pain caused by excessive Wii play. Fortunately, it is not serious and resolves with rest.

The benefits of Wii and similar systems may extend even beyond the heart. Recent studies show that games that require strategic thinking boost both heart rate and cognitive abilities and memory. Intrigued by this finding, the National Science Foundation has awarded a $1.2 million grant to determine how video games improve mental capability. So, no matter what your age, you can spice up your exercise routine by including action video games in your program. As far as screen time goes, this certainly beats *SpongeBob SquarePants* (kids) or reruns of *Wheel of Fortune* (adults).

Aerobic exercise has a graded effect on your heart health, meaning that more is better. Increasing exercise duration and intensity are associated with greater reductions in blood pressure, decreased insulin resistance, and prevention of cardiovascular disease, as well as decreased risk of stroke. So if you are able to progress beyond the prescription of walking thirty minutes per day, go for it. Increase your walking time to one hour per day, or replace walking with a more strenuous exercise such as jogging, rowing, bicycling, swimming, or use of an elliptical trainer, stair climber, or cross-country ski machine.

Exercises that make you sweat will enable you to make the most dramatic strides in your physical and cardiovascular fitness. If you opt for these more strenuous routines, you need to begin with a five-minute aerobic warm-up to prepare your cardiovascular system for the exertion to come and reduce the stress on your heart. This can be the same activity (jogging, cycling, etc.) simply performed at a slower pace.

This leads us to a couple of comments on stretching. Static stretching before aerobic exercise has been the standard for decades, but don't do it. Static stretching neither reduces injuries nor prepares your cardiovascular system for exertion. When you bend over to touch your toes or stretch your legs by leaning against a wall, you often cause the muscles to tighten rather than relax. In addition, studies demonstrate that static stretching before playing a sport is associated with diminished performance. An aerobic, movement-oriented warm-up is best.

Make sure to take five minutes to cool down at the end of your workout. This usually consists of walking. Never stop abruptly after the endurance part of your workout, as this can cause shifts in blood pressure leading to fainting, abnormal heart rhythms, and reduced blood flow to the heart. After cooling down, your final step is stretching.

Resistance Training

We have spelled out the aerobic or cardio component of your prescription. Now we will add resistance training to the program. You may want to consider resistance exercises—usually this means weight lifting—twice a week. The old myth that resistance training puts too much strain on the heart and causes sustained high blood pressure is simply untrue. Like aerobic training, resistance exercises are probably good for your cardiovascular system.

Two meta-analyses have demonstrated that resistance training actually lowers resting blood pressure. Furthermore, the addition of resistance training to aerobic exercise is associated with improved blood sugar control, and in observational studies it has been linked to a reduced risk of developing diabetes.

Resistance training can also aid in weight loss and help offset the age-related gains in body fat that occur almost imperceptibly but add up over the years. Because resistance training increases muscle mass, the metabolic rate increases, meaning that a person burns more calories during the day. For every pound of muscle added, a person burns an additional

DO YOU NEED A TARGET HEART RATE TO GET A GOOD WORKOUT?

Fitness companies include heart rate monitors with treadmills, elliptical trainers, rowing machines, and stationary bicycles, promising to help people achieve heart rates that put them in their "fat-burning zone," "fitness zone," or some other yet-to-be-defined zone. Do these heart rate targets help you get a better workout? Does safety mandate that you purchase the latest iPhone app to track your heart rate during exercise? For the most part, the answer to these questions is no.

When people talk about heart rate and exercise, they generally refer to their maximum heart rate. The maximum achievable heart rate is the heart rate that a person would have at full exertion, and is easily estimated using a simple formula:

Maximum heart rate in men = 220 – age
Maximum heart rate in women = 206 – (.88) x age

Doctors use these calculations to evaluate results of exercise stress tests. While some cardiologists have extended this concept, recommending that their patients exercise to reach a particular heart rate—often 65 percent to 85 percent of the calculated maximum heart rate—the data supporting this practice are inconclusive.

You don't have to use some arbitrary percentage of your maximum calculated heart rate to guide your workouts. The truth is that you can have an excellent workout at both relatively low and relatively high heart rates, depending upon your exercise regimen and your own personal cardiac characteristics. Tailor your workout to how you feel, and make sure that you exert yourself—evidence of a good workout will be obvious as the sweat begins to flow. The real key to exercising effectively is to make sure that you are exercising consistently. As one researcher noted, the most important calculation related to exercise is not your maximum heart rate; it's determining where in your busy schedule you can fit a daily workout.

10 calories per day; this limits weight gain and facilitates weight loss. In addition, by increasing lean muscle mass, resistance training targets what Mayo Clinic researchers have termed "normal-weight obesity"—people who appear slim but have a high ratio of fat to muscle. Weight training increases the percentage of lean muscle mass at the expense of fat, which reduces the risk of heart disease.

In older people, resistance training has additional benefits. It prevents loss of bone density, helping to ward off osteoporosis. Of course, resistance training also increases strength. Adults lose an average of 1 pound of muscle mass per year after age forty, and resistance training helps to prevent this loss. Maintaining muscle increases functional capacity and strength, reducing the risk of falls and fractures in the elderly.

While resistance training is safe for most heart patients, a few conditions make this sort of exercise dangerous, including aortic valve stenosis, uncontrolled high blood pressure, aortic dissection, and Marfan syndrome. In many cases, once the condition is treated, resistance training is permitted.

INTERVAL TRAINING: MORE BENEFIT IN LESS TIME

"I can't find the time to exercise!" We hear this complaint daily. People want to exercise, but between work, family, doctor's appointments, and other commitments, they just can't find the time. That's where interval training can help. Once reserved for competitive athletes, interval training is a real option for all of us. With this approach, you can squeeze your workouts into shorter time periods, and possibly derive even greater benefits from them.

The principle of aerobic interval training is to vary the intensity of your activity, alternating periods of strenuous exertion with periods of recovery. For the runner, this may mean alternating four-minute sprints with three-minute walks, using the walk to recover from the heavier exertion. Nearly every aerobic activity, from running to swimming, biking, and even Rollerblading, can be approached in this fashion. Adapting this strategy to walking, an interval workout would alternate four minutes of rapid walking with a three-minute recovery period at a more leisurely pace, repeating the pattern two or three times.

How does aerobic interval training produce more benefits in less time? Compared to standard, steady exercise, interval training produces greater increases in endurance, oxygen use, and general fitness and in some patients may cause larger increases in HDL cholesterol. In addition, studies show that interval training has beneficial effects on body weight and blood pressure.

One final benefit of interval training: patients report that varying their exercise increases their interest and motivation, helping them to stick with the program.

STAYING IN THE GAME

Fewer than half of those who begin an exercise program stick with it. Here are a couple of tips to help you stay in the game. First, think about how you feel after each workout. Savor your sense of well-being and accomplishment. Remind yourself of those good feelings each time you are tempted to skip a session. Second, invest $2 in a notebook and record your workout daily. This will help engrain the habit of daily exercise.

This sounds like a lot of effort, but let's put it into perspective. Finding thirty minutes per day to work on heart health is the best investment you are ever going to make. Maybe your brisk walk can be a standard part of your day. Walk to work, walk to lunch, walk to a meeting—just walk. Join a health club or buy yourself a set of light dumbbells. You can keep the weights under your bed, so they won't take up space.

Exercise provides great social opportunities. Sign up for a class; whether you take up kickboxing, Zumba, or the next new fad, you will have fun with friends and get a good workout. On weekends, play tennis with your spouse or kids. If you play golf, walk the back nine holes instead of riding in the cart; arrive at the nineteenth hole refreshed, and have a healthy snack instead of chips and soda.

DO YOU NEED TO SEE A DOCTOR BEFORE YOU START EXERCISING?

You need the answer to this question before beginning an exercise program, but doctors themselves argue about it. The bottom line is that we want to make sure that exertion is safe for you. We think we can do that without sending each and every person to the doctor for an exercise permission slip.

Preexisting Coronary Heart Disease or Symptoms

Let's start with the people who really do need to drop by the doctor's office. If you know that you have coronary heart disease, you should see a doctor before beginning an exercise program. This means that if you have had a heart attack, a stent, angioplasty, or bypass surgery, you need medical clearance before exercising.

SITTING: BAD FOR THE HEART

We spend more time sitting than we do standing or walking. Many of us sit at a computer all day at work. We then sit in our cars as we drive home to our televisions, eager to settle in for two hours of sitting while we watch a game. Sitting is second only to sleep as the "activity" that occupies most of our time. Sitting does not sound like a high-risk activity, but it is.

Multiple observational studies suggest that the more time you spend sitting, the greater your risk of developing heart disease and the shorter your life will be. A recent study examined the link between watching screen-based entertainment, death from all causes, and cardiovascular events. Studying a population of 4,500 Scottish adults, researchers found that more than four hours of daily sitting for recreational screen time (television, computer) was associated with an increased risk of developing cardiovascular disease and substantial excess mortality.

Why is sitting associated with poor cardiovascular health? One likely explanation is that men and women who sit for prolonged periods—behind a desk at work or in front of a screen at home—have unhealthy lifestyles in other ways, such as a poor diet or smoking. In addition, studies suggest biological costs specifically tied to prolonged sitting, including increased inflammation, abnormal lipid metabolism, elevated blood glucose levels, and decreased metabolic rate, which can lead to weight gain. In a surprising finding, research suggests that you can't offset hours of sitting during the day by exercising in the evening. Inactivity researcher Marc Hamilton notes that "exercise is not a perfect antidote for sitting."

Don't sit for prolonged periods. Walk around the office. Visit a co-worker. Get a drink of water or a cup of coffee. Get up!

People who have symptoms that may be coronary heart disease—chest, neck, or arm pain or shortness of breath with exercise—should also see a doctor for evaluation. In this scenario, the doctor will often order an exercise stress test, which involves walking on a treadmill at different speeds and inclines. This test determines the level of exercise that is safe for your heart. The results guide your doctor or trainer as he or she builds an exercise program for you.

YOUR HEART RATE: A SIMPLE HEART TEST AT HOME

Measuring your pulse (heart rate) gives you important information about your fitness and heart health. If you don't have a heart rate monitor, you can take your pulse the old-fashioned way. Place two fingers on the front of your neck. Pressing gently, move your fingers to one side of the neck until you feel a pulsation; that is your carotid artery, pounding with each heartbeat. Count the number of beats in thirty seconds and multiply by 2. The product is your heart rate.

Now you can determine two numbers that give you valuable information about your heart health—your resting heart rate and your heart rate recovery. A lower resting heart rate—the heart rate while you are sitting quietly—is associated with better health and longer life. If your resting heart rate is 60–80 beats per minute, this is good news. If it is greater than 90, you might want to see your doctor for a heart checkup. Heart patients with an elevated resting heart rate face an increased risk of dying over a five-year period.

The second number to measure is heart rate recovery. This number can be determined only if you exercise vigorously. Check your heart rate just before you finish a tough workout and remember the number. Then recheck your heart rate when you are 1 minute into your cool-down walk. Your heart rate should drop by at least 12 beats during the first minute of your cool-down. A smaller drop in heart rate is a warning sign and should lead to a doctor's appointment. The good news? Once you begin an exercise program, you will see improvement in both of these heart rate indices.

No Known Coronary Heart Disease and No Symptoms

If you don't have coronary heart disease or any of its symptoms, things are much simpler, particularly at the low-intensity end of the exercise spectrum. People without known coronary heart disease can begin a program of walking without a visit to the doctor.

If you plan to do more vigorous exercises—the kind that make you sweat, such as running and cycling—doctors disagree about the need for pre-exercise screening. The American Heart Association suggests that asymptomatic men over forty-five and asymptomatic women over fifty-five should consider having a stress test before beginning vigorous exercise. We disagree.

The problem is the inaccuracy of stress tests in people who are unlikely to have heart disease. In people with no risk factors for heart disease, a stress test will produce at least twenty false positive results for every true positive. This means that on the way to identifying one person who actually has coronary heart disease, twenty people will be told incorrectly that they have it, too. These twenty healthy people will then undergo a variety of expensive, and sometimes risky, tests that ultimately turn out to be unnecessary. We want to minimize unnecessary medical tests and the complications that they cause.

"HONEY, CAN YOU SHOVEL THE DRIVEWAY?"

Don't answer yes too quickly. Shoveling snow can be hazardous, sending more than 11,000 people to the hospital every year. While most of the medical problems are orthopedic, 7 percent are cardiac, and deaths attributable to snow shoveling are usually traceable to the heart. In fact, when blizzards occur, deaths from coronary heart disease spike.

How does shoveling snow trigger a heart attack? First of all, it's hard work. In one study, when shoveling heavy snow people reached heart rates of 173 beats per minute and systolic blood pressures of 200; these changes put enormous stresses on the heart and can cause a plaque in an artery to rupture, leading to a heart attack. In addition, cold air causes blood vessels to constrict as the body tries to prevent heat loss, and this can reduce blood flow to the heart. To ensure your safety, follow a few simple rules: (1) dress warmly, (2) use an ergonomically designed shovel and push the snow instead of lifting, (3) start slowly (a warm-up), and (4) every ten minutes take a two-minute break in which you stand up straight and walk for a minute, then rest. Some people get a free pass: if you have coronary heart disease or if you have two or more risk factors for coronary heart disease (see list below), don't shovel snow without your doctor's permission.

We do think there are some people who should drop by the cardiologist's office on the way to the mall to shop for their first pair of running shoes. We base our recommendations on a person's cardiovascular profile. Yes, we profile our patients. And we are much better at it than airport security guards.

RISK PROFILE FOR CORONARY HEART DISEASE

Diabetes

Smoking

High blood pressure

High cholesterol

Family history of early heart disease (before age 50)

If you are middle-aged or older and have two or more of these risk factors for coronary heart disease, see your doctor before beginning to train for that marathon that has been on your to-do list ever since you turned forty. On the other hand, if your profile puts you at low risk (one or none of the risk factors), begin training today.

MITRAL VALVE PROLAPSE, YOUR HEART VALVES, AND EXERCISE

So far, we have focused on the relationship between exercise and coronary heart disease, the most common heart problem. What about people with heart valve issues? Should they exercise? The answer depends upon the type of problem they have. The most common heart valve abnormality is mitral valve prolapse; 2 to 3 percent of the population has this condition. It is not dangerous. Mitral valve prolapse means that the mitral valve is a little bit floppy or elastic; in most people with prolapse, the valve works just fine. People with mitral valve prolapse can and should exercise. The common misconception that exercise will make the prolapse worse is incorrect.

The only people with heart valve problems who need to be careful about exercising are those people with aortic stenosis, a condition in which the aortic valve, which separates the heart from the rest of the body, becomes severely narrowed. This places a tremendous workload on the heart. People with moderately severe or severe aortic stenosis should not exercise strenuously. Most people with severe aortic stenosis will undergo heart valve replacement, after which they can exercise without limitation.

THE COMPETITIVE ATHLETE

In the second week of January 2010, Americans were stunned when two competitive athletes in peak condition, Chicago Bears defensive end Gaines Adams, age twenty-six, and Southern Indiana center Jeron Lewis, twenty-one, died with no warning. They joined a tragic list that includes Flo Hyman (Olympic volleyball), Hank Gathers (NCAA basketball), Pete Maravich (NBA), and Korey Stringer (NFL). All were world-class athletes who died suddenly of heart disease.

These events are not as rare as you might think. Hundreds of other athletes have suffered similar fates. Each year in the United States, 200 to 300 young athletes suffer sudden cardiac death. Basketball and football players account for most of the deaths in the United States, while soccer is the more common predisposing sport in Europe. Men and boys are affected nine times as often as women and girls, and African Americans are affected five times as frequently as Caucasians.

Newscasters highlight the emotional impact of these events, the lives and careers cut short. There is usually little discussion of the causes, and only recently have the media focused on their prevention. The fact is, we know why these tragedies occur, and for the most part we can determine in advance who is at risk.

First, let's talk about the causes. When middle-aged and older people die during or after exertion, the cause is usually a heart attack triggered by coronary heart disease that has developed over a lifetime. Such is not the case with competitive athletes. Athletes who experience sudden cardiac death usually have an underlying heart condition that has been present since birth, a problem that we ought to be able to identify beforehand. In peak physical condition, these athletes train and play hard, exposing their hearts to extraordinary stresses. These stresses can aggravate unsuspected heart abnormalities, creating risks that might not occur in others with the same abnormality who perform less strenuous exercise. When a young athlete dies, the immediate cause is usually an abnormal heart rhythm, brought on by the combination of a structural heart problem and intense physical activity. An exception to this rule is the athlete with Marfan syndrome. In patients with this condition (Flo Hyman had it, and Abraham Lincoln probably did, too), sudden death is caused by rupture of an aortic aneurysm.

In the United States, the most common underlying condition that causes sudden death in athletes is hypertrophic obstructive cardiomyopathy. People with this condition have overgrowth of part of the heart muscle, and the heart rhythm tends to be unstable. It is not rare—about one in five hundred people has it. It is so common, and so dangerous, that the NFL recently announced that it will start screening players for this condition.

Sudden Cardiac Death in Athletes		
CAUSE	INHERITED?	DIAGNOSED BY
Hypertrophic cardiomyopathy	Yes	EKG, echocardiogram
Right ventricular cardiomyopathy	Yes	EKG, echocardiogram
Marfan syndrome	Yes	CT scan, MRI scan, echocardiogram
Abnormal coronary artery	Yes	Stress test, CT scan

We all agree that any individual known to have one of these conditions needs a cardiac workup before participating in strenuous sports. The key question is, why don't we identify young athletes with these problems *before* they die? In the United States, high school and college athletes are screened by a perfunctory history and physical examination. This protocol misses many critical heart problems, and the tragic consequences are reported on the front page of your local newspaper.

The situation differs dramatically in other countries. In Italy, all competitive athletes twelve to thirty-five years old must participate in a mandatory national screening program and undergo a detailed history and physical examination, as well as an annual EKG. If any abnormality turns up on these tests, they undergo further examination, which frequently includes an echocardiogram. The International Olympic Committee endorses this more intense screening strategy, recommending that athletes have an EKG every two years.

The reason that the IOC supports this approach is that it seems to work. Since more rigorous screening was instituted, sudden deaths in athletes have dropped by nearly 90 percent in Italy. After adopting the Italian protocol, Dutch doctors found that for every 143 athletes screened, doctors identified 1 athlete who had a potentially lethal heart problem. They could actually count the lives saved.

Why don't we do this? Some claim that this approach is too expensive for the United States. We don't agree. Italy spends $40 per athlete for the screening. In the United States, a school can buy a portable EKG machine for $500, and the cost of interpreting each EKG is about $5. So expense is not the issue.

Others argue that the accuracy of screening is imperfect. It is certainly true that widespread screening will produce some false positives— people who appear to have something wrong but are found to be normal on echocardiogram or CT scan. These athletes will lose a few days of training while doctors figure out that they are okay. While this is inconvenient, we don't think it should block efforts to save the lives of our young athletes.

Noting that we don't mandate other kinds of screening tests of undisputed value, such as colonoscopies and mammograms, some researchers question how we can argue for cardiac screening in athletes. In the case of these athletes, we are talking about performing noninvasive tests to prevent deaths among children and young adults. We have a societal obligation to ensure the health of our young. This is fundamentally different from the unenforceable (but medically sound) recommendation that all adults age fifty or above undergo colonoscopy; we can't force adults to have this invasive test. But we can mandate that we protect our children.

All competitive athletes of high school age or older should invest a couple of hours in a detailed personal and family history, a physical examination, and an EKG. At a minimum, the history should search for specific warning signs or red flags. If you have a young athlete in the family, look at this checklist; you'll likely be able to determine if any of these factors apply. If any of them do, a visit to the cardiologist is imperative.

SCREENING ATHLETES FOR HEART DISEASE

Family History

Early heart disease in family (in a relative less than 50 years old)

Sudden cardiac death or sudden death of unknown cause

Family member with hypertrophic cardiomyopathy, Marfan syndrome, or other inherited heart disease

Personal History

Heart murmur

High blood pressure

Fainting spells

Chest pain with exercise

Excessive shortness of breath with exercise

Unusual fatigue

It is also important to pay attention to warning signs in athletes. Twenty percent of young athletes who die experience symptoms during the week before the tragedy. Common complaints are chest pain, feeling faint, indigestion or heartburn, increasing fatigue, and profound shortness of breath. If any of these occurs, especially if it represents a change, don't write off the symptoms as the result of a tough workout. Investigate. Save a life.

At the end of the day, is screening athletes for heart disease cost-effective? Maybe not. But is it worth it? We think so.

MARATHON RUNNING: GOOD FOR THE HEART?

Nearly half a million Americans finish a marathon each year. Marathon running is gaining in popularity—and, unfortunately, in notoriety. Every year, we read at least one story describing an athlete who died during or shortly after a marathon. It turns out that the actual risk of dying as a result of running a marathon is between 1 in 50,000 and 1 in 100,000. This is exceedingly low. Heart problems in older marathoners are almost always the result of coronary heart disease; in younger athletes, they're the result of inherited heart defects. Following the screening guidelines we have provided can identify these conditions and ensure the runner's safety. In particular, remember that exercise does not erase damage from years of smoking, high cholesterol, or high blood pressure.

Recently, the media have reported stories that have complicated the picture for runners. When runners undergo blood tests and an echocardiogram just after completing a marathon, the tests reveal mildly abnormal heart function. Within two weeks, the heart returns to normal. While this suggests a potential cardiac cost to marathon running, the benefits of long-distance running—including decreased body fat, decreased heart rate, lower blood pressure, and excellent lipid profiles—far outweigh these transient cardiac changes. In addition, athletes who train harder and run more than 45 miles per week have fewer abnormalities on these tests, demonstrating a benefit to preparing appropriately. Overall, long-distance runners have greater cardiovascular fitness than people who do not exercise. The message here: if you decide to run a marathon, see a doctor first if you fall into a category for which we recommend screening, and take the time to train.

RX: EXERCISE

Exercise basics:

How much

- At least 30 minutes per day
- Five days per week

What type

- *Aerobic*
  Brisk walking at a minimum
  Fun alternatives—basketball, Frisbee, bicycling
  Vigorous exercise that causes you to break a sweat if you can
  Heart rate monitor is generally unnecessary

- *Resistance*
  Two days per week
  Light weights or machines
  After aerobic exercise

- *Warm-up*
  Before each exercise session: movement-based, like a light jog

- *Cool-down and stretching*
  After completing the workout

See a doctor before you start a strenuous exercise program if:

You have coronary heart disease

You have chest pain or shortness of breath with exertion

You have two or more risk factors:

- Smoking
- Diabetes
- High blood pressure
- High cholesterol
- Family history of early heart disease

CHAPTER 8

EMOTION AND YOUR HEART: YOU *CAN* BE SCARED TO DEATH

THE BIG PICTURE

Do stress and negative emotions such as anger, anxiety, and depression cause coronary heart disease? Is emotional stress dangerous for patients who already have heart disease?

We heart doctors tend to focus on the patient's plumbing, often ignoring his or her emotional state. We address heart disease with high-tech medical imaging, expensive medicines, and complex procedures. But researchers are increasingly focused on the mind/body relationship, particularly the connection between emotional stress and coronary heart disease. The evidence supporting this link is building, and it is increasingly clear that heart patients will benefit if we—and they—pay a little more attention to their emotions, stressors, and social support networks.

Studies suggest an association between emotional stress and the development of heart disease, but the effect of emotional stress on patients who already have heart disease is even more important. If you have coronary heart disease, your emotional well-being could make a major difference in your heart health. So how can you prevent a heart attack brought about by the emotional roller coaster of life or the unrelenting stress of your job? The medical literature and the media are filled with misleading and controversial answers to these questions. Like our patients Bob and Mary Linder, most people do not understand the interplay between emotion and the heart, and these misconceptions put their health at risk.

THE HEART AS THE SEAT OF EMOTION

Shakespeare knew it. Seventeenth-century poet John Donne wrote about it. And anybody who has experienced the pain of deep loss or the joy of unconditional love has felt it. The strong connection between your emotions and your heart has been a central theme in art and literature for centuries. Both in literature and in life, negative emotions can hurt the heart. In Shakespeare's thirty-nine plays, ten characters die as a result of strong emotion. In one of theater's most memorable scenes, King Lear, nearly mad with grief after the death of his daughter Cordelia, suffers from symptoms that seem remarkably like those of a heart attack and literally dies of a broken heart. Today, we understand how grief and intense feelings affect the heart, and we have pinpointed the particular emotions that jeopardize heart health.

"I KNEW YOU WERE GOING TO HAVE A HEART ATTACK!"

Armed with a clipboard, the emergency room nurse asked fifty-five-year-old Bob Linder a series of questions about his health, his life, and his profession. Flat on his back and staring at the ceiling, Bob tried to ignore the crushing pain in his chest as he explained that he was vice president at a telecommunications company. Calm and unruffled, his wife, Mary, quickly chimed in, "Bob is an overachiever. He is complete type A. He travels all the time, always has a deadline, and never relaxes. With that kind of schedule, I'm not surprised we wound up here." Bob told us that his last doctor's visit showed that he had a normal cholesterol level and normal blood pressure. He believed that these good test results protected his heart—but his EKG said otherwise. Bob's heart was not getting enough blood flow. He was having a heart attack.

We took Bob straight to the cardiac catheterization laboratory. He had severe narrowing of all three arteries on the heart, and one of the arteries was almost completely blocked by a blood clot that had formed on top of a plaque. There was only one option: emergency bypass surgery to limit the damage and prevent what might become a massive heart attack.

At the operating room doors, Mary kissed Bob goodbye and told him that she loved him. Watching him being wheeled into the operating room, she broke down in tears. "I always knew you were going to have a heart attack," she whispered.

Bob's surgery was progressing well. We had completed two of the bypasses and were just about to start the third when the phone in the operating room rang. Mary Linder was having chest pain in the waiting room. Her EKG looked threatening. Actually, it looked a lot like Bob's.

The cardiology team took Mary to the very same cardiac catheterization laboratory that Bob had visited three hours before. Her catheterization revealed a near total blockage of her left anterior descending coronary artery—another impending heart attack in the Linder family. She was lucky; a stent in the artery resolved her problem, and surgery was not necessary.

After the procedure, the team told Mary that she had to spend the night in the hospital. She requested that she be placed in a room on a different floor than Bob—she did not want to hinder Bob's recovery by causing him further emotional distress.

Bob and Mary Linder both recovered and did well. Before leaving the hospital, they asked us about the role that stress had played in their heart problems. We explained the myths and realities about emotion, stress, and heart disease. Bob's type A personality had not caused his coronary heart disease, although his frequent bouts of anger and frustration at work may have contributed. At the other end of the spectrum, Mary's calm demeanor hadn't protected her from coronary artery disease. Her high cholesterol and high blood pressure were the culprits—and since she rarely went to the doctor, she did not know she had these problems. The acute emotional stress she experienced at the hospital probably triggered Mary's heart attack. Mary's belief that emotional stress can harm people with heart disease was correct. Keeping the news of her stent from Bob for a few days was probably a good idea.

After fixing their plumbing, we armed the Linders with the information they needed to stay healthy once they left the hospital. Much of this focused on medicines, diet, and exercise. But we also explained the role of emotional health in heart patients, emphasizing the risk of developing depression after hospital discharge and discussing how certain emotional triggers can increase the risk of heart attack and death in people with heart disease.

Bob and Mary first came to the hospital in 1997. Years later, they are still doing well. Bob finds that jogging regularly relieves his stress. Mary runs with him and does yoga three times per week; her high blood pressure and cholesterol levels are easily managed with medicines.

DO NEGATIVE EMOTIONS AND STRESS CAUSE HEART DISEASE?

After receiving the diagnosis of heart disease, one of the first questions is always "Why did I get coronary heart disease?" We all know the traditional risk factors for heart disease: high cholesterol, smoking, obesity, poor diet, diabetes, family history, lack of exercise. Should we add stress and negative emotions to this list? Even after hundreds of scientific studies on this topic, the question still generates controversy and, in some cases, intense emotion.

While causality is unproven, there appears to be an association between coronary heart disease and anger, anxiety, and depression. Some suggest this could be due to the damaging behaviors that often accompany negative emotions (e.g., smoking, poor diet, lack of exercise), or the physiological effects that emotions can have on the heart and blood vessels (e.g., high blood pressure). Later, we will delve more deeply into how emotional stress affects the heart. For now, we will present the evidence suggesting an association between development of heart disease and two negative emotions, anger and anxiety.

Anger

The relationship between the heart and the constellation of emotional traits that includes anger, hostility, and cynicism has been examined extensively in observational studies. Although such studies are not considered the highest level of evidence, the findings are so consistent that they can't be ignored.

For some of us, anger and frustration begin early in the day. *Cut off by the guy in the Pinto. Then stuck behind a slow truck—what is wrong with that guy? Got around the truck, but still missed every single light. Almost there, but reached the final intersection just as road construction began—why do they have to do this during rush hour, anyway? Spilled the coffee reaching for the parking pass. Why can't they have automatic parking gates? Arrived at work ten minutes late, frustrated and mad at the world.* If this is your typical morning, you are not going to like what we have to say next.

Repeated bouts of anger are associated with thickening of the arteries and development of plaque, possible precursors to heart attacks. Over time, people who are frequently angry appear to have an increased risk of developing coronary heart disease. The stronger and more frequent the bouts of anger, the greater the risk of heart disease.

Some scientists argue that expressing anger, rather than holding it in, is better for the heart. This is unproven. Yelling might make you feel better for a moment, but it will probably endanger your job or your relationships—leading to further stress and anger. A more effective strategy includes avoiding situations that trigger anger, and managing anger when it does occur.

People who anger easily are frequently also pessimistic and cynical, and pessimism is bad for your heart. In an observational study of nearly 100,000 women, those with a pessimistic, cynical disposition developed more coronary heart disease, had more heart attacks, and died earlier than optimists. Cynical women were also more likely to develop cancer.

TYPE A PERSONALITY AND RISK OF DEVELOPING HEART DISEASE

The term *type A behavior pattern* was coined by cardiologists Meyer Friedman and R. H. Rosenman in 1959. They defined a personality type encompassing a chronic sense of urgency, impatience, competitiveness, anger, hostility, and the need to maintain control. Initial studies suggested that people with type A personality had increased risk for development of coronary heart disease. But further research suggested that it was the hostility and anger components specifically, not the personality type as a whole, that were potential drivers increasing the risk of heart disease. A personality characterized by hostility and frequent, intense anger is associated both with the development of coronary artery disease and with the progression of disease in people with known coronary heart disease.

Anxiety

Like anger, anxiety may forecast the development of coronary heart disease. We all know the tight feeling that we get in the chest when we become very anxious, so we should not be surprised to learn that this emotion can affect heart health. The circumstantial evidence supporting anxiety as a marker of heart risk is strong. In an observational study of 50,000 eighteen- to twenty-year-old Swedish men, those with high levels of anxiety substantially increased their risk of developing coronary heart disease over the next thirty-seven years. A recent meta-analysis incorporating twenty studies and nearly 250,000 individuals also found that anxiety is associated with development of coronary heart disease.

Once again, the more frequent and intense the anxiety and worry, the more likely the development of heart disease. Veterans with post-traumatic stress disorder, which is characterized by intense anxiety, tend to have more calcium (a marker of coronary blockages) in their hearts' arteries than do soldiers without the disorder. On the civilian front, people who suffer from panic disorders face an increased risk of developing heart problems.

Stress

While acute emotional stress can precipitate the broken heart syndrome (see box on next page), Mary Linder blamed her husband's heart disease on the chronic stress of his job. Does this sort of unremitting chronic stress really lead to heart disease? This is one of the most controversial questions in the study of emotion and the heart, but evidence from large, population-based studies supports a connection.

Stress is pervasive. In a 2010 survey, three-quarters of respondents reported that they had experienced unhealthy stress levels in the preceding year. When asked to pinpoint the primary sources of stress, the three most common issues were money (76 percent), work (70 percent), and the economy (60 percent). When it comes to examining the link to heart disease, work stress has received the most attention.

While dissecting the elements of stress in the workplace, researchers have focused on three elements: job strain, effort-reward imbalance, and justice. High job strain refers to being in a position where high demands are made upon you, but you have low decision-making capability. In one observational study, high job strain was associated with a substantial in-

THE BROKEN HEART SYNDROME: OUR BEST EVIDENCE LINKING EMOTION TO THE DEVELOPMENT OF HEART DISEASE

In 2005, Johns Hopkins researchers stunned the American public with their description of a condition called stress cardiomyopathy, a potentially life-threatening heart problem brought about by intense emotion. After their report was published in the *New England Journal of Medicine,* the American media christened this illness "broken heart syndrome."

Hopkins doctors studied nineteen people who suffered acute chest pain and catastrophic heart failure after sudden emotional stress. The most common precipitating event was death of a loved one, but in two cases the life-threatening event was a surprise party. (Maybe that party for Mom's sixty-fifth birthday isn't such a good idea after all....) None of these people had preexisting heart disease, but they all had heart failure by the time they reached the hospital. The researchers postulated that stress cardiomyopathy is caused by abnormal blood vessel behavior coupled with a sudden and massive release of major stress hormones such as adrenaline. In most people, stress causes arteries to dilate. In these patients, emotional stress caused the arteries to constrict or shrink, thereby reducing blood flow to the heart and impairing heart function.

This understanding of stress cardiomyopathy—or broken heart syndrome—represents our best scientific evidence of a biochemical link between emotional stress and heart disease. Interestingly, almost all of the patients with stress cardiomyopathy were women. We don't yet understand why women may be more vulnerable than men. But we do know that this story has a happy ending: all of the patients recovered.

crease in the risk of developing serious cardiovascular disease. Similarly, jobs with high demands and low financial reward have been linked to progression of atherosclerosis and development of cardiovascular disease.

Another key variable is perceived justice at work—when employees feel that their supervisors consider their viewpoints, involve them in decision making, and treat them fairly. In a study of more than 6,000 male British civil servants, employees who perceived a lack of justice at work had nearly double the risk of developing heart disease over a period of nine years. Additional research has shown that the way employees cope with unfair treatment turns out to be as important as the treatment itself. When people practice "covert coping," they don't let their supervisor or co-workers know that they feel they have been treated unfairly. This turns out to be a costly approach. Men who frequently practiced covert coping had a higher risk of experiencing a heart attack or dying of heart disease.

WORKED TO DEATH

While American studies of work-related stress and heart disease focus primarily on the quality of the work environment, others have examined the relationship between the quantity of work and heart health. In one recent British study, researchers found that employees working three or more overtime hours per day substantially increased their risk of heart-related problems over a ten-year period. The risk was particularly high among overtime workers with low decision-making capability and high job strain. While the study did not tease out the cause of increased heart disease among overtime workers, researchers noted that employees who worked longer hours were more likely to smoke, had less favorable cholesterol profiles, and had less time for leisure-time exercise than their co-workers.

In Japan, the concept that excess work portends bad health is old news. The Japanese have a legendary work ethic, which has created a new problem and a new word: *karoshi,* translated as "death from overwork." Coined in 1982, the term is well known in Japanese culture. Japanese society recognizes that excessive work, meaning more than sixty hours per week, can cause a variety of health problems and may even lead to death, often from heart disease. The Japanese Ministry of Labor has legitimized this concept, allowing workers' families to apply for monetary compensation after *karoshi.* Alas, compensation is difficult to obtain: the government pays only twenty to sixty families per year.

The cardiac impact of stress extends far beyond the workplace. Marital dissatisfaction is associated with development of atherosclerosis. By contrast, happily married individuals seem to enjoy some protection from heart disease, with married men in particular facing a lower lifetime risk of cardiovascular disease than their unmarried counterparts.

The stress of caregiving can also predispose people to heart disease. In the Nurses' Health Study, nurses who were caring for a sick spouse markedly increased their risk of having a cardiac event over a four-year period. At the same time, we all know people who experience profound satisfaction from caregiving. Closer analysis suggests that people who feel stressed by caregiving are the ones most likely to develop health problems of their own.

If you are a primary caregiver for a parent, spouse, or other loved one, make sure that you have your own support systems in place. Caregiver support groups, blogs in which caregivers share challenges and solutions, or even a weekly lunch with friends can help to relieve stress. Remember, just as on a plane a parent must put on her oxygen mask before her child's, if you do not take care of yourself, then you will not be in a position to care for someone else.

GOOD VIBRATIONS: DO POSITIVE EMOTIONS PROVIDE CARDIAC PROTECTION?

If negative emotions and chronic stress are potentially dangerous, are a cheerful disposition and the absence of stress protective? Researchers from the University of Pittsburgh set out to answer this question by studying the effect of emotional vitality in more than 6,000 men and women. Emotional vitality includes a sense of energy and well-being and the ability to regulate emotions effectively. Individuals with the greatest emotional vitality are the kind of happy, calm people we thought existed only on certain television shows from the 1960s. It turns out that a strong sense of emotional vitality is associated with a substantially lower risk of developing coronary heart disease.

LONGER LIFE WITH A SMILE

The idea that happier people live longer is intuitively appealing. While we can't offer proof that happiness helps people avoid the ravages of heart disease, several studies support the power of a smile. Wayne State researchers analyzed photos of 230 major-league baseball players who played before 1950, grading the players' smiles on a scale from 1 to 3—a score of 1 indicated no smile, 2 a slight smile, and 3 a full smile. They then correlated the quality of the smile with the length of that player's life. The result—? The better the smile, the longer the life. Average life expectancies were seventy-three years for a score of 1, seventy-five for a score of 2, and eighty for a score of 3. Boston slugger Ted Williams, who was known to have a brilliant smile, lived to eighty-three. Even if you are a Yankees fan, we hope that these results brought a smile to your face.

DEPRESSION

Of all negative emotional states, depression has received the most attention from cardiologists. There is strong circumstantial evidence linking depression both to the development of coronary heart disease and to a poor prognosis in people with existing coronary heart disease.

Clinical depression and cardiovascular disease are the two leading causes of disability worldwide. They frequently coexist in the same patient, creating a synergy that makes both conditions worse. At any given time, about 5 percent of people in the general population are suffering from depression. Unfortunately, we have more bad news for them. Depression is associated with increased risk of developing coronary heart disease over time. For depressed people who already have heart disease, without treatment the outlook is unfavorable.

Heart patients are prone to depression. Twenty to 30 percent of all patients with heart disease develop depression—a startling figure that has led many physicians to assume that depression is normal in people with heart disease. After all, they reason, anybody would be upset and depressed to discover he had heart disease. They also assume that the depression will get better on its own with time. But both of those beliefs are wrong. Depression is common in people with heart disease, but it is not normal.

When people with heart disease develop depression, they fare poorly, experiencing more heart attacks and a higher risk of death than their non-depressed counterparts. After a heart attack, depression substantially increases the risk of having another heart attack and the risk of dying within six months. People who develop depression after bypass surgery are more likely than their counterparts to die within the next two years. Even people with stable coronary heart disease do not live as long if they are depressed. And just as with stress and other negative emotions, the worse the depression, the sooner and more severe the cardiac events.

Despite these chilling statistics, doctors and nurses routinely ignore heart patients' complaints of feeling sad, empty, and listless. Patients and their families often attribute these feelings to their heart problems, failing to recognize that they are depressed. It is crucial that people with heart disease pay close attention to these symptoms of depression, and seek help.

HEART ATTACK TRIGGERS:
THE HEART PATIENT AND EMOTIONAL STRESS

There is no question that depression is a bad omen in the heart patient. Other emotions are dangerous for heart patients as well, and some of them can actually trigger a heart attack. Anger, one of the most common emotional triggers, precedes 2 percent of all heart attacks—meaning that anger could cause 30,000 heart attacks per year in the United States. In people with coronary heart disease, a bout of intense anger dramatically increases the risk of a heart attack. Anger can also trigger dangerous heart rhythms in heart patients. In people with implanted defibrillators, 15 percent of the rhythms that cause sudden death follow a period of anger.

The idea that anger can trigger a heart attack has been around for centuries. We often tell the story of John Hunter, a prominent eighteenth-century Scottish surgeon who frequently experienced chest pain during moments of anger or stress. Although he didn't understand coronary heart disease as well as we do today, he did recognize the triggers of his chest pain well enough to proclaim that his life was "in the hands of any rascal who chose to annoy or tease me." These words were prophetic. He collapsed and died—most likely of a heart attack—in a fit of rage during a heated argument with his hospital administrators.

One of the most common questions people ask after a heart attack is "When can I return to work?" The answer is usually four weeks. But patients with established heart disease should be asking an even more important question: "How will my job affect my heart?" After a heart attack, returning to a job with excessive stress increases the risk of heart attack or death from heart disease. People who have had a heart attack should try to minimize the stress associated with work, even if this means finding a new job.

While we can control many potentially stressful situations, such as avoiding people who may trigger our anger, or choosing a job that does not stress us unduly, some events are unpredictable and uncontrollable. Major public stressors such as natural disasters, wars, and terrorist attacks take a cardiac toll on vulnerable people in the population.

On January 17, 1994, the Northridge earthquake devastated parts of southern California. That day, the number of deaths from coronary heart disease in Los Angeles County nearly doubled. The greatest death toll was recorded closest to the epicenter of the earthquake, with the number of patients dying from heart attacks decreasing in proportion to distance from

THE MOST WONDERFUL—AND DANGEROUS—TIME OF YEAR

Everyone looks forward to Christmas and New Year's. But adults with heart disease must beware of what Dr. Robert Kloner termed "The Merry Christmas Coronary" and the "Happy New Year Heart Attack." Across the country, heart attack deaths peak on Christmas Day, with December 26 running a close second and New Year's Day coming in third. For people with coronary heart disease, Christmas is the most dangerous day of the year. This is not simply a result of cold weather (although it is true that more deaths from heart disease occur in winter than in summer)—the holiday heart attack peaks occur in balmy Los Angeles as well as in frigid Boston. Possible explanations include emotional stress, changes in diet, increased alcohol consumption, and delays in seeking medical care. Many also point to the unusual stressors that can accompany the holiday season: family arguments, travel, long lines at the airport, finding money to buy gifts, and preparing meals for large numbers of people. Recognize your sources of stress. If seeing your in-laws causes you chest pain, consider making a different holiday plan for next year. It could save your life. And if you experience chest pain during the holidays, don't ignore it. Get to the emergency room.

the epicenter. In the two weeks following the earthquake, the number of people dying from heart attacks was unusually low, in part because many of the most vulnerable people had already died.

Hurricane Katrina has had a long-term impact on the heart health of New Orleans residents. Tabulating the heart risk four years after the storm, Tulane University researchers found a persistent increase in the risk of heart attack. Researcher Dr. Anand Irimpen hypothesized, "Chronic stress and how people deal with it—overdoing those things that are detrimental to health (such as smoking, alcohol, substance abuse, overeating, and not yet resuming exercise habits)—appear to play an ongoing role." He cautioned that we should pay careful, long-term attention to those affected by major natural disasters, including people affected by the 2011 earthquake and tsunami in Japan.

Man-made disasters also endanger heart patients. At the beginning of the first Gulf War, Israeli citizens were under constant and enormous stress, wearing gas masks and continually running for safety as Scud missiles rained down on Tel Aviv. The first days of the war saw a dramatic increase in heart attack admissions to local hospitals. As in the case of the Northridge earthquake, this rate decreased after a few days—the war continued, but the most vulnerable patients had had their heart attacks in the initial days of the fighting. In addition, people eventually became somewhat accustomed to the constant sounds of sirens and the stresses of war.

For Americans, the stress associated with the terrorist attacks of September 11, 2001, was qualitatively different from the stress experienced by communities during earthquakes and rocket attacks. True, there was a local increase in the number of heart attacks in New York and Washington, as had been the case with the Northridge earthquake. But the stress associated with 9/11 was longer-lasting and had a far greater geographic reach. In addition to heart attacks, people experienced dangerous heart rhythms (arrhythmias), which peaked ten to twelve days after the attacks and remained high for about a month. The entire country was affected: the risk of abnormal heart rhythms was as elevated in Miami as in New York City. The constant barrage of images and news stories from Ground Zero made this event real for citizens across the country, creating a prolonged period of intense collective stress.

TYPE D PERSONALITY AND THE DISTRESSED HEART

While the link between type A personality and heart disease has recently been discredited, a new link has been proposed between heart disease and type D personality. Coined by Dutch researcher Johan Denollet in 1995, the term *type D personality* refers to a "distressed" personality profile that includes frequent negative emotions coupled with social inhibition. The typical type D person experiences anger, anxiety, tension, depression, and worry, but because he feels inhibited in social situations, he does not easily share his emotions with others. Although causality is not proven, heart patients with type D personality are more likely to suffer heart attacks and death, and they do worse after receiving coronary artery stents. In the latter instance, having a type D personality profile seems to negate the benefits of the high-tech stents used to keep coronary arteries open. Unfavorable behaviors probably contribute to these poor outcomes—type D patients are more likely to forgo exercise, eat poorly, smoke, and skip prescribed medicines. Doctors and families should pay particular attention to ensuring that type D heart patients focus on a heart-healthy lifestyle and comply with lifesaving therapies.

SPORTS AND STRESS: SPECTATORS BEWARE!

The year 2006 was a dream come true for German soccer fans. Germany hosted the World Cup and finished third before a television audience of more than 1 billion people. German fans were passionate about their team—to the point of danger. The *New England Journal of Medicine* reported that on days of the German team's matches, the number of people falling victim to cardiac emergencies in Munich more than doubled. While the risk of cardiac events increased in both men and women, men had nearly twice as many problems as women. Blood tests in these people revealed that the excitement of the games caused high levels of proteins that increase blood pressure and inflammation, which likely contributed to the heart attacks.

The riskiest match occurred on June 30, when Germany beat Argentina after a dramatic penalty shootout. That day saw a large spike in heart attacks. Recent studies in the United States find a similar phenomenon with American football, with Super Bowl Sunday doubling as heart attack day in emergency rooms across the country.

The message here: men with coronary heart disease need to be careful when watching emotionally charged sporting events. If you are watching a game and experience chest pain, turn off the television, chew an aspirin, and call 911 if you are not better in a few minutes.

HOW DO STRESS AND NEGATIVE EMOTIONS AFFECT THE HEART?

We have presented a great deal of evidence (primarily from observational studies) supporting a relationship between emotional stress and heart disease. So why are so many doctors still skeptical about this connection? The evidence is available, but the case is still not airtight.

The link between the heart and emotions is complicated, and scientists are far from having all the answers. But we do have a pretty clear understanding of the basic mechanisms involved. Emotional stress can affect heart health through two different pathways: changes in your body's physiology and changes in your behavior.

The Physiology of Stress

The studies we have discussed do not definitively prove that negative emotions cause or worsen coronary heart disease, because we still don't understand the precise mechanisms by which emotional stress affects the heart. The only instance in which we have exact causes nailed down is the case of stress cardiomyopathy, or broken heart syndrome. Still, doctors and scientists do have quite a bit of evidence that emotional stress affects your cardiovascular system.

It doesn't take a medical degree to know there is a connection between your emotions and your heart's function. If you step out into a crosswalk and see a truck bearing down on you, your fight-or-flight instinct kicks in. You jump back onto the curb, and your heart suddenly feels like a jackhammer in your chest. Your breathing is quick and shallow. You are hyperalert. In a fraction of a second, your brain has communicated with your heart and the rest of your body, preparing you to deal with danger. How does this happen?

The fight-or-flight mechanism illustrates the changes in the body's physiology that are precipitated by extreme emotion. Confronted with danger, your brain and nervous system send out a rapid-fire series of messages. The adrenal glands (located near your kidneys) flood the bloodstream with

THE STRESS OF THE BIG CITY

We love New York City and don't want to pick on The Big Apple. But data are data. A 1999 study suggested that living in New York City—or even just visiting—increases your risk of dying from a heart attack. Compared with people who live in other cities, New York City residents have a substantially higher risk of a fatal heart attack. Visitors to New York have an increase in the chance of dying from a heart attack during their visit. However, when visitors return home, their risk returns to normal. This effect holds true for New Yorkers— their risk of heart attack plummets when they leave the city. Interestingly, these effects are unique to New York City, consistent with the hypothesis that New York is more stressful than other large cities. Our advice? When you are in New York City, counter the stress by taking some time to relax. Visit the parks. Have a nice (healthy) meal at an excellent restaurant. See a Broadway show. Make sure that you have some fun.

adrenaline, cortisol, and other chemicals and hormones that prepare your body to deal with acute stress. Whether the stressor is emotional or physical, your body responds the same way.

These nerve impulses, hormones, and chemicals activated by stress or danger have direct and significant effects on your heart. Heart rate and blood pressure rise. Blood becomes thicker and platelets are activated, making the blood more likely to clot. Inflammatory proteins are mobilized to help heal impending physical injuries. These responses are meant to protect you and help the body deal with danger and injury. If you are young and healthy, your body tolerates these events and soon returns to its normal state. But in the wrong person or the wrong circumstance, these responses to stress can spell danger for your heart.

The stress response can also cause problems with the heart's electrical conduction system. In most people, emotional stress increases the heart rate (the number of beats per minute); that's why we commonly speak of a racing heart. But in some people, stress also changes the heart rhythm, which reflects the pathways of electrical impulses inside the heart. Dangerous heart rhythms caused by the fight-or-flight response include ventricular fibrillation, ventricular tachycardia, and atrial fibrillation. The first two—ventricular fibrillation and ventricular tachycardia—usually require quick action with a defibrillator to save a life.

Like heart rhythm, your heart's arteries can also experience abnormal, dangerous responses to certain emotional stressors. Normally, the arteries on your heart and in other parts of the body enlarge whenever extra blood flow is needed. Think of the arteries in your legs when you are out for a run: they are maximally dilated to bring oxygen and glucose to your hardworking muscles. Your heart's arteries have a similar response when the heart is called on to pump faster and harder. This is a standard response to physical or emotional stress. But in people with coronary heart disease, the heart's reaction to stress is often abnormal. Sometimes the heart's arteries don't dilate at all, and in other cases they actually constrict, reducing much-needed blood flow to the heart and causing chest pain or even a heart attack.

Even relatively small, everyday stressors can be dangerous for people with heart disease, raising blood pressure and heart rate and increasing blood clotting and blood vessel dysfunction. Many people are afraid of public speaking, and laboratory studies show that when speaking in front of an audience many people suffer inadequate blood flow to the heart. So, heart-wise, it may be a good idea for people with coronary heart disease to

THE HEARTBREAK OF SOCIAL REJECTION

Difficult social relationships, particularly family relationships associated with high demands and excessive worry (think parenthood), have long been linked to angina. But interactions with strangers can also influence heart health. Dutch researchers examined the acute cardiovascular effects of social rejection in college students. Twenty-two subjects provided photographs of themselves and were told that these photographs would be shown to students at another university for a study examining first impressions (in fact, the photos were not shown to anybody). A few weeks later, the subjects' heart rates were monitored as they were shown pictures of the fictional other students and then informed whether or not the students had liked their photograph. The revelation that a subject was *not* liked caused a pronounced and sustained drop in heart rate. While the researchers did not discover an antidote for the pain of rejection, they demonstrated a convincing link between emotion and the heart.

avoid public speaking if it gets them worked up. Even the stress associated with challenging math problems—say, counting backward from 1,000 by sevens while somebody is trying to distract you—can affect blood flow to the heart in people with heart disease.

Like acute stress caused by specific events or experiences, chronic stress—particularly job stress or marital stress—can affect your heart and blood vessels. With chronic stress, you don't walk around with a heart rate of 150 and a blood pressure of 220 over 130, as happens with the fight-or-flight response. But chronic stress does activate the same systems in your body and can take a toll over time. Increased blood pressure, inflammation, and endothelial dysfunction may harm the inner lining of the heart's arteries, setting the stage for the development of atherosclerosis and obstructing plaques. Additionally, chronically high levels of the stress hormone cortisol contribute to the development of diabetes, which, as you know, increases the risk of heart problems.

HOT RESPONDERS

People react to stress differently. We envy those fortunate people who never get frustrated, flustered, or angry. Their emotional stability may protect them from the damaging effects of stress on the heart's arteries. At the other end of the emotional spectrum are those individuals who are particularly susceptible to the hormonal and chemical onslaughts caused by stress. Researchers call them "hot responders." Hot responders have an exaggerated fight-or-flight response when stressed, resulting in excessive increases in heart rate, blood pressure, and blood clotting. At least three different genes have been identified that predispose people to becoming hot responders, and there may also be a genetic component to one's likelihood of developing dangerous heart rhythms in response to stress. One interesting note regarding those fortunate few who always seem emotionally stable and stress-free: people who are generally happy and have an optimistic outlook on life have lower baseline levels of cortisol, and also appear to have a reduced biochemical response to stress. The genetic basis for this—is there a "happiness" gene?—has not been elucidated.

Stress and Behavior

In addition to acute physiologic changes affecting the heart and blood vessels, emotional stress also threatens your heart through the damaging behaviors that often follow in its wake. A variety of stress-induced behaviors can cause heart disease, including poor diet, lack of exercise, smoking, excess alcohol consumption, and not taking prescribed medications. Which hurts heart health more, the changes in physiology or the stress-induced behaviors? Doctors argue quite a bit about this question, but the answer is irrelevant. When it comes to devising a plan to manage emotional stress, they are a package deal. The best strategy is to reduce emotional stress *and* avoid the unfavorable behaviors that accompany it.

How Does Emotional Stress Trigger a Heart Attack?

Now that we understand the physiology of the stress response, we can explain how acute emotional stress poses a serious threat of triggering a heart attack in people with coronary heart disease. Severe stress of any sort is particularly dangerous for those who also have what we call "vulnerable" plaques—those that are unstable and prone to rupture—obstructing their arteries. When vulnerable plaques rupture, blood clots form on top of them, blocking the artery on the heart. The cardiac muscle cells that are supplied by that blocked artery die, and a heart attack results.

Unfortunately, there is no reliable way to tell who has vulnerable plaques. But we *can* tell who has coronary heart disease through a doctor's visit and some simple noninvasive tests. If you know that you have coronary heart disease, we recommend that you take precautions as if you do have vulnerable plaque.

In the stressed patient with coronary heart disease and vulnerable plaque, strong emotions lead to potentially fatal changes in the heart and blood. Fueled by anger or excitement, blood pressure and heart rate increase. The increased blood pressure hammers away at the vulnerable plaque, causing it to rupture. Compounding this problem, stress causes the blood to become thicker and activates the blood clotting system, increasing the chance that a large blood clot will form at the site of the ruptured plaque. This raises the risk of heart attack even further.

How can you prevent this scenario? First, try to avoid extreme emotional stress, both by limiting exposure to stressful situations and by developing coping strategies that reduce your response to stress. The second approach is to use medicines. Beta-blockers can prevent increases in heart rate and blood pressure, and aspirin can prevent blood clotting. If you have coronary heart disease, your doctor has probably prescribed these medicines. Stick with the program.

TREATMENT: WHERE EMOTIONAL AND HEART HEALTH MEET

If we accept that stress and negative emotions are associated with heart disease, the next question is clear: what can we do about it? The answer depends upon whether or not you already have heart disease.

If you do not have heart disease, your goal is to avoid its development. The best way to prevent heart disease is to reduce traditional risk factors through a heart-healthy lifestyle including exercise, a good diet, and abstaining from smoking. Although preemptive stress management and emotional regulation therapies do influence heart rate and blood pressure,

YOUR SOCIAL NETWORK, YOUR DOG, AND YOUR HEART

When compared to people with a strong social network, those with low levels of social support—social loners—are at increased risk of developing heart disease and of suffering from its complications. For example, happily married people experience fewer cardiac events than do single people and people with marital stress. Scientists hypothesize that a strong social network prevents the emotional highs and lows that are associated with heart disease.

Pets can also play an important role in the life of a person who is single, widowed, or simply lonely. Studies of heart patients suggest that pet ownership confers many of the same benefits as person-to-person social interaction. When hospitalized patients are visited by therapy dogs, their levels of stress and anxiety diminish, as do blood pressure and blood levels of stress hormones. At Cleveland Clinic we use canine greeters to put patients and their families at ease. This concept even bridges the gap between the medical and legal professions: students at Yale Law School can "check out" Monty, a therapy dog, to provide them with thirty minutes of stress relief.

For heart patients, canine companionship can produce long-term benefits. In one large study of heart attack survivors, both pet ownership and a high overall level of social support were associated with a greater chance of survival at one year. The pet benefit was observed only in dog owners, though; cat lovers actually had slightly decreased survival rates. This anomaly may relate to the exercise dog owners get from walking their pets.

there is little evidence that they reduce the risk of developing heart disease. Nevertheless, we certainly favor stress management if it makes people feel better and improves quality of life. After all, there are scientific reasons to believe that reducing the frequency and intensity of the chemical onslaught of the fight-or-flight response is a good thing.

What about people who already have heart disease? Here we are on more solid ground in recommending a variety of measures to enhance emotional health. Because we know that outbursts of intense emotion and anger can trigger heart attacks, people with coronary heart disease should avoid placing themselves in predictable high-stress situations. If you have coronary heart disease and know that you get very worked up watching your favorite team in the playoffs, wait for the evening news to get the result.

We realize that it is impossible to go through life avoiding all stressful situations. But heart patients with a tendency to get intensely angry or emotionally worked up must develop coping skills, recognizing their personal triggers and learning to respond to them calmly. In his book *The Power of Full Engagement,* Tony Schwartz emphasizes the importance of identifying emotional triggers and provides a variety of techniques for managing them, ranging from deep breathing exercises to forcing a smile to ward off anger. There is no single strategy that is right for everybody. The key is to figure out what works for you.

Understandably, skepticism remains about the utility of this sort of therapy in heart patients. Stress management and effective coping skills certainly make people feel better. But do they really prevent heart attacks and prolong life? The waters here are a bit murky, but evidence supporting a benefit does exist.

Cognitive Behavioral Therapy

Cognitive behavioral therapy (CBT) teaches patients to reframe stressful situations so they don't trigger a cascade of negative emotions. For example, CBT would have taught the man trapped in his Pinto and late for work to have a markedly different response to his challenging commute. Facing slow-moving trucks, road construction, and traffic lights that seem to plot against him, he might think: *I am going to be a little late today. But traffic is still moving, and I will be able to catch up quickly once I get to the meeting.*

This will not be a big problem. I'm glad that I left the house on time. Meanwhile, I can use this delay to my advantage. I can finally finish that book on tape and find out how Tom Clancy's latest thriller ends. With this approach, stress and frustration melt away, replaced by relaxation and a sense of accomplishment.

When patients with coronary heart disease are given instruction in stress management and CBT, heart rhythm and blood vessel function improve more than in patients receiving only routine medical care. In fact, researchers from Duke University found that the impact of stress management training on heart health was similar to the benefit obtained from an aerobic exercise program. In addition, stress management training made patients feel better, reducing their tendency to feel depressed or emotionally stressed. Similarly, a Canadian study found that identifying and helping heart attack patients who exhibited high levels of distress improved their psychological function and appeared to reduce their risk of dying from heart disease.

In the best study to date, Swedish physicians performed a randomized controlled trial examining the impact of a year-long cognitive behavioral program in patients who had been hospitalized for coronary heart disease. After hospital discharge, treated patients attended twenty 2-hour sessions on reducing and managing emotional stress. Over the next eight years, training in emotional coping and stress management reduced the risk of a recurrent heart attack by 45 percent. Patients who attended the greatest number of sessions had the fewest heart problems. The researchers calculated that for every ten heart patients who took the course, one heart attack would be prevented. The message here is clear: a well-constructed stress management program, included in the context of standard medical care, can be beneficial for heart patients. Ask your doctor about this option.

Transcendental Meditation

Although perhaps best known for entrancing the Beatles, Transcendental Meditation is vying for a position as a mainstream technique for stress reduction in heart patients. A small, preliminary study of people with coronary heart disease suggested that Transcendental Meditation reduced heart attacks, strokes, and deaths. In a subsequent sixteen-week randomized controlled clinical trial, heart patients practicing Transcendental Meditation had reductions in blood pressure, heart rate, and insulin resistance. Study authors concluded that Transcendental Meditation can reduce the body's response to stress and may improve heart disease risk factors. Intrigued by these studies, the NIH has committed millions of dollars to the further study of Transcendental Meditation in heart patients.

Yoga, Biofeedback, and Guided Imagery

Each of these relaxation techniques has a following, and has shown to be effective at reducing stress. In addition to improving flexibility and balance, yoga is associated with reductions in blood pressure, drops in circulating adrenaline levels, and better heart rhythm control. Biofeedback, which enables people to control their physiologic reactions to stress, shows promise in the management of patients with cardiovascular disease. And guided imagery is an effective technique for reducing anxiety; it is widely used to help patients relax before heart surgery.

Although the impact of these three therapies on hard cardiovascular endpoints such as heart attack is not yet clear, preliminary studies suggest that they are certainly not harmful. We do not discourage heart patients from adding them to the usual medical care; at the very least, if they make people feel better and reduce their stress, that is still an important benefit.

Exercise for Stress Relief

Each heart patient should choose a method of stress relief that works for him or her. Our recommendation is exercise. You can couple exercise with any of the other therapies, but it needs to be a component of your program for emotional and heart health. As we explained in Chapter 7, exercise is proven to improve your cholesterol profile and blood vessel health, but it is also an excellent stress reducer. If you are a heart patient, get yourself started on the right exercise track by enrolling in a cardiac rehab program. You will manage your traditional risk factors and feel better—and less stressed—as a result of the combination of exercise and social support.

PRAYER, RELIGION, AND YOUR HEART

Scientists have conducted hundreds of studies examining the impact of prayer and religion on heart health, and this research has sparked more than a few spirited debates. In their search for a relationship between religion and the heart, investigators have focused on religiosity (a person's level of religious involvement) and prayer.

A recent study of more than 90,000 women made headlines in the *New York Times* with its conclusion that the more religiously oriented an individual, the more likely the person was to be alive a decade later. While most studies find no specific relationship between religiosity and heart health, many have corroborated the observation that religious people tend to live longer. Possible non-theological reasons behind this finding include benefits of membership in a strong social network and a general tendency toward "clean living" among religious people.

What about prayer? Before wheeling a patient into the operating room, family members often say, "I'll be praying for you." Does prayer work? Scientists have conducted several trials of intercessory prayer, or prayer on the behalf of others. A recent review of the ten best randomized controlled trials including more than 7,000 patients could discern no clear evidence that such prayer improved health outcomes. However, there was no harm, either. Although religious observance and prayer do not appear to open blocked arteries or fix leaking heart valves, personal prayer and visits by a clergy member often provide emotional comfort to patients. We therefore offer these to our heart patients through our Healing Services Program. Combining these healing services with our traditional medical approaches to the heart helps us to move beyond the plumbing and treat the whole patient.

Treating Depression in the Heart Patient

Finally, let's turn back to depression, the most common psychological problem in heart patients. Since depressed patients fare worse than patients who are not depressed, it seems logical to assume that treating depression will improve heart outcomes. Two large randomized controlled studies have tested this hypothesis. In the largest study, depression treatment improved heart patients' quality of life and medication adherence but had no impact on cardiovascular outcomes.

It was a huge disappointment to find that treating depression did nothing to help heart health. Subsequent review of the data suggested a possible silver lining, however: patients receiving certain antidepressant drugs (selective serotonin reuptake inhibitors such as Zoloft and Lexapro) appeared to have a reduced risk of heart attacks, possibly as a result of the medications' effect on blood clotting. While this provides some cause for optimism, there is no conclusive evidence that treating depression is good for the heart itself. But depression in heart patients should definitely be treated, because it will improve quality of life.

The first step in treating depression is to figure out who has it. This part is easy. The American Heart Association recommends that everyone with heart disease should be screened for depression with two simple questions.

DEPRESSION SCREENING: TWO SIMPLE QUESTIONS

1. *During the past month, have you frequently felt down, depressed, or hopeless?*

2. *During the past month, have you felt little interest or pleasure in doing things?*

CHOOSING A MOVIE: LAUGHTER IS GOOD MEDICINE

Laughter is good for you, and we have the science to prove it. Cardiologist Michael Miller examined the impact of emotionally charged movies on blood flow. He had subjects watch two different movies—the World War II movie *Saving Private Ryan,* with its many violent scenes, and *Kingpin,* a comedy. The stressful and disturbing scenes in *Saving Private Ryan* caused reduced blood flow in 70 percent of subjects. In contrast, funny scenes from the comedy were associated with improved blood flow in 95 percent of people. Miller concluded that laughter is good for your blood vessels. Other studies suggest that laughter is associated with decreased levels of stress hormones and platelet clumping and can even serve as exercise when combined with yoga and deep breathing. The average adult laughs fewer than ten times per day, compared to three hundred episodes of daily laughter for many children. Do yourself and your heart a favor and treat yourself to a comedy or uplifting movie. Put laughter back in your life.

If you or a loved one has heart disease—newly diagnosed or chronic—see your doctor for help if the answer to either one of these questions is yes. You will be glad that you did.

EMOTIONAL STRESS AND THE HEART: START THE CONVERSATION

We cannot prove that negative emotions cause heart disease, but we believe that they are associated with worse outcomes in heart patients. Traditional medicine concentrates on physical health and completely ignores emotional factors. This is a mistake. If you are a heart patient, make sure that you discuss your emotions and the stress in your life with your doctor. Doctors frequently fail to ask patients about their emotional well-being, so you may need to be the one to broach the issue. As University of California psychiatrist Dr. Joel Dimsdale wrote in a recent editorial, "Physicians are frequently timid about assessing emotional symptoms. It is odd that we thread catheters, ablate lesions, and give rectal exams but are uncomfortable asking our patients about their lives."

Help your doctor over his or her discomfort and start this conversation. Complete treatment for the heart patient means looking inside the heart—literally and figuratively—to treat the whole patient, both mind and body.

RX: EMOTION, STRESS, AND YOUR HEART

If you don't have heart disease:

    Realize that emotional stress may contribute to the development of heart disease

    Don't let stress cause unhealthy behaviors

    Exercise for stress relief and heart health

If you do have heart disease:

    Discuss your emotional state and sources of stress with your doctor

    Recognize emotional triggers and avoid them if possible

    Choose one or more methods for stress reduction

- Exercise (our favorite)
- Cognitive behavioral therapy
- Transcendental Meditation
- Yoga
- Guided imagery
- Biofeedback

    Take the simple screening test for depression

    Remember that depression is not normal in the heart patient

    Don't ignore depression—get help and you will feel better

CHAPTER 9

HOW TO TELL FACT FROM FICTION: SORTING THROUGH THE MEDICAL EVIDENCE

THE BIG PICTURE

Joan Stoddard is a seventy-two-year-old woman with coronary heart disease who sees us every year for management of her cardiovascular risk factors. At her last visit, she voiced an alarming concern. She had recently watched a television news program describing an important scientific study that "proved" that taking calcium supplements increases the risk of developing heart disease. Joan was terribly worried because, on the advice of her family physician, she had been taking calcium supplements for many years for her osteoporosis, a condition in which bone density is decreased. Postmenopausal women are particularly vulnerable to this condition, so doctors often recommend calcium supplements to try to maintain bone strength and ward off fractures.

Joan's favorite anchorman had relayed the study's findings, complete with a graphic of a bottle of calcium pills with a giant question mark superimposed on it. His two-minute story made Joan question five years' worth of calcium supplements. Had she hurt her heart by taking calcium to strengthen her bones and try to avoid a hip fracture? Did the new study mean that she should discard her calcium pills and risk letting her bones become brittle? Answering Joan's many questions, we explained that the link between calcium supplementation and the development of heart disease is relatively weak. She should continue to take calcium to protect her bones: in Joan's case, the benefit to her fragile bones outweighed the possible small risk to her heart.

Like Joan, thousands of patients face daily dilemmas created by media reports of "new studies" and "startling scientific findings." We live in an era of nearly instantaneous mass communication, where quick headlines containing "important" health information are considered vital commodities. Media headlines such as the following captivate huge audiences:

♥ *"Stem Cells Ready for 'Prime-Time' to Repair the Damaged Heart"*

♥ *"Study Shows That Eating Fish Is Good for You, Even When It's Fried"*

♥ *"Vitamin D Cuts Heart Disease by 47 Percent"*

Citing "compelling" study results, media reports create both excitement and anxiety. But are these studies correct or misleading? If you do some careful investigation, you will find that many of the new studies have unheralded counterparts that show exactly the opposite findings. And you will often uncover debates and disagreements between respected experts on each side. How can you decide what to believe?

To illustrate the challenge, let's look at the controversy and misinformation surrounding vitamin D. Doctors agree that adequate vitamin D intake (600 to 800 IU per day, depending upon age and gender) is important for bone health. Based upon recent scientific studies and media attention, today there is great interest in a potential relationship between vitamin D and heart health. A recent news report describing the favorable effects of vitamin D on heart disease states, "The results of a study presented to the American College of Cardiology show that correcting deficient vitamin D blood levels can reduce the risks associated with coronary artery disease." Later the article goes on to claim, "Deficient levels of Vitamin D are responsible for millions of needless deaths and much suffering each year. Extensive research has shown exactly how this mega nutrient works on the cellular level to provide lowered risk from many lethal conditions including cancer and heart disease." The story makes you feel you should drive immediately to the nearest pharmacy and buy a bottle of vitamin D. We have no doubt that many people who read the story did just that.

Two months after this study was presented, the Institute of Medicine (IOM) issued a report with its own recommendations for vitamin D. The IOM is a highly respected national organization that serves as the health arm of the National Academy of Sciences, originally chartered under President Abraham Lincoln. Composed of world-class experts, the IOM frequently has the last word on health issues.

In this instance, recognizing tremendous public confusion and conflicting scientific evidence, the American and Canadian governments charged the IOM with assessing the available data on the health impacts of vitamin D. Members of the IOM looked at more than a thousand studies, not just the single study featured in the mass media. In its report, the IOM stated, "The committee . . . found that the evidence supported a role for these nutrients [vitamin D and calcium] in bone health but not in other health conditions." Finding that the majority of Americans and Canadians already receive adequate amounts of vitamin D in the food they eat, the IOM concluded that most people do not need vitamin D supplements. Addressing a concern that the media had not covered, the IOM noted potential side effects of megadoses of vitamin D, including hypercalcemia, a condition in which blood levels of calcium rise to toxic levels, leading to nausea, constipation, vomiting, and even kidney failure. The bottom line: don't take extra vitamin D to try to protect your heart.

This sort of story plays out every week. Vitamin D, fish oil, red wine, long-distance running, heart scans—one day they are touted as good, and weeks later media reports warn against them. Faced with such contradictory evidence, how can you make rational health decisions? The answer lies in understanding how to interpret and judge the scientific evidence. Not all studies are created equal, and not all evidence carries the same scientific weight. Like a good detective, you must learn to judge the *quality* of the evidence. We will help you earn your gold shield as a medical detective, explaining how you can determine the strength of the evidence you are reading.

Medical research commonly employs three kinds of study designs: observational studies, randomized controlled trials (RCTs), and meta-analyses. There is a distinct hierarchy in the strength of evidence provided by these three sources of data. Observational studies are about as reliable as a little old lady who claims that she can identify the perpetrator of a crime because she saw him through the rain from her window two blocks away. In other words, they provide weak evidence. A randomized controlled trial produces the strongest evidence: data from an RCT are like a video showing the crime, with a clear shot of the criminal's face. Meta-analyses are somewhere in between. A good meta-analysis, which compiles and evaluates the findings of multiple studies, is like strong circumstantial evidence—police found the weapon used in the crime at the suspect's house, and footprints at the scene match the suspect's tennis shoes.

To understand the hierarchy of medical evidence, you need a bit of insight into how doctors perform these three types of studies and the terminology they use to describe results.

JUDGING THE STUDIES: THREE KEY QUESTIONS

Before we explain the three types of medical studies and their respective pros and cons, we need to arm you with a few statistical tools to employ every time you look at a new medical report.

There are three important questions you should ask of every medical study, and for each question a simple statistic provides the answer:

1. *What are the odds that the study results are incorrect, or simply due to chance?*

2. *How large is the treatment's effect?*

3. *How many people would we need to treat to see a benefit of the therapy?*

The Role of Chance

Whether a study is a full-fledged RCT or an observational study, you must always ask, "Could the results be explained simply by chance?" Actually, the answer to this question is always yes. There is *always* the possibility that the findings are the result of chance alone. So the real question is, "What is the *likelihood* that the results of a study were caused by chance alone?" Put another way, what is the probability that the study results are wrong?

Scientists use a number called the P-value to describe the probability that the study findings are incorrect, a result of chance. This number is featured prominently in all medical reports. If the P-value of a study is 0.01, there is a 1 percent, or 1 in 100, probability that the results are incorrect. If the P-value is 0.05, the likelihood that study results are erroneous is 5 in 100, or 5 percent, and so on. The smaller the P-value, the lower the probability that the study results are just a matter of chance. When the

FDA evaluates a study of a therapy—a medication or medical device—it requires that the P-value be less than or equal to 0.05: it wants a 5 percent or less probability that the study is incorrect. Sometimes the FDA even requires two separate studies with P-values less than 0.05 before it will approve the therapy. Medical websites will often include the P-value when they report study results, but news reports almost never do. We recommend that you consider a study potentially believable when the P-value is 0.05 or less.

How Large Is the Treatment's Effect?

The second important piece of information we need when evaluating clinical studies is the magnitude of the benefit of a medicine or therapy. Of course we have numbers for this, too. One important measure is known as the hazard ratio, or HR, which defines the extent to which the therapy increased or decreased the particular health risk being studied. An HR of less than 1 indicates that the risk is decreased; for example, most studies of cholesterol-lowering statin drugs tend to show an HR of 0.75 for heart attacks, meaning that these drugs reduce the risk of a heart attack by about 25 percent. On the other hand, an HR greater than 1 means that the therapy *increases* the risk. When hormone replacement therapy was studied in postmenopausal women, the HR for the development of new heart disease was 1.29, meaning that the therapy actually increased the risk of heart disease by 29 percent. Like the P-value, the hazard ratio is often reported by medical websites, but less often in the popular media.

How Many People Would We Need to Treat to See a Benefit?

As we've seen, the P-value tells you if the study results are likely to be correct and not merely the result of chance, and the HR describes the magnitude of the benefit. But be careful, as such numbers may distort the real extent of any benefit.

Consider this example: A new anti-heart-attack drug is assessed in an RCT of 20,000 people. Ten thousand patients get the drug, and 10,000 patients receive a placebo. Two of 10,000 placebo patients suffer heart attacks over a five-year period, while only one of 10,000 patients receiving the drug has a heart attack. Study organizers report that the study drug reduces the risk of heart attack by 50 percent (the HR is 0.50). Media reports herald this as a wonder drug—it cuts the risk of heart attack in half.

Let's consider this result carefully. We need to treat 10,000 people with this medicine to prevent a single heart attack over a five-year period. In the statistics of medicine, this way of measuring benefit is called the "number needed to treat." In this case, the number of people we would need to treat in order to see a benefit is very large—too large unless the drug has absolutely no side effects and is very inexpensive. When you examine reports describing wonder drugs and spectacular new therapies, look for this statistic.

OBSERVATIONAL STUDIES

Now that you have the statistical knowledge to judge a study's validity, it's time to look at the studies themselves. Most studies covered by the media are observational studies. Observational studies do not describe the results of a scientific experiment; that is, investigators do not assign therapies to patients and then measure the outcomes in these different groups. Instead, observational studies typically involve a retrospective design, which means they look at events that occurred before the study began. Observational studies often include very large numbers of people, ranging from the hundreds to the hundreds of thousands. Because of these large numbers, observational studies often appear definitive to the unsophisticated interpreter (or media outlet). But as the recent vitamin D discussions reveal, observational studies often contain serious flaws that are overlooked in the race to generate headlines.

Vitamin D and Heart Disease:
D Stands for "Don't Get Fooled Again"

In the study claiming that vitamin D prevents heart disease, researchers examined the medical records of 41,000 subjects. Sounds impressive, doesn't it? The investigators divided the patients into three categories: people with normal vitamin D levels, people with moderate deficiency, and people with severe deficiency. Next, the researchers identified the people who had experienced a heart attack or stroke. The finding? Patients with severe vitamin D deficiency were much more likely to have suffered a heart attack or stroke. So there you have it: low levels of vitamin D are associated with heart attack or stroke, and everyone should take vitamin D supplements to prevent these catastrophic disorders, right? In an interview with WebMD, the author of this study provided exactly this interpretation: "There is enough information here for me to start treatment based on these findings." Case closed.

Can you see the flaws in this study? Do you understand why it is too unreliable to drive medical decision making? A closer look reveals that the study did not *prove* that vitamin D deficiency causes heart disease. Nor did the investigators test whether administration of vitamin D lowered the risk of heart disease. The study authors merely described an "association" between low vitamin D levels and subsequent development of disease. But this does not necessarily mean that vitamin D deficiency *causes* heart disease. It is easy to build a plausible alternative explanation for the association. For example, we know that vitamin D is produced in the skin after exposure to sunlight, so being indoors results in low vitamin D levels. What if the people with low vitamin D were deficient because of other health problems that kept them inside? And because these people were in poor health, maybe they didn't exercise—and we know that lack of exercise increases the risks of heart attack and stroke.

So what if the higher level of heart disease in these patients is related to their lack of exercise, rather than a lack of vitamin D in their diets? In this example, the low levels of vitamin D may be a marker for less outdoor exercise, but it is the lack of exercise that is responsible for the increased risk of heart disease, not vitamin D deficiency. Supplementing vitamin D in such individuals will not cause them to exercise.

Based upon this explanation, we would say that vitamin D deficiency is *associated* with heart disease, but we would add the caution that *causality* is unproven.

Observational Studies and the Problem of Confounding

We say that an observational study is "confounded" when other factors may provide alternative explanations for the findings (in the vitamin D case, for example, it may be lack of exercise, rather than vitamin D deficiency, that is a cause of heart disease). The most sophisticated observational studies attempt to adjust for all of the confounders that can be measured. For example, researchers may check blood pressure and cholesterol levels, ask patients about their exercise habits, check to see whether they have diabetes, and determine their smoking histories—basically examining known risk factors for coronary heart disease. Then, using statistics, researchers adjust for these confounding factors in an effort to determine whether patients with low levels of vitamin D actually do have a higher risk of heart disease—that is, whether vitamin D levels are independently associated with the risk of heart disease. Sometimes adjusting for confounding factors makes the initial association completely disappear.

Trying to account for other possible variables and explanations is a laudable goal. Unfortunately, most observational studies do not have access to the entire medical history and all of the physical characteristics of every patient in the study. Instead, they typically assess patient histories and characteristics by using administrative data—information that was obtained from Medicare or health insurers, which originally collected the information as part of the process of paying medical claims. In administrative databases, no systematic effort is undertaken to assess every possible cardiovascular risk factor, so adjustment for confounding factors is almost always incomplete.

The best—or worst—example of the problem with confounders occurred with hormone replacement, where initial observational studies led to incorrect prescriptions and affected the health of millions. Throughout the 1980s and 1990s, observational study after observational study showed that hormone replacement therapy (HRT), which supplemented estrogen or estrogen and progesterone in postmenopausal women, was associated with a lower risk of coronary heart disease. The logic of this practice seemed inescapable. Young women suffer less heart disease than men, but following menopause they gradually catch up. Researchers showed that estrogen favorably affects several important cardiovascular risk factors, including cholesterol levels. The final piece of apparently definitive evidence was a series of enormous observational studies showing that postmenopausal women who took estrogen had a lower incidence of heart disease. Soon gynecologists, family physicians, and cardiologists began treating nearly every middle-aged woman with HRT.

However, in 1991 the National Institutes of Health (NIH) proposed a bold research program known as the Women's Health Initiative, which included randomized controlled trials of hormone replacement therapy in postmenopausal women. One of the centerpiece projects was an RCT comparing hormone replacement therapy with a placebo in postmenopausal women.

Between 1993 and 1998, 16,608 women were enrolled in the study. Half received a placebo and the other half received HRT (estrogen plus progesterone). Physicians were "blinded," which means they did not know which of their patients were receiving the treatment and which were receiving the placebo. In this study, as in all good RCTs, an independent group of scientists called the Data Safety and Monitoring Board had access to the clinical trial data as it was accumulated. This oversight is necessary because a study may show statistically significant benefit (or harm) for a therapy prior to study completion. In such cases, the study leadership is informed and the study is stopped prematurely.

On May 31, 2002, the Data Safety and Monitoring Board stopped the estrogen-plus-progesterone HRT trial three years early because patients assigned to HRT had a 26 percent higher incidence of invasive breast cancer. Furthermore, there were statistically significant increases in coronary heart disease (a 29 percent increase), blood clots in the lungs (a 113 percent increase), and stroke (a 41 percent increase). There were a few benefits of HRT, including a reduction in hip fractures (which was expected) and a decrease in the incidence of colon cancer (an unexpected result). But despite these favorable effects, the study authors concluded that "overall health risks exceeded benefits from use of combined estrogen plus progestin." Two years later, the NIH stopped a similar large patient study using estrogen alone because of a 39 percent increase in risk of stroke.

After the shock of these two studies abated, many researchers asked what had gone wrong with the earlier observational studies that apparently had "proved" the benefits of HRT. The problem, as you probably guessed, was confounders. The observational studies failed to account for the other health habits of women who just happened to take HRT. Such women tended to be affluent, educated, and particularly health conscious. In the observational studies, women who took HRT had less coronary heart disease because they were healthier in many other ways compared with women who did not take HRT.

Despite this example, observational studies continue to dominate medical research, primarily because they are far easier and less expensive to perform than RCTs. Though observational studies have flaws, when they are performed properly they *can* yield important clues and useful medical insights that may help formulate hypotheses for subsequent testing using a proper RCT. For that reason, observational studies are considered "hypothesis-generating," meaning that they raise questions, rather than provide answers to important scientific issues.

When you hear reports of observational studies, it is important to ask the right questions. What were the sources of data and what was their reliability? Did the authors make good-faith efforts to adjust for measured confounders? Do the authors properly describe the limitations of their study, or do they tend to overinterpret the findings?

How to Recognize and Interpret Observational Studies

Media reports usually fail to distinguish between observational studies and RCTs. However, certain clues in the report should alert you to the likelihood that a study is observational rather than a more definitive RCT.

CLUES SUGGESTING THAT A STUDY IS OBSERVATIONAL

♥ *Study is not planned in advance (before therapies are given)*

♥ *Administrative data are used (data from Medicare, a health plan, or a state or national database)*

♥ *No intervention is tested*

♥ *Participants are not randomly assigned to therapies*

♥ *Very large numbers of patients*

♥ *Association reported (instead of causality)*

Because observational studies are retrospective, often use data collected for other reasons, and cannot account for all confounders, experienced physician-scientists recommend viewing them with caution unless they show a large treatment effect—at least a doubling of benefit or a halving of risk, which corresponds to a hazard ratio of greater than 2 or less than 0.5. Therefore, if you read a news report about a study showing that people taking vitamin D experienced a 25 percent reduction in the incidence of heart disease, you should not rush out to buy vitamin D. Approach these results with the skepticism of an experienced scientist and consider them as interesting preliminary findings that may warrant further study. Otherwise you will find yourself forever running from one trendy therapy to another.

RANDOMIZED CONTROLLED TRIALS

Randomized controlled trials are the gold standard of evidence-based medicine. When performed properly, this sort of study offers the opportunity to systematically determine which of several alternative therapies produces the best outcomes for patients.

THE OLD TESTAMENT, DANIEL, AND THE FIRST CLINICAL TRIAL

The first known clinical trial was described by Daniel of Judah in the Old Testament in approximately 600 BCE. According to the Book of Daniel, Daniel and the children of Israel were required to accept a diet of meat and wine by the Babylonian king Nebuchadnezzar. Preferring a different diet, Daniel lobbied for vegetables and water. He was eventually able to convince the king to perform a clinical trial.

For ten days, Daniel and the Israelite children received a diet rich in vegetables and water, while other children ate the king's rich foods. The results are reported clearly: "At the end of ten days, it was seen that they [the children who consumed vegetables and water] were better in appearance and fatter in flesh than all the youths who ate the king's rich food. So the steward took away their rich food and the wine they were to drink and gave them vegetables."

While this was not a randomized trial, it successfully tested a therapy—a vegetarian diet—and had both a control group and an experimental group. The intervention is clearly described, as are the trial duration and outcomes. (And this trial was published in one of the few "journals" that has a greater impact than the *New England Journal of Medicine*—the Bible.)

The modern era of RCTs began in 1836, when French physician Pierre Charles Alexandre Louis conducted a fascinating study to determine whether bloodletting was effective in the treatment of pneumonia. In the nineteenth century, doctors believed that circulating blood-borne factors were responsible for many diseases, and that removing the "bad blood" would help the patient improve.

Louis studied seventy-seven pneumonia patients. He divided them into two groups, with those in one group receiving bloodletting during the first four days of their illness while those in the other group were not initially treated by bloodletting. The results were shocking. Among the group receiving early bloodletting, 44 percent died, whereas patients in the group in which bloodletting was withheld experienced only a 25 percent mortality rate. Unfortunately, Louis's discovery that bloodletting was harmful was completely ignored. In addition, the scientific methods he proposed for conducting an RCT were largely overlooked for the next 110 years. He was ahead of his time.

What critical features enable the RCT to serve as our key building block in evidence-based medicine? First, the study must be prospectively designed. This means that the scientific questions are formulated in advance, the experiment is designed in a systematic fashion, no data are collected until the design is finalized, and the design generally is not changed during the course of the study.

Another important element of a high-quality RCT is the random assignment of patients to treatment groups. Why is randomization so important? To be a truly fair test, the treatment groups must be very similar in patient characteristics, so that the only important difference between groups is the treatment being examined. For example, if one group contains more older patients or more who are seriously ill, the outcome may be influenced by those differences rather than by the treatment itself. By randomizing patients, almost all factors (known or unknown) that might influence the outcome are present in equal proportions in the various treatment groups. This approach virtually eliminates the confounders that make observational studies so unreliable.

A third feature of high-quality RCTs is the blinding of all participants, including both patients and their caregivers (usually physicians), so that none of the participants know which therapy is being delivered to individual patients. If both patients and health care providers are blinded, the trial is said to have a double-blinded design. Why is blinding so critical? If either the patients or their physicians know who is receiving a treatment, their own expectations may strongly influence the results. If a patient believes that a treatment is likely to be helpful, he may actually perceive a benefit. If physicians believe that a therapy is beneficial, they may find better outcomes in the patients who they know received that therapy. The best example of expectations influencing outcomes occurs with the placebo effect: if you administer a placebo to a hundred patients with a headache, thirty to forty of them will report excellent pain relief.

Obviously, an unblinded trial design (also known as an open-label trial) represents a particularly high-risk approach when the outcome involves a subjective assessment by either the patient or the physician. In heart disease studies, for example, subjective outcomes might include the duration and severity of chest pain, shortness of breath, or ability to exercise without pain. Such studies should nearly always be blinded. If they are not, their conclusions should be viewed with skepticism.

LIMITATIONS OF RCTS

Ascertainment Bias and Studies That Aren't Blinded

Although blinding of participants is considered a cornerstone of high-quality RCTs, sometimes blinding is not feasible. Several years ago, a group of doctors conducted a study to assess the effectiveness of a left ventricular assist device (LVAD) in prolonging survival in patients with advanced heart failure. LVADs are small implantable pumps that take over some of the workload of the heart in patients whose own hearts have been weakened by disease. In this important LVAD study, patients were randomly assigned to receive medical therapy (drugs) or an LVAD pump. Obviously, since the LVAD is a surgically implanted device, it was impossible to blind either patients or their doctors.

In this case, researchers were trying to determine whether the LVAD had any impact on the likelihood of death—a result that is free of bias, of course. But in the LVAD study, physicians also reported on two measures of improvement in heart failure. The first was relatively objective and involved measuring patients' exercise performance on a treadmill. The other was a subjective assessment by physicians concerning whether patients had general improvements in functional capacity. There was no improvement in exercise capacity as measured on the treadmill, but according to doctors' assessments of functional capacity, there was a statistically significant improvement. Which result do you believe?

In this LVAD trial, the study designers made a fatal but common error: they assigned the surgeon who implanted the LVAD to determine the functional status of the LVAD patients. Do you think the surgeon who implanted the device was an unbiased observer in determining the effectiveness of his therapy—the LVAD—in improving patients' symptoms?

We call this type of error an ascertainment bias, because it reflects the inherent biases of participating physicians in ascertaining the results of the study. A proper trial design would have employed completely independent observers to assess the functional status of *both* the medical and surgical treatment groups.

Selection Bias in Enrollment

If an RCT is going to help us make decisions in the day-to-day practice of medicine, it must include the sorts of patients that we see routinely. The randomized study participants must represent a cross-section of patients eligible to receive the therapy being studied. However, there are many examples where patients' or physicians' inherent biases prevented typical patients from getting into a clinical trial, distorting the results and limiting our ability to apply the findings to a broad population.

Let's say we want to do a study comparing coronary artery stenting to bypass surgery in patients with chest pain brought on by physical exertion. The physicians enrolling such patients are often interventional cardiologists (who perform stenting), so they may have well-established beliefs about which patients are likely to benefit from bypass surgery versus stenting. They might send the sickest patients to surgery and the healthiest straight to angioplasty and stenting, thus enrolling only a small percentage of potentially eligible patients in the trial. Therefore, the conclusions cannot be generalized to include all patients with stable chest pain, since neither the sickest patients nor the healthiest ones were enrolled. This type of problem in an RCT is known as selection bias.

Dropout

Dropout means exactly what you think it means. If an RCT is designed to compare outcomes for treatments given over a period of years, it is inevitable that some patients or their physicians elect to stop the assigned treatment or end their participation in the trial. This phenomenon can have a major impact on the results of RCTs. Dropout is almost never random; it often relates to side effects of the assigned therapy. In a long-term clinical trial, some patients may experience complications from the therapy and stop taking the drug within days or weeks.

To minimize the effect of dropout, properly designed RCTs use an approach known as "intent to treat" (ITT) to analyze results. An ITT analysis includes all patients in the analysis of outcome regardless of whether they stopped taking the drug during the trial. Basically, investigators include a patient in the final analysis of the effects of a drug even if he stopped the drug on the second day of the study. Since patients who stop the drug cannot experience benefits, ITT is a conservative approach because it actually biases the study results *against* the active therapy.

This is the best way to present trial results. If a study began with 10,000 patients and the final analysis reports only on the 7,000 who completed the study, this should raise a red flag. The study authors have not analyzed the data correctly, and we should question their conclusions.

Straying from the Primary Endpoint

In evaluating the results of a clinical trial, investigators must focus on the primary outcome that they said they wanted to study—the one they specified before the study began. We call this outcome the primary endpoint. Generally, an RCT has only one primary endpoint, and this outcome is the single most important focus of the trial. Why do we focus on only one outcome? Remember that we consider P-values significant at a level of 0.05 or less, meaning that 5 percent of the time (or less) a positive result will be erroneous. If we allowed an RCT to specify twenty primary endpoints, there would be a high likelihood that at least one of these results would be positive, just as a result of chance.

Given these statistical nuances, planners of RCTs designate a single outcome as the primary endpoint and all other outcomes as secondary or tertiary endpoints. For example, a study of a new drug for heart failure might specify death as the primary endpoint: how many deaths were there among people taking the drug, compared to the number of deaths among people taking the placebo? Secondary endpoints might include quality of life, hospitalization for heart failure, and distance walked during six minutes of exercise. If, when the study is completed, there is no reduction in the risk of death, we consider the study negative. Even if the study shows improvement in the secondary endpoints, the drug maker and study investigators should not claim that they have proven benefits. When a drug or device improves secondary endpoints, these findings are "hypothesis-generating"—they must be confirmed in another trial where these purported benefits are the primary outcome of interest.

Although these rules for RCTs may seem harsh, this type of discipline is absolutely necessary to avoid declaring a therapy "better" or "superior" when this has not been firmly established. Unfortunately, physicians and companies reporting clinical trial results frequently confuse primary and secondary endpoints, often deliberately. The media report study results just as the study leaders describe them, often misleading the public about the benefits and risks of a therapy. In the worst examples, the study authors report benefits for outcomes that were never even considered in designing the trial. This type of misreporting is sometimes disparagingly described as "data mining," although the formal term is "post-hoc analysis." When you hear about results of an RCT, always consider whether the described benefits are related to the primary endpoint or to some other secondary outcome.

Surrogate Endpoints

In evaluating clinical trials, we always pay careful attention to the primary endpoint. Many cardiovascular RCTs are what's called morbidity-and-mortality trials, typically defined as studies that use a combination of death, heart attack, and stroke as the primary endpoint. However, many studies use endpoints that are much less serious—for example, comparing the effectiveness of various therapies at improving blood levels of cholesterol.

The rationale for such trials is the belief that improving cholesterol will ultimately result in reductions in morbidity and mortality. We say that improvement in cholesterol levels serves as a surrogate for the outcomes we really consider important, which is a reduction in heart attack and stroke. Other common surrogates include blood pressure measurement or improvements in blood sugar levels. An increasingly popular surrogate for heart disease is the assessment of plaque accumulation in arteries of the neck. In theory, a treatment that slows progression of plaque buildup would be expected to reduce heart attacks and strokes. But we don't know this for sure.

Although surrogate endpoints are useful for exploring hypotheses, using them to make decisions regarding the superiority of alternative therapies is risky. Several years ago, a major drug company developed a drug that raised good cholesterol (HDL) by more than 60 percent, an effect superior to that of any existing drug. The company then launched a major RCT to determine if the drug reduced morbidity and mortality. Two years into the study, the Data Safety and Monitoring Board stopped the trial because patients who received the HDL-raising drug experienced a 58 percent increase in mortality. The medicine raised HDL, which should have been good. But it also actually increased the number of deaths.

Unfortunately, there are many similarly dramatic examples of trials that have misled the medical community. Studying surrogate endpoints can help investigators to better select therapies or drug dosages for formal morbidity and mortality trials, but such research can never substitute for properly designed studies that measure more important outcomes.

Subgroup Analyses: Keep Looking Until You Get a Positive Result

A particularly vexing but common problem involves analyzing outcomes for multiple subgroups of patients within an RCT. A subgroup is any arbitrary population within the trial, such as men (instead of both men and women), older patients (instead of patients of all ages), or patients with diabetes (instead of both diabetics and non-diabetics). Subgroup analyses make it hard to interpret clinical trials, because if you study enough subgroups, there is a high likelihood that one of these groups will have a positive response by chance alone. A subgroup analysis is like a fishing expedition—cast a line and see what you reel in. A world-renowned statistician who's a friend of ours said, "Let me study enough subgroups and I'll show you a positive trial." He wasn't joking.

For example, in an infamous study that compared aspirin and a clot-dissolving drug for treatment of heart attack, physicians decided to demonstrate to the medical community the unreliability of subgroup analyses. They examined the results of the study in subgroups categorized by the astrological signs of the patients. And what did they find? Aspirin increased mortality by 9 percent in people born under the sign of Libra or Gemini but decreased mortality by 28 percent in all other astrological subgroups.

Be wary of large studies that report positive outcomes only in patients with very specific characteristics (e.g., diabetic men over the age of seventy); this sort of result usually comes from fishing for a positive outcome in the various subgroups.

Misreporting of Clinical Trials: Follow the Money

Although we consider RCTs the most reliable source of scientific evidence, they are not always reported in an appropriate and scientifically unbiased fashion. Major clinical trials of drugs and medical devices are usually funded by commercial entities, typically pharmaceutical companies or medical device manufacturers, which have strong economic incentives to report favorable results. A recent review of clinical trials revealed that industry-sponsored RCTs were nearly twice as likely to report favorable findings compared with RCTs of the same therapies conducted by non-profit groups. A separate study showed that medical journal articles reporting results for industry-sponsored RCTs were more than five times as likely to recommend the therapy compared with studies funded by not-for-profit groups.

How are the results of clinical trials influenced by the funding sources? Their influence begins during the design phase. An RCT is theoretically designed to answer a clinically important scientific question, but the study sponsor initiating the trial has the opportunity to specify which question is asked. This is not exactly like fixing a baseball game, but it does mean that study designers can increase the odds of a favorable result.

A well-known example illustrating the way that trial design can be tilted to benefit the manufacturer involved a study of drugs to prevent acid reflux. The first drug from this class to be approved was effective, but its patent was going to expire soon, opening the door to low-cost generics. So the manufacturer decided to preserve its income stream by introducing a "new" drug that was really only a slightly altered version of the original compound. The company launched a clinical trial designed to determine whether the new drug was more effective at relieving symptoms than the older drug. Unsurprisingly, the study reported superior results with the new drug. But there was a major problem: the dosage of the older drug used in the RCT was 20 mg, whereas the dosage of the new drug was 40 mg. Despite this obvious source of bias, the new drug for reflux rapidly gained market share and remains the best-selling drug in this class.

META-ANALYSES

A meta-analysis is an important type of study that uses complex mathematical formulas to combine several RCTs to create a larger data set. The hope is that it will help researchers answer questions that could not be addressed using any other approach.

Scientists conduct meta-analyses because it is not possible to perform a large randomized trial for every possible treatment. One reason might be cost: a typical cardiovascular RCT enrolls thousands of patients and can cost several hundred million dollars. Or sometimes an important safety question will arise about a widely used drug and no single existing RCT can provide an adequate answer. In essence, meta-analyses combine small studies in order to simulate what might be observed if all the patients in those smaller studies had been included in a single larger RCT.

The most important strength of this method is its ability to bring together all the RCT data available for a particular therapy. Its weaknesses include the hazards of combining studies that enrolled different patient populations, administered therapies for different lengths of time, or may have had different primary endpoints. Although meta-analyses are more reliable than observational studies, they can sometimes produce incorrect results.

Because of the complex methods employed, the conduct of a meta-analysis always deserves careful scrutiny. How were the studies identified? Did the authors miss important RCTs that would have contributed important data? Did the authors have access to the original raw data from the studies they included, or did they only use those outcomes reported in published accounts? Using only published material may be influenced by a phenomenon called publication bias, also known as the "file drawer" problem. Sometimes studies that fail to show the benefits of a therapy are never published—they remain in the authors' file drawer. For example, one meta-analysis showed that administration of magnesium was beneficial in patients who were having a heart attack. A subsequent large RCT showed no benefits. The meta-analysis produced the wrong answer because investigators in prior magnesium studies had published only RCTs with favorable results, while negative studies—those that showed no benefit to magnesium—sat in researchers' file drawers, inaccessible to the authors of the meta-analysis.

Because of these limitations, most authorities consider meta-analyses intermediate in reliability: more useful than observational studies, but less definitive than a properly designed RCT. Nonetheless, meta-analyses can have a huge impact. We published a meta-analysis in 2007 that reported a 43 percent increase in the incidence of heart attack in patients treated with the diabetes drug Avandia. Although controversial at the time of publication, this meta-analysis eventually resulted in a complete ban on the drug in Europe and severe restrictions on its use in the United States.

DEALING WITH PUBLICATION BIAS

Publication bias, as we've seen in our discussion of meta-analyses, can have a catastrophic effect on the reliability of medical research. In 1997, this problem finally received the attention of Congress, which established an online registry for keeping track of all randomized clinical trials (http://clinicaltrials.gov). The concept was simple: if everyone was aware of the existence of a clinical trial, public pressure to release its results would make it much less likely that only positive results would be published, with negative ones buried.

Initially, the website had limited impact. Registration was voluntary, and there was no enforcement to ensure participation. However, an association of medical journal editors subsequently adopted a policy that any clinical trial that had not been registered before the research began would not be accepted for publication. And in 2007, Congress added some teeth to the law, passing legislation requiring drug makers to register clinical trials and report results on the website. These requirements have definitely helped reduce the vexing problem of publication bias.

CONSIDER THE SOURCE:
WHICH JOURNAL PUBLISHED THE STUDY?

When evaluating a medical study, you need to assess the quality of the journal that published the findings. The best journals employ a rigorous process for vetting publications. Submitted manuscripts are reviewed by several experts who carefully scrutinize the study, looking for flaws in design or conduct. Authors are generally given the opportunity to respond to the criticism. If the responses are inadequate, the journal declines to publish the article.

The finest medical journals publish fewer than 5 percent of submitted articles, but most rejected studies eventually find homes in less well-established journals, which are far less demanding in their reviews of proposed manuscripts. The most prestigious journals include the *New England Journal of Medicine*, the *Journal of the American Medical Association*, and a British journal, the *Lancet*. Articles published by these sources are generally considered reliable. A second tier of general medical journals is also quite solid, including the *Annals of Internal Medicine*, the *Archives of Internal Medicine*, and the *British Medical Journal*. In the field of cardiology, two specialty journals dominate: *Circulation*, published by the American Heart Association, and the *Journal of the American College of Cardiology*, published by the American College of Cardiology, the professional society representing U.S. cardiologists.

If a scientific study is referenced in the media, check to determine where it was originally published. If it was published in one of the above journals, it is probably a reasonably well-conducted study. However, there are still no guarantees. Even the most prestigious journals make mistakes, sometimes publishing manuscripts they eventually retract. This has been a particular problem with the *Lancet,* which has retracted more than its share of high-profile manuscripts. In 2010, for example, it retracted a very well-known—and fraudulent—study it had published in 1998 suggesting a link between autism and childhood vaccinations.

ABSTRACTS: DON'T BE FOOLED

Not all research cited in the media is actually published. The study mentioned earlier in this chapter, extolling the benefits of vitamin D in preventing heart disease, was presented as an abstract at a scientific meeting. In most cases, abstracts and presentations have not been fully peer-reviewed and are viewed by physician-scientists as preliminary data. The level of reliability increases if the abstract is eventually published as a fully peer-reviewed scientific paper. But many abstracts never actually reach publication, and even fewer eventually appear in top-quality journals.

You will notice the media reporting large numbers of heart-related abstracts, presentations, and studies every March and November; these months correspond to the annual meetings of the American College of Cardiology and the American Heart Association, respectively. At each meeting, upward of 20,000 attendees gather to hear more than 1,000 abstracts, and the media pick up on the most interesting presentations.

OUR APPROACH

As we explore heart health with you, we answer your questions by reviewing the available evidence. After reading this chapter, you will recognize that the quality of this evidence varies. In some cases, we have gold-standard randomized controlled trials to guide our recommendations (e.g., taking statins prevents heart attacks in people with high LDL cholesterol). In other instances, particularly when it comes to lifestyle interventions such as diet and exercise and their relationship to heart health, we often have only observational studies, a weaker level of evidence. For each topic—from the potential impact of red wine on your cardiovascular system to the essential role of angioplasty and stenting in certain heart attack victims—we point out the level of evidence and provide our best recommendation based upon careful examination of the available information.

STAYING INFORMED

Now that you understanding the various types of medical studies, you are a better-informed patient and can ask the right questions. If you have concerns about a specific medication or treatment your doctor proposes, it is entirely appropriate to ask him what scientific evidence leads him to believe that this treatment is right for you. Is the recommendation based upon an observational study, an RCT, or a meta-analysis? Did the study assess morbidity and mortality, or did it focus on surrogate outcomes? Don't hesitate to read the study on your own, either.

However, it is important to understand that high-quality scientific studies do not exist for every therapy that we use. It's fine for a physician to say that a recommendation is based upon personal opinion or personal experience, but if your physician is reluctant to share information about why he or she recommends a particular therapy, you might consider finding another doctor.

RX: JUDGING THE MEDICAL EVIDENCE

Don't jump to conclusions every time you hear of a new study

Be a detective: ask questions about the study

Consider the study likely to be reliable if:
  It is a randomized controlled trial (RCT)
  It has been published
  It appears in a top journal

The study is less reliable if:
  It is an observational study or meta-analysis
  It has been presented only in abstract form
  It does not appear in a top journal

Before changing therapies based upon the results of a new study, ask your doctor if the study applies to you and if it appears reliable

CHAPTER 10

WHICH HEART TESTS DO YOU NEED?

THE BIG PICTURE

Your neighbor Bob—who is slightly overweight and spends much of the summer "exercising" on his riding lawn mower—brags that he passed his annual stress test. Your friend at work got a clean bill of heart health based upon a cardiac CT scan. Actors in television commercials gleefully discuss their cholesterol tests, proclaiming that a popular cereal has improved their levels. These people are reassured, even smug, as they report their favorable test results. Perhaps you should share in their satisfaction and schedule a battery of medical tests. But which heart tests, if any, are right for you?

From high-tech, three-dimensional CT scans that reveal the state of the heart's arteries in minutes to a basic cholesterol assessment that helps to determine your future heart attack risk, we have tests to examine every aspect of both your heart itself and your risk factors for developing heart disease. With each passing year, our repertoire of heart tests grows. Sometimes new tests add valuable information, as did the move from measuring total cholesterol to the current standard of assessing different cholesterol and lipid fractions. In other cases, our "advances" raise questions, create controversy, and even increase patient risk, as we'll discuss in regard to routine CT scanning of the heart.

We rely on data to formulate a testing strategy that fits your cardiac situation. We don't order expensive or risky tests simply to provide reassurance; we will reassure you when we sit down to talk. When we choose medical tests, we keep key principles in mind—principles you should apply as well. Paramount among these: *you should have a medical test only if the test result will cause a change that will secure or improve your health.* If you are experiencing chest pain with exertion—a classic symptom of coronary artery disease—an exam to assess your heart's arteries is in order. On the other hand, routine exercise stress testing in people with no symptoms of heart disease—a common practice—is generally a bad idea.

Before you demand, or submit to, a test of your heart's health, use our guidance to determine whether the test is right for you. Don't let media stories determine your testing regimen. You don't need a CT scan of your heart just because President Obama had one (he probably did not need this test, either). Use our scientifically based advice to go beyond the headlines and develop a program that provides the information you need without creating confusion, subjecting you to unnecessary risk, or emptying your wallet.

THE WRONG TEST, A MEDICAL CATASTROPHE, AND A HEART TRANSPLANT

One misstep—an unnecessary test performed just to provide extra reassurance that her heart was okay—put Janice Levin on a treacherous path that caused so much damage to her heart, she required a heart transplant.

A fifty-two-year-old nurse, Janice was appropriately concerned when she developed chest pain. With hypertension and a few extra pounds around the middle, she had noticed occasional brief twinges of stabbing pain around her left shoulder. Having recently embarked on an exercise program and diet, she decided to get her chest pain checked out.

Janice's doctor diagnosed "atypical chest pain most likely of musculoskeletal origin." Typical chest pain arising from coronary heart disease tends to include a pressure-like sensation that comes on with exertion and subsides with rest. Janice's pain did not fit this profile for a cardiac source. Her doctor initially made all of the right moves. He performed a physical examination, which was normal except for a slight elevation in blood pressure. Blood tests revealed a favorable cholesterol profile and low levels of C-reactive protein, a marker of inflammation. Janice's EKG was also normal.

Her doctor was correct in his diagnosis of atypical, or non-cardiac-related, chest pain. Janice required nothing more than reassurance and a plan to manage her risk factors; with weight loss and exercise, her blood pressure would fall and her long-term risk of heart disease would diminish from its already low level. But Janice got much, much more than conversation and reassurance.

Deciding to go the extra step, Janice's doctor ordered a coronary CT angiogram examination to rule out the possibility of coronary artery blockages. This is a relatively new test, rapidly growing in popularity, in which images of the heart's arteries are created using an advanced type of CT scanner.

Janice suffered no direct complications from the CT scan of the heart. The contrast dye did not affect her kidneys (as it sometimes does), and she did not sense the radiation (equivalent to more than a hundred chest X-rays) as it penetrated her heart and outlined her arteries. Unfortunately, the study suggested that she might have some coronary heart disease. Two arteries contained mild blockages. Calcium in a third artery made it hard for her doctors to see inside it, and they thought there was probably an important blockage there.

Already on a road filled with expensive and increasingly invasive tests, Janice's doctors scheduled yet another examination, a cardiac catheterization. It sounded reasonable when Janice's doctors explained that they wanted to be certain and to reassure her.

During the study, doctors placed catheters (plastic tubes) in the heart to inject contrast dye and visualize the artery in question. The angiograms showed that the blockages seen on the coronary CT angiogram were trivial and did not need treatment. But then the procedure went dangerously out of control. Janice developed sudden and intense chest pressure. Her heart rate increased dramatically and her blood pressure plummeted. The next picture of Janice's arteries showed that one of the catheters placed in her heart had torn her aorta, the main blood vessel carrying blood to the body. This is a potentially fatal complication. Janice's aortic tear extended into the left main coronary artery, the most important artery feeding blood to the heart. This interfered with blood flow in the artery and caused an immediate and life-threatening heart attack.

Barely conscious, Janice was rushed to the operating room for emergency open heart surgery. Doctors performed coronary artery bypass surgery, routing critical blood flow around the torn artery to the blood-starved heart muscle. Janice survived the surgery and was discharged two weeks later. The episode caused significant heart damage, cutting her heart function in half. But at least she was alive.

Unfortunately, within six months of the emergency surgery, Janice's bypass failed. She had stents inserted to prop open her arteries, but they failed, too. Doctors had run out of conventional options. Janice needed a whole new heart. She was sent to the Cleveland Clinic, where we performed an urgent heart transplant. We would say that Janice did well with her heart transplant. But when we consider the entire story, it is hard to feel good about her outcome.

Janice began with a normal heart and atypical symptoms completely unrelated to her heart. She underwent tests that she did not need, leading to risky procedures. Although the risk of a real catastrophe was small, it happened. Janice's experience, reported in a major medical journal, illustrates the hazards of the inappropriate use of sophisticated medical tests (the cardiac CT scan) and emphasizes the need for restraint in applying new technologies in patient care. Medical tests can be powerful diagnostic tools, but if misused, they can cause serious harm. More tests and more procedures are not always better.

BASIC TESTS YOU SHOULD HAVE

When we discuss tests to assess heart health, we divide them into two broad categories: tests that assess risk factors for heart disease and tests that detect the actual presence of heart problems. As a general rule, we recommend certain tests for risk factors in virtually everybody, reserving examinations to detect heart problems for those patients in whom we have good reason to suspect cardiac issues.

Tests for risk factors are simple, inexpensive, and very low risk. They include blood pressure measurement, obesity screening with body mass index, a lipid panel (cholesterol test), and, in those at risk for diabetes, assessment of blood glucose.

Blood Pressure Measurement

♥ *What it is: Measure of the pressure of blood against the walls of your arteries*

♥ *Who should have it:*
- All adults: at least once every two years
- Those with hypertension or cardiovascular disease: every few months

Every adult should know his or her blood pressure. The test is simple and noninvasive. We place a cuff around the upper arm, and as the cuff inflates and deflates we get two numbers that reflect blood pressure. The higher number, systolic blood pressure, is the pressure in your arteries when the heart contracts, or squeezes. The lower number, diastolic blood pressure, is the pressure in your arteries when the heart relaxes between contractions. We report your blood pressure with the systolic number first. So a blood pressure of 120 over 80 (120/80) means that the systolic pressure is 120 and the diastolic pressure is 80.

If the systolic number is 140 or greater or the diastolic number is 90 or greater, you have high blood pressure, also called hypertension. A systolic pressure of 121 to 139 or a diastolic pressure of 81 to 89 is defined as pre-hypertension. Prehypertension is a call to action, alerting you to the opportunity to prevent the development of full-fledged hypertension. A normal blood pressure is less than or equal to 120/80.

Should you check your blood pressure at home or with the machine at the gym or in the back of the pharmacy? This is not necessary if your blood pressure was normal at your doctor's visit. However, if you have high blood pressure, checking at home can confirm that lifestyle and medical therapies are working.

If you decide to measure your blood pressure at home, we have a few tips to ensure that you get accurate readings. Don't measure your blood pressure right after you wake up; blood pressure tends to be highest in the morning. Similarly, wait at least 30 minutes before checking your blood pressure if you have just exercised or consumed anything with caffeine. When you are ready to measure your blood pressure, sit quietly for a couple of minutes. Then get your first reading. Wait two or three minutes and then recheck to confirm your first result. Keep a log of your blood pressure and take it to your next doctor's appointment.

If you check your blood pressure at the drugstore or supermarket, make sure the machine has been calibrated recently. Also, the machine at the store works best in those with average-sized arms. If your upper arms are smaller or larger than average, the blood pressure reading from one of these machines may be inaccurate.

WHITE COAT HYPERTENSION

Do you get a little bit nervous when you go to a doctor's appointment? If you do, you are not alone. For many of us, a visit to the doctor causes emotional stress, and your body responds by activating your fight-or-flight response. This releases adrenaline and other hormones into your bloodstream, increasing blood pressure. We call this doctor-induced increase in blood pressure "white coat hypertension."

If your doctor determines that you have high blood pressure based upon a reading at the office, make sure that this is not simply white coat hypertension. Buy your own blood pressure monitor and check your pressure at home under less stressful conditions. If your resting blood pressure at home is normal (120/80 or less), you have white coat hypertension. Although white coat hypertension does not require treatment, many studies suggest that patients with white coat hypertension are not completely normal, and many develop sustained hypertension within a few years, particularly if they fail to adopt a healthy lifestyle. If you have white coat hypertension, stay on top of your blood pressure (frequent blood pressure checks, exercise, good diet) to limit your chance of developing real hypertension in the future.

Obesity Screening and BMI

♥ *What it is: Body mass index, or BMI, is an assessment of weight that takes height into account (weight in kilograms divided by height in meters squared)*

♥ *Who should have it: Everybody*

As you are aware from Chapter 4, BMI helps to determine if you are overweight or obese. In most cases, you can tell whether you are overweight just by looking in the mirror. But doctors increasingly use the BMI to supplement weight assessment. You can determine your BMI by entering your height, weight, age, and gender at the website www.nhlbisupport.com/bmi. An ideal BMI is 20 to 25. A BMI between 25 and 30 almost always indicates that a person is overweight. A BMI greater than 30 meets the medical definition of obesity.

If you are very muscular, you may have a slightly high BMI without having excess body fat. On the other hand, if you recognize that you are overweight, you can use your BMI to guide weight loss. You don't need to check your BMI (or your weight) daily, but reassess your BMI at least once per year, or when you have significant weight changes.

Lipid Profile/Cholesterol Test

♥ *What it is: A blood test that includes your total, LDL, and HDL cholesterol and triglyceride levels*

♥ *Who should have it: Every adult starting at age twenty*

All adults should have their lipids assessed. The LDL cholesterol is the single most important value. We suggest a lipid panel every five years beginning at age twenty. If any values are abnormal or if you have established cardiovascular disease, you'll need the test annually. Most patients on statins should have a lipid panel every six months. Today, only half of young adults have undergone cholesterol screening. Find the time in your schedule and have this simple blood test. It could save your life.

Fasting Blood Sugar

♥ *What it is: A blood test for glucose performed in a person who has not eaten for at least eight hours*

♥ *Who should have it: Patients with known diabetes and those with abdominal obesity, a risk factor for diabetes*

Most people without diabetes do not require routine blood glucose screening. However, those who are overweight and have abdominal obesity face a

C-REACTIVE PROTEIN: DO YOU NEED THE NEW BLOOD TEST?

When it comes to heart-related blood tests, C-reactive protein (CRP) is getting a lot of attention. Proponents maintain that we should measure CRP levels in all patients and use the results to guide therapies designed to help prevent coronary heart disease. There are equally vocal opponents of routine CRP testing.

CRP in the blood provides a general indication of inflammation in the body. In the presence of inflammation, CRP levels go up. Because coronary heart disease is an inflammatory process, it is associated with increased CRP. A person with a higher CRP level faces an increased risk of future cardiovascular events. As with any test, the question centers on what we do with test results. How can we use them to improve health?

We measure CRP levels in some, but not all, patients. Specifically, we use CRP levels to help us decide for or against a statin prescription in patients with cardiovascular risk factors but normal or only slightly elevated cholesterol. A large clinical trial demonstrated that patients with high CRP values and normal LDL levels benefited from statin therapy. On the other hand, if you have established coronary heart disease or a clearly elevated LDL, you require a statin anyway, and CRP testing may be unnecessary. Don't request this test just because it has gained media attention. Instead, ask your doctor if this test will help formulate your medical plan.

high risk of developing diabetes, and we recommend an annual blood glucose test in such individuals to enable early detection of diabetes. A normal fasting blood glucose is less than 100 mg/dL.

TERMINOLOGY OF TESTING

Before we move on to a discussion of more advanced cardiovascular testing, we need to cover a few key terms, which will go a long way toward helping you to determine whether a medical test is right for you.

TERM	DEFINITION
Pretest likelihood	Likelihood that you have the condition the test assesses
Sensitivity	Ability to detect the disease, if it is present
Specificity	Likelihood that a positive test is correct

Pretest Likelihood

We should order an advanced test (one that is risky, that is expensive, or that involves radiation) only if we think that a person has a high likelihood that the test will lead to a change in the diagnosis or guide more effective therapy. For example, an emergency room doctor might obtain an X-ray of your son's arm if it is very swollen and extremely tender after a collision in a soccer game. In this case, there is a high likelihood that the arm in broken and will require a cast. On the other hand, if your child only has a small bruise and feels well enough to keep playing, both you and an emergency room doctor would judge that an X-ray is unnecessary. The pretest likelihood of a broken arm is low, and exposing your son to an X-ray is neither cost-effective nor likely to change the outcome.

What should be the pretest probability of finding an abnormality before we order a test? That depends upon the test, its risks, and its costs. Measuring blood pressure has no associated risk and minimal cost, so we do it in everybody. A lipid panel has virtually no risk and a very small cost, so again we recommend this in all adults. On the other hand, a cardiac catheterization to examine the heart's arteries is invasive and expensive, and it should be performed only when we think there is a high likelihood of identifying coronary heart disease that might require stenting or bypass surgery.

Sensitivity

The sensitivity of a test refers to the ability of the test to detect the disease if the person does have the condition. Virtually no test is 100 percent sensitive. But you want to make sure that a test has a sensitivity that is high enough to improve your physician's ability to make the right diagnosis.

Specificity

The specificity is the probability that a positive test is correct, meaning that the person actually has the condition we are assessing. Again, we want this number to be high. When the test comes up positive but the person does not have the disease, we call the result a "false positive." A false positive result—we incorrectly think that the person has a problem—can lead to further testing and invasive procedures. This is exactly what happened with Janice Levin. A test that results in a lot of false positives is said to have a low specificity.

QUESTIONS TO ASK BEFORE YOU HAVE A HEART TEST

Correctly applied, cardiac tests identify disease, permit early treatment, prevent heart attacks, and save lives. But they are also overused and can expose patients to unnecessary risks. Before you undergo any medical tests beyond a blood pressure measurement and a lipid profile, get answers to six questions to make sure that the test is right for you.

♥ *What condition are we looking for?*

♥ *What is the pretest likelihood that I have the condition?*

♥ *What is the sensitivity of the test in me (the test's ability to detect the condition)?*

♥ *What is the specificity of the test in me (the chance that a positive test is correct)?*

♥ *What are the risks of the test?*

♥ *What are the benefits of the test?*
  • How will it change my therapy?
  • Will it improve my health?

ADVANCED CARDIOVASCULAR SCREENING IN THE ASYMPTOMATIC PATIENT

Everybody should know their blood pressure, blood cholesterol levels, and BMI. But do you need more information? If you have no known heart disease, wouldn't it be helpful to have a stress test or a CT scan in order to reassure yourself that your arteries are okay? The answer is almost always no. There is considerable debate when it comes to cardiovascular screening of the asymptomatic patient: should we assess risk factors to estimate the probability that a person has coronary heart disease, or should we obtain an advanced imaging study or stress test in everybody in order to determine whether they actually have coronary heart disease?

The American College of Cardiology and the American Heart Association recommend the use of risk factor scores in asymptomatic patients, reserving more sophisticated and invasive testing only for those with concrete signs and symptoms of coronary heart disease. We can get a pretty good idea of the likelihood that a person has or will develop coronary heart disease based upon simple measures such as age, gender, smoking history, blood pressure, lipid values, presence of diabetes, and family history. A few superaggressive fringe groups, most with a vested interest in imaging, urge high-tech imaging studies to assess the presence of atherosclerosis in virtually all asymptomatic patients. We side with the American College of Cardiology and the American Heart Association in the view that it would be irresponsible, harmful, and expensive to subject every adult to a battery of cardiovascular imaging studies. The rate of false positive studies is high enough in asymptomatic individuals that most patients with no symptoms but abnormal imaging studies will *not* have any significant coronary disease revealed by cardiac catheterization.

Remember why we get medical tests in the first place. As the editors of the prestigious *Archives of Internal Medicine* point out, we don't perform them "to reassure," "just in case," or "just to know." We order medical tests in order to guide therapy. These editors therefore recommend that we subscribe to the principle "less is more": "if a test is not sufficiently accurate to change clinical management in a particular setting, it should not be done."

Let's say we see a sixty-year-old man who has no chest pain or other symptoms of heart disease. But he does have risk factors, including diabetes, high blood pressure, and elevated LDL cholesterol. We are going to recommend a heart-healthy diet, exercise, medical treatment for his high blood pressure, and a statin to lower his LDL cholesterol level. Some practitioners will also obtain a cardiac CT scan to determine whether he actually has coronary heart disease. This test requires administration of intravenous contrast (which can cause allergic reactions and kidney problems) and exposure to radiation (which increases his long-term risk of cancer). In addition, it is expensive.

Suppose we obtain the CT scan, and it shows that the patient does have coronary heart disease. We would still prescribe a heart-healthy diet, exercise, medical treatment of the high blood pressure, and a statin—exactly what we recommended based upon his risk factors. In this asymptomatic patient, the CT scan neither changed therapy nor improved prognosis. It did lighten his wallet—insurance companies rarely cover the $500 to $1,000 price tag of the test.

The ultimate goal of screening asymptomatic people for coronary heart disease would be to prevent clinical disease and deaths, and we have no evidence right now that screening offers any benefit to asymptomatic patients. Our colleagues in other areas of medicine have made similar observations: screening tests do not prevent deaths from melanoma or prostate cancer, either. Why is this the case? Two key problems are overdiagnosis and overtreatment. The tests may tell us if a person has a disease, but they cannot tell us whether this person, if left alone, will actually die from the disease. So we perform additional tests and procedures on everybody who screens positive, exposing them to risk. We cannot recommend routine imaging of the heart's arteries in asymptomatic people when there is no evidence proving its benefit.

Now we turn to individual tests. Use this section to understand tests that your doctor recommends. Before you undergo *any* test, remember to get answer to the six key questions to help you determine if the test is right for you.

Electrocardiogram

♥ *What it measures: The heart's rhythm and rate*

♥ *Who should have it: Anybody with chest pain or suspected heart disease*

One of the oldest tests in modern medicine, the electrocardiogram (EKG or ECG) remains useful more than a century after its development. You can't walk down a hospital cardiology corridor without encountering a technician wheeling around a portable EKG machine.

The EKG consists of twelve distinct electrical signals recorded from different sites. This provides twelve different views of the heart's electrical activity, almost like looking at a sculpture from different angles in order to appreciate the entire work. If you are in a hospital, your EKG monitor will generally display two or three of these views, providing enough information for the nurses and doctors to know if your heart rate and rhythm change.

What can we learn from the EKG? An electrocardiogram can confirm that the heart's natural pacemaker is functioning normally and that the heart's electrical system conducts the impulses in a normal way. If the electrical impulse is delayed or blocked during conduction through the heart, the patient is diagnosed as having heart block and may need an implantable pacemaker. If the heartbeat is irregular, an arrhythmia is present; the EKG can determine whether the abnormality affects the heart's upper chambers (atria) or lower chambers (ventricles).

We diagnose atrial fibrillation, the most common atrial arrhythmia, when we observe rapid and irregular impulses on an EKG. The EKG also reveals when a patient suffers from ventricular tachycardia, a potentially lethal condition in which the lower chambers (ventricles) beat too rapidly. We can also use the EKG to detect premature ventricular contractions (PVCs), one of the most common abnormal heart rhythms. Once thought to represent a serious disorder, we now know that most PVCs are not serious or life threatening, although they may cause palpitations, an awareness of the extra heartbeats.

Because arrhythmias often occur at unpredictable times, we sometimes order a test called a Holter monitor to catch an arrhythmia that we may have missed with a routine thirty-second EKG. The Holter monitor consists of EKG electrodes and a portable recorder that the patient wears for twenty-four to forty-eight hours. Patients keep a diary describing symptoms so that we can correlate EKG abnormalities with symptomatic episodes. Sometimes the arrhythmia is so infrequent that the Holter monitor does not catch an episode this period. In such cases, we often equip the patient with an event recorder, a device worn for days or even weeks. Whenever he or she feels a symptom, the patient activates the recorder to capture the event on the EKG.

The EKG is our most important tool in the diagnosis of a heart attack (myocardial infarction). When a patient presents to the emergency department with chest pain, an EKG should be obtained within five minutes.

Characteristic changes in the EKG enable us to diagnose an acute heart attack and may indicate the need for an emergency heart catheterization to open a blocked coronary artery. If EKG changes are more subtle, we may admit the patient to the hospital for blood tests and monitoring to rule out a heart attack.

After a major heart attack, the EKG usually remains permanently abnormal. This creates a problem for some patients because, during a future visit to the ER, a physician may misinterpret old EKG changes as indicative of a new heart attack. If you have had a heart attack, we recommend carrying a miniaturized version of your EKG in your wallet to enable physicians to compare new EKGs with the older tracing.

Today the EKG remains an essential tool in cardiac diagnosis, enabling physicians to diagnose heart rhythm disturbances, heart attacks, and a host of other conditions. Plus it's inexpensive and can be obtained within a few minutes in almost any setting. Although supplanted by more modern tests for some applications, the simple EKG will likely be around a hundred years from now.

ECHOCARDIOGRAMS AND THE SHIPYARD

In May 1953, two Swedish scientists, a physician and a physicist, had a terrific idea. What if you could bounce sound waves off the heart and use the returning sound wave echoes to construct a visual image of the moving heart? They paid a visit to a local shipyard in Malmo, Sweden, where a company had received an instrument that used ultrasound, or high-frequency sound waves, to test materials for manufacturing defects. Using their charm, the scientists persuaded the company to loan them the ultrasound equipment for the weekend.

The physician, Dr. Inge Edler, placed the industrial ultrasound device on a patient's chest and looked at the screen. He was astounded! He was able to see reflections from structures within a beating heart. Nobody had ever seen anything like it. At that moment, echocardiography was born. The scientists had to return the ultrasound equipment at the end of the weekend, but cardiologists soon had their own echo machines. Six decades after this discovery, we have better ultrasound equipment than the average shipyard, and echocardiography is one of our most important tests in cardiovascular care.

Echocardiography

♥ *What it assesses: The heart's structure and pumping ability and heart valve function*

♥ *Who should have it: Anybody with a heart valve problem or murmur, reduced heart function, or history of a heart attack*

Echocardiographic equipment has evolved considerably in the decades since Edler first placed an industrial scanner on a patient's chest wall. Modern echo machines generate incredibly detailed pictures of the heart chambers, valves, and other cardiac structures. Typically, a fist-sized imaging device, known as a transducer, is placed on the chest, sending and receiving high-frequency sound waves. Since sound waves are poorly transmitted by air, we coat the transducer with a jelly-like fluid to ensure good transmission of the ultrasound energy to the chest wall. Patients roll onto their left side to bring the heart closer to the chest wall. The echo technician presses firmly, placing the transducer at several locations to get different views of the heart; this procedure may produce slight discomfort. Ultrasound waves are reflected by cardiac structures back to the transducer, and a sophisticated electronic system generates a moving video image of the heart's four chambers: the right and left atria, and the right and left ventricles. Of these, the left ventricle is most important because it functions as the main pumping chamber of the heart. Because the ultrasound pictures of the heart are moving images, we can assess contraction of specific walls of the heart and identify regions damaged by a heart attack. The location of a wall motion abnormality tells the cardiologist the specific location of previous damage by a heart attack or other disease.

If you remember one number from your echocardiogram, it should be your ejection fraction, which reflects the overall function of the left ventricle by measuring the percentage of blood it expels during each heartbeat. Normally, about 60 percent of the blood in the left ventricle is ejected during each cardiac contraction; the lower limit of a normal ejection fraction is approximately 50 percent. An ejection fraction in the range of 35–45 percent is considered moderate dysfunction, and values less than 35 percent represent more severe impairment. In patients with congestive heart failure or valvular heart disease, we follow the ejection fraction closely over time with periodic echocardiograms. In heart failure patients, a low or falling ejection fraction may indicate the need for additional drug therapy, or trigger us to place an implantable cardiac defibrillator to treat the dangerous heart rhythms that often occur in patients with severe heart damage. In patients with valvular heart disease, a decrease in the ejection fraction often indicates that it is time for surgical valve repair or replacement.

Echocardiography plays a unique role in the diagnosis of heart valve problems. We assess the structure and motion of heart valves using an adaptation of cardiac ultrasound known as Doppler echocardiography. Doppler echocardiography and some fancy physics allow us to determine the presence and size of leaks through heart valves and the severity of narrowing of valves. These insights help us to decide when to recommend heart valve surgery.

Although we can acquire reasonably good echo images in most patients, several factors limit the quality of echocardiographic examinations, including the distance between the transducer at the chest wall and the heart. Obese patients and those with severe lung disease (COPD) pose particular challenges. To improve echo image quality, physicians needed to find a way to place the ultrasound transducer in a fluid environment closer to the heart. The esophagus, passing directly behind the back of the heart, is an ideal location. By placing small ultrasound transducers on scopes designed to traverse the esophagus, doctors invented the procedure known as trans-esophageal echocardiography. We perform this test when we need high-resolution images of cardiac structures. For example, if the routine echocardiogram suggests that a valve leaks, but we can't quite determine if it leaks enough to warrant surgical repair, we may perform a trans-esophageal echocardiogram to get a better quality image. We sedate the patient and numb the throat with a local anesthetic, then pass an echo transducer through the mouth, into the esophagus, and direct it toward the heart. The images we obtain provide incredibly detailed pictures of heart structures. Although patients are often apprehensive about undergoing this test, most do not find the experience particularly unpleasant. In most cases, the quality of the diagnostic information is worth the minimal discomfort.

Echocardiography is indispensable to modern cardiologists and heart surgeons. One of the most important reasons echocardiography is so popular is that it can generate detailed cardiac images without radiation. As any woman who has been pregnant knows, ultrasound is safe. There are no known adverse effects of exposing human tissue to ultrasonic energy of the type and intensity used in echocardiography.

Despite its immense value, echocardiography is significantly overutilized in many cardiovascular practices. Because the procedure is generously reimbursed, many physicians have purchased echo machines for their offices and perform ultrasound examinations without adequate clinical reasons to do so. It is challenging for an individual patient to know whether an echo exam is appropriate or inappropriate, but we encourage you to ask directly why the study is necessary and how the findings will influence your future care.

Stress Testing

♥ *What it assesses: Likelihood that a person has blockages in coronary arteries*

♥ *Who should have it*:
- Patients with chest pain and a moderate risk of having coronary artery disease
- Patients who have had a heart attack (before resuming full activity and exercise)

After a standard electrocardiogram, stress tests are probably the most common tests used in patients with known or suspected coronary disease. In its simplest form, an exercise test involves walking on a treadmill while the physician and/or technician monitors a continuous EKG to see how the heart performs under the stress of exercise.

How We Perform a Standard Stress Test

We follow a standard algorithm when we stress the heart. The most common approach, known as the Bruce protocol, begins with the treadmill set at 1.7 miles per hour and a 10-degree slope. At three-minute intervals, we increase both the treadmill speed and slope, making the heart work harder. The Bruce protocol has ten discrete steps, with the highest level reaching 7.5 mph and a slope of 28 degrees. No patients attain Stage 10, a level reserved for world-class athletes. Reasonably fit individuals typically reach Stage 4 or 5, which represents a speed of 4.2 or 5.0 mph, respectively, with a slope of 16 or 18 degrees. For people with severe impairment in exercise capacity, we modify the Bruce protocol by starting at 1.7 mph, but with a zero degree slope.

Doctors use different criteria to decide when to stop the stress test. Bring your tennis shoes to the test. But don't worry; nobody is going to let you keep going until you collapse from exhaustion in a puddle of sweat. Some physicians prefer a "symptom limited" test in which the patient exercises as long as possible, stopping only if chest pain develops (but short of exhaustion). Other testing laboratories end the test when a patient reaches a target heart rate, typically 85 percent of the maximum predicted heart rate for the patient's age and gender. This number declines with age—an older patient simply cannot reach the heart rate that he may have achieved at a younger age.

Whether the treadmill test is symptom limited or heart rate limited, the principal goal is to stress the heart to determine if coronary blockages are present. A stress test has three possible outcomes: positive, negative, or equivocal. We deem a stress test to be positive (abnormal) if certain EKG changes occur during exercise that are usually associated with the presence of coronary blockages. In determining whether the test is positive, the physician may also consider whether the patient experienced chest pain similar to the symptoms that the stress test was originally ordered to evaluate. However, strictly speaking, only the presence of EKG changes, not symptoms, is considered strong evidence of an abnormal stress test.

Positive findings suggest that obstructed coronary arteries cannot supply enough blood flow to meet the exercising heart's demand. If no chest pain is provoked and no EKG changes occur, we say that the test is negative (normal). We reserve a third category, equivocal, for tests with subtle EKG changes that aren't quite definitive enough to judge whether a coronary blockage is present.

Limitations of Stress Tests

Stress tests are frequently wrong. Understanding their limitations is essential for well-informed patients, because an incorrect test can lead to serious unintended consequences. Remember our previous discussion of testing terminology. We can apply those principles to identify the limitations of stress tests and to determine when their use is appropriate.

In patients with significant blockages in the coronaries, only about 65 percent will have a positive (abnormal) stress test; this means that the sensitivity of the test is only 65 percent. Therefore, 35 percent of patients with major blockages in the coronaries will have a negative stress test (a false negative). Conversely, when the stress test is positive, this finding is correct only about 70 percent of the time. So the specificity of a stress test is 70 percent. For the 30 percent of patients with a positive stress who are later shown not to have blockages, the stress test resulted in a false positive. As you remember from Janice Levin's story, a false positive result is the most problematic type of error, because it can lead to additional testing and serious complications.

Because stress testing has a relatively low sensitivity and specificity, we must be careful how we apply it. But doctors order stress tests too often in situations where the test is not very useful. Consider a forty-five-year-old man with no symptoms, normal LDL cholesterol, and normal blood pressure levels who consults his physician before starting an exercise program. The physician orders an exercise test to make sure that it is safe for the patient to exercise vigorously. The stress test is abnormal, and both the physician and patient are faced with a dilemma—what to do next?

In this situation, most doctors opt for a heart catheterization, which usually shows no blockages. The beaming physician delivers the good news, and the patient is reassured. But let's step back for a moment. The patient underwent an unnecessary and invasive test (thankfully without complications) that cost thousands of dollars. Doctors repeat this scenario hundreds of thousands of times every year.

Remember that the usefulness of a test is determined by its sensitivity, its specificity, and the pretest likelihood that the patient has disease. The problem with this particular patient is a low pretest likelihood of coronary heart disease. With no symptoms or risk factors, our forty-five-year-old man has less than a 2 percent likelihood of having coronary disease, yet he still underwent stress testing. Fortunately, he did fine. Let's say, though, that we encounter 100 men just like him. Based upon their risk factor profiles, only two will actually have significant coronary blockages. But if we perform stress tests on all 100, thirty of them will have a positive (abnormal) stress test. Why? You will recall that the specificity of stress testing is only 70 percent (a 30 percent false positive rate). Furthermore, with a sensitivity of 65 percent, only one out of the two men who actually has the disease will have a positive stress test. Therefore, if we stress-test 100 forty-five-year-old men who have no symptoms or risk factors, thirty-one men will have positive tests, but only one of them will actually have coronary artery blockages; for the other thirty, the result is wrong. Worse yet, many of these patients will subsequently undergo additional unneeded procedures such as heart catheterization.

Now let's consider the opposite example, an exercise stress test in a person who has a high likelihood of having coronary artery disease. It makes more sense to do the test in this person, right? Wrong! Consider a fifty-five-year-old man with chest pain during exertion. He smokes, and he has diabetes, high cholesterol, and high blood pressure. His pretest likelihood of coronary disease is greater than 80 percent before you put him on the treadmill for a stress test. If we have 100 such men, eighty of them will have coronary heart disease. Based on what we know about the sensitivity and specificity of stress testing, the procedure will correctly diagnose coronary disease in fifty-two, fail to detect real disease in twenty-eight, and be falsely positive in another six—not a very good performance, considering that based upon symptoms and risk factors alone, we already knew that 80 percent of these men would actually have coronary blockages.

You can see from these two examples that stress testing performs poorly in patients with either a low pretest likelihood of having coronary blockages or a high pretest likelihood of coronary disease. Stress testing is most valuable for patients with an intermediate likelihood of coronary disease. In such patients, approximately half will actually have disease and half will not. If the stress test is positive, we often proceed with further testing because the abnormal stress test increases the likelihood that coronary disease will be found. In those with a normal stress test, we can judge that their likelihood of having coronary disease is low.

While stress testing is rarely necessary for individuals without symptoms or patients with a high likelihood of disease, there are some exceptions. We recommend stress testing for people in certain professions where a sudden heart attack would put the public at risk, such as commercial airline pilots and school bus drivers. For everyone else, we limit stress testing to individuals with symptoms and an intermediate likelihood of coronary disease.

Stress Testing After a Heart Attack

After a patient has a heart attack, we perform a modified stress test. A full symptom-limited test that pushes a patient to 85 percent of the predicted maximum heart rate is not considered safe in the first few days or weeks following a heart attack, but a modified stress test that stops when the patient reaches 70 percent of the maximum heart rate has proven very useful. We use this test to convince both ourselves and the patient that it is safe to leave the hospital and return to the normal activities of daily living. For most individuals, common activities such as walking, bathing, or sexual activity rarely raise the heart rate beyond 70 percent of the predicted maximum. Therefore, successful completion of a stress test limited to 70 percent of the predicted maximum heart rate suggests that a person will not develop chest pain or other symptoms after discharge. Then, about six weeks following the heart attack, we perform a full stress test, either symptom-limited or terminating at 85 percent of the maximum predicted heart rate, to confirm that the patient can engage in unlimited activity.

Stress Testing After Bypass Surgery or Stenting

Some physicians perform routine annual stress tests in patients with known coronary disease who have undergone an angioplasty (stenting) or bypass surgery, in order to determine if coronary disease has recurred. We do not recommend this approach. Annual stress tests in these patients will result in some false positives, leading to unnecessary heart catheterizations and, in some cases, unnecessary angioplasties. In addition, since all post-angioplasty or post-bypass patients should already be receiving aspirin and medications for cholesterol and blood pressure, a positive stress test will not guide medical therapy. An approach of watchful waiting after bypass or stenting is more prudent than repeated annual stress testing. We carefully interview these patients about the presence or absence of symptoms, and reserve stress testing for individuals who develop new chest pain.

Special Stress Tests

Nuclear Stress Tests

Several decades ago, recognizing the limitations of standard stress testing, leading researchers developed methods to improve the accuracy of the stress test. Monitoring the EKG during the treadmill test is an indirect approach to detecting a deficit in blood flow to the heart muscle, so physician-scientists sought a way to directly visualize the perfusion of blood in the walls of the heart. Eventually, methods using radioactive isotopes emerged as the most accurate method to "see" blood flow in the heart muscle.

Known as a nuclear stress test, this procedure begins with exercise on a treadmill (or sometimes a bicycle) just like a standard stress test. Then, at the peak of exercise, a small amount of a radioactive isotope (tracer) is injected through an IV, and the patient is immediately placed in a scanner. The tracer travels via the blood and passes through the coronary arteries, where the heart muscle takes up the radioactive isotope. The more blood flow received by an area of the heart, the more radioactive tracer deposited in that region of the heart. Areas of impaired blood flow during exercise don't take up tracer and appear as "cold" spots in the scan.

There are two principal reasons why an individual might show a cold spot on a first nuclear scan. First, the area with little or no tracer uptake could represent a scar from an old heart attack. In that case, the heart muscle in that zone is not living tissue and won't ever take up the tracer. Alternatively, the cold spot on the first scan might represent an area of living muscle with decreased blood flow from a coronary blockage. In that case, the heart muscle is alive, but it's not getting enough blood flow during exercise to take up the radioactive tracer.

In order to distinguish between these two possibilities, we perform a second scan after the patient recovers from exercise to see what happened within any areas that had a deficit in blood flow during the first scan. If the cold spot represents permanently damaged heart muscle (an old heart attack), the second scan continues to show absence of tracer uptake in this zone. If, however, the cold spot represents living tissue that is not adequately supplied with blood during exercise, the cold spot fills with tracer on the second scan. We call a permanent cold spot a "fixed" defect and an area that takes up tracer in the second scan a "reversible" defect. Differentiating fixed from reversible defects is very valuable to both cardiologists and cardiac surgeons. Restoring blood flow via a stent or bypass surgery won't benefit a fixed defect, but it will likely help substantially if the defect is reversible.

PET Scans

Occasionally we are fooled by a nuclear stress test. In some cases, coronary blockages are so severe that an area of the heart shows up as a fixed defect on the second scan even though the heart muscle in the region is alive. Identifying such areas is pivotal because restoring blood flow through bypass surgery may allow the heart muscle to function again. If we suspect this scenario, we perform another type of nuclear scan, known as positron emission tomography (PET). This type of scan identifies living tissue in the heart even if it has a poor blood supply. An area with poor blood flow but with increased uptake of a special PET tracer represents living heart muscle that may begin to contract normally if supplied with blood. We use this scan in patients with severely reduced heart function to determine whether increasing coronary blood flow by stenting or bypass surgery will improve heart function.

Echo Stress Tests

We can also use echocardiography to improve stress test accuracy. We perform an echocardiogram at rest, followed by exercise on a treadmill or stationary bicycle, with a second echo performed during the peak of exercise. Rather than imaging blood flow as in a nuclear stress test, an echo stress test looks for areas of heart muscle that function well at rest but contract poorly during exercise. Heart muscle with a limited blood supply doesn't contract vigorously when stressed by exercise. Therefore, areas that contract poorly during the exercise part of the echo examination are likely supplied by a coronary artery with a blockage.

Chemical Stress Tests

During development of nuclear and echo stress tests, a dilemma arose: what about patients who cannot exercise due to arthritis or other limitations? The solution involves administering drugs that simulate the effects of exercise, a procedure known as a chemical stress test. The details about how these drugs work are not important, but there are a few concerns you need to understand. One of the drugs used in a chemical stress test can exacerbate asthma, so make certain to inform your doctor if you have lung disease. Also, caffeine can block the effects of the drugs, so don't drink caffeinated beverages for twenty-four hours prior to the test. If you smoke, don't use nicotine-containing products (including smokeless tobacco) for eight to twelve hours before the test. Keep in mind that an exercise stress test is superior in accuracy to a chemical stress test, so don't opt out of exercise unless you really are incapable of walking on a treadmill or using a stationary bicycle.

Are Nuclear and Echo Stress Tests Better?

Are nuclear and echo stress tests superior to old-fashioned EKG-based tests? Yes, but the improvement is modest. When compared to each other, echo and nuclear stress tests are similarly accurate, provided that the team performing each test is skilled and experienced. Some hospitals and practices rely more on one or the other. If you need a stress test, get the type that your doctors use routinely. Most important, do not consider either test infallible. Both echo and nuclear stress testing are somewhat better that regular EKG stress testing, but they are still frequently wrong.

We can minimize mistakes by ordering these tests in the right patients. But, as with standard stress testing, doctors drastically overuse nuclear and echo stress tests. The stimulus for overuse is primarily economic; both types of studies are generously reimbursed. In fact, testing in general is so lucrative that many cardiologists derive a substantial portion of their income from these imaging procedures.

There are other important downsides to consider. Nuclear studies expose patients to enough radiation to measurably elevate the risk of cancer, according to some experts. For either echo or nuclear stress testing, a false positive examination can lead to further procedures, some of them invasive, such as cardiac catheterization. Be cautious and carefully discuss the advantages and disadvantages of undergoing an imaging stress test, particularly if the study is performed in your physician's office. You should be particularly wary of repeated nuclear studies, because these expose you to higher cumulative doses of radiation with a corresponding increase in the lifetime risk of cancer.

CARDIAC CATHETERIZATION

♥ *What it assesses: Blockages in coronary arteries*

♥ *Who should have it:*
- Patients with chest pain thought to be from coronary artery disease
- Patients having a certain type of heart attack

Every year, we perform more than 2 million heart catheterizations (commonly called "caths") in the United States. For a patient undergoing a heart cath for the first time, it can seem like a scary proposition—the insertion of long tubes (catheters) into the heart chambers and coronary arteries. However, patients who have undergone this procedure will tell you that it's not particularly uncomfortable.

Before a cath, we give patients a mild sedative. We then inject local anesthetic in the groin area (or the wrist if we are going to use the radial artery at the wrist to gain access to the body's arteries). Once the area is numb, we insert a variety of different types of tubes (catheters) into the artery and advance them under X-ray guidance into the heart and its arteries.

CARDIAC CATHETERIZATION, ANGIOPLASTY, AND STENTING: LEG OR ARM?

For decades, we have relied upon the femoral artery in the leg as our standard approach to enter the circulation and get our catheters into the heart. Although common, this approach has drawbacks. There is some discomfort with this procedure. In addition, patients must be careful after the procedure, often having to lie flat for hours, so that they do not disrupt the puncture site in the leg. This can be very uncomfortable, especially for people with back pain. Even with precautions, about one out of every 200 patients bleeds from the femoral artery or nearby vein as a result of the procedure.

In order to improve patient safety and comfort, European cardiologists now perform the majority of their cardiac catheterization and stenting procedures through the wrist. Introducing catheters into the radial artery in the wrist (this is the artery where you can feel your pulse) lowers the risk of bleeding to less than 1 percent. However, the procedure is more challenging for the cardiologist. It also involves greater radiation exposure, although scientists estimate that the increased radiation is equivalent to twenty chest X-rays, representing only a small risk to the patient. We are amazed by the rapid recovery associated with the radial artery procedure. If a patient has the cath in the morning, he looks completely normal (except for a Band-Aid at the wrist) by lunchtime.

Today, fewer than 10 percent of procedures in the United States are performed via this technique, versus 60 percent in Europe. If you are scheduled to have a catheterization or stenting procedure, ask your cardiologist if it can be done through the wrist. You should also ask if the physician is experienced in performing this type of procedure.

We often begin the catheterization procedure by obtaining a picture of the left ventricle, the heart's main pumping chamber. We inject iodine-containing contrast dye into the pumping ventricle and record an X-ray "movie" as the heart squeezes and ejects the dye. Although the heart pumps out all of the dye within a few beats, this short video provides enough information for us to assess heart function and to calculate the ejection fraction. We also get some idea of mitral and aortic valve function, although heart valves are best examined with an echocardiogram.

THE FIRST CORONARY ANGIOGRAM: A SERIES OF FORTUNATE EVENTS

The era of routine cardiac catheterizations with coronary angiograms (X-rays of the heart's arteries) began by accident. On October 30, 1958, an obscure and crotchety Cleveland Clinic cardiologist, Dr. Mason Sones, was performing a heart catheterization to examine a man's leaking aortic valve (echocardiography was not yet available). At the time, it was forbidden to inject contrast dye into the coronary arteries. Doctors believed that putting iodine-containing contrast into the coronary arteries would cause ventricular fibrillation, a fatal heart rhythm abnormality.

During the procedure, Dr. Sones's catheter accidentally slipped into the opening of the right coronary artery just as he injected contrast dye. He pumped the dye directly into the artery. Horrified, Dr. Sones prepared to make an incision and open the patient's chest to save his life. The team watched the monitor anxiously. The dye produced a clear picture of the patient's coronary artery. Then the heart began to slow, and eventually stopped. Disaster! But a moment later, the heart started to beat again. The patient recovered and did just fine.

Most normal doctors of the time would have collapsed with relief, thankful that they had not killed the patient and vowing never to make the same mistake again. Not Sones. Recognizing that he could generate pictures of the coronary arteries without harming patients, he began to deliberately inject dye into the heart's arteries to diagnose coronary artery disease. He convinced others of the procedure's safety and diagnostic power. Thanks to his efforts, a revolution in medicine was born. And millions have benefited from his fortunate mistake.

The procedure pioneered by Dr. Sones is now known as coronary angiography. Catheters with special curves are inserted through the groin, passed through the aorta, and inserted into the openings of the coronary arteries. The cardiologist injects contrast dye into a coronary artery while X-raying the heart. Although modern contrast dye is much less toxic than the material used by Dr. Sones, it still sometimes causes the heart to slow. The cath operator may therefore ask you to cough, which helps to clear dye from the coronaries and restore a normal heart rate. A typical cardiac catheterization may take only fifteen to thirty minutes, although the preparation adds about a half hour. After the procedure, the catheters are removed and the physician holds pressure on the artery to stop bleeding. In some cases, we insert a special plug in the artery to prevent bleeding.

To interpret coronary angiograms, we review the video images and grade the severity of any blockages, reported as the percentage of narrowing. Thus, we say that a completely blocked artery has 100 percent stenosis, while a partially blocked artery may have 50 percent stenosis. Under most circumstances, blockages less than 75 percent are not considered flow-limiting because exertional chest pain (angina) does not usually occur until the artery has a 75 percent or greater obstruction. Visual grading of the arteries' narrowings is imprecise and subjective, and there is large variability in interpretation between different observers. For this reason, whenever possible, and particularly if you have concerns, get a second opinion on the interpretation of your coronary angiogram.

Though somewhat invasive (it includes puncture of an artery and passage of catheters into the heart), cardiac catheterization in the contemporary era is very safe.

Risks of Cardiac Catheterization	
TYPE OF RISK	**DEGREE OF RISK**
Death	1 in 1,000
Stroke	1 in 1,000
Kidney failure (temporary)	1 in 300
Bleeding	1 in 200
Allergic reaction	1 in 200

Allergic reactions to contrast dye are uncommon and rarely serious. In mild cases, patients develop hives. In more severe cases, swelling in the throat can cause blockage of the windpipe, which requires emergency treatment. Pretreatment with antihistamines and cortisone can prevent some of these reactions. Those allergic to shellfish face an increased risk of a reaction to contrast dye. Tell your doctor if you have an allergy to shellfish, or if you have had a reaction to a previous X-ray test that included dye administration.

Contrast dye can also cause kidney damage. This complication is usually reversible, but it may delay discharge from the hospital. Factors predisposing to kidney problems include diabetes, preexisting kidney disease, and dehydration. In high-risk patients, we often administer intravenous fluids overnight prior to heart catheterization, and nearly all centers give IV fluids for a few hours after the procedure to wash out the dye. Your doctor can minimize the risk of kidney problems by limiting the volume of contrast used during the procedure. Make sure to tell your doctor if you have diabetes or kidney problems, and ask if he or she will be able to limit your exposure to potentially harmful contrast material.

Doctors perform too many cardiac catheterizations. Some cardiologists elect to perform angiography in most patients with chest pain, regardless of whether the symptoms are typical or atypical of angina. Cardiologists who are quick on the trigger to perform catheterization often scare patients by warning of dire consequences if the cath is not performed promptly.

In reality, not every patient with chest pain requires a cardiac catheterization. Urgent catheterization is needed only in patients suffering from an acute heart attack. For most other patients, we recommend a more deliberate decision-making process. Don't let yourself be rushed into a procedure that you may not need. If you have stable chest pain, particularly if you are not hospitalized, ask questions about the risks and benefits of the procedure. If you have doubts, don't hesitate to seek a second opinion. Don't forget that catheterization and coronary artery stenting in stable angina patients do not reduce the risk of death or heart attack, so you can take the time to discuss all options with your cardiologist and/or family physician.

CT Scans of the Heart

We Americans love our CT scans. We now perform more than 80 million CT scans per year in the United States, with cardiac scans representing a

TOO MANY HEART CATHS

When a patient is having a large heart attack, urgent cardiac catheterization with assessment of the coronary arteries is critical. The goal is to get the blocked artery open as quickly as possible, and we actually measure the "door-to-balloon time," which is the number of minutes from the moment the patient hits the hospital doorway until we have an angioplasty balloon inflated in the heart in order to open up the blocked artery. Wasted minutes kill heart muscle cells, and rapid catheterization saves lives.

We don't do such a good job when we perform elective (non-urgent) diagnostic catheterization in patients with suspected, but not confirmed, coronary heart disease. Duke University researchers recently reviewed elective cardiac catheterizations in nearly 400,000 patients. In each case, doctors judged that the evidence for coronary heart disease was strong enough to justify this invasive procedure. How often were they correct? Thirty-eight percent of the time. Just over one-third of patients had obstructive coronary artery disease.

Can we do better? Yes. Before ordering a cardiac catheterization, we need a thoughtful and honest appraisal of the likelihood that a person really has coronary artery disease. Is the chest pain typical? Does the person have risk factors for coronary heart disease? Would a noninvasive stress test help with the decision? Both your doctor and you should ask some questions before an elective trip to the cardiac cath lab.

growing proportion of this total. Apparently healthy people with no symptoms of heart disease are lined up for radiation-laden CT scans, seeking reassurance that there is no silent killer lurking in their chests. CT, or computed tomography, employs X-rays and sophisticated computers to create high-resolution, three-dimensional views of the body. While it has been used for decades to examine the brain, lungs, and abdominal organs, CT scanning of the moving heart is a relatively new phenomenon.

The key problem with CT scans of the heart is that we are not yet sure how test results should influence therapy. Some doctors claim that finding coronary artery disease will cause them to add a statin or an aspirin. Others use the test to determine whether a cardiac catheterization is necessary. Thus far, we have no strong evidence to support either practice. Nor do we have evidence that cardiac CT scans result in treatment changes that prevent heart attacks or prolong life. Despite these limitations, CT scanning of the heart is spreading like a wildfire—and, like a wildfire, producing significant damage.

Doctors use the CT scanner for two different types of heart tests: calcium scanning and coronary CT angiography.

Calcium Scanning

Coronary plaques tend to accumulate calcium, a process described by the term "hardening of the arteries," an antiquated moniker for coronary heart disease. One of the first applications for cardiac CT, coronary calcium scanning, detects calcium in the heart's arteries. The more calcium in the coronaries, the more plaques and disease. Based on the norms for their age and gender, patients receive a coronary calcium score, which can range from zero (no calcium) to more than 400 (dense calcium, sometimes associated with coronary blockages).

Patients with higher calcium scores tend to have an increased risk of experiencing a heart attack. Therefore, they require strong efforts at risk factor modification. But we generally recommend such steps—quitting smoking, regular exercise, Mediterranean diet, appropriate medicines—no matter what the calcium score. So we have to ask how a high calcium score changes a patient's habits and management. If the person already follows a heart-healthy lifestyle and sees a good doctor, the answer is that it doesn't.

Nevertheless, coronary calcium scanning has developed an almost cult-like following. Purchasing their own CT scanners, entrepreneurial cardiologists aggressively promote coronary calcium scoring. Many patients undergo annual tests in order to track their calcium scores, This serial or repeat scanning has no value and should be avoided. In the worst abuses, billboards advertise things like "Valentine's Day Specials," offering a discount when "you and a loved one" both get scanned. This sort of snake oil promotion, coupled with a lack of data proving a benefit to the scans, has soured thoughtful cardiologists on this technology. Our advice: avoid this test for now.

Coronary CT Angiography

With coronary CT angiography, doctors obtain pictures of a person's coronary arteries using a specialized high-speed, high-resolution CT scanner, rather than a cardiac catheterization. Instead of injecting contrast dye directly into the coronaries, they administer the dye intravenously and obtain CT images as the dye passes through the coronary arteries, With no groin

A CARDIAC NURSE MAKES THE COVER OF *TIME*

A forty-nine-year-old registered nurse, Michael Fackelman helped thousands of patients recover from heart disease. Grateful patients and families recognized him in the hospital hallways and showered him with gratitude. But it was not until his own heart problems came to light that Fackelman gained national recognition. On September 1, 2005, Fackelman the patient—not Fackelman the nurse—landed on the cover of *Time* magazine.

A former collegiate swimmer, Fackelman exercised regularly and followed a healthy diet. When a Cleveland Clinic cardiologist asked Fackelman to do him a favor and serve as a subject to test a new type of cardiac CT scanner, he agreed. After all, he expected the test to show images of perfectly clean coronary arteries. Instead, the test revealed a tight blockage in his left anterior descending coronary artery. Doctors described it as "a heart attack waiting to happen." Fackelman underwent angioplasty and stenting to prop open the blocked artery.

In the *Time* story, author Christine Gorman commented, "The favor Fackelman did may well have saved his life." This makes a great story line, and it undoubtedly added to the enthusiasm for this high-tech test. But was Fackelman really "a heart attack waiting to happen?" Did the CT scan truly save his life? Should you rush out and pay $500 to $1,000 for one of these advanced scans?

No. Placing stents in the coronary arteries of asymptomatic people neither saves lives nor prevents heart attacks, although, as in Janice Levin's case, such procedures *can* cause serious complications. Resist your craving for sexy, high-tech medicine. If you don't have symptoms of heart disease, you don't need a coronary CT angiogram. And if you do have chest pain or diagnosed heart disease, this is probably not the right test for you, either. At this point, the coronary CT angiogram is still a test looking for solid evidence.

puncture and no catheters advanced into the heart, this test is less invasive than a standard cardiac cath. High-tech and less invasive: what's not to like?

We'll tell you. The images generated by this test vary widely in quality, but they are never as clear and crisp as those from a standard coronary angiogram. As a consequence, scans often result in false positive studies, in which a blockage is incorrectly diagnosed or overestimated in severity. The presence of coronary calcium renders the scans difficult to interpret, and the scans don't perform well in patients with irregular heart rhythms such as atrial fibrillation. Despite these limitations, proponents of the technique claim that it has a low false negative rate, making it useful in ruling out coronary disease in low-risk patients.

Critics, including ourselves, point to widespread and inappropriate use of this technology to screen patients with a low pretest probability of disease, thereby increasing health care costs. In addition, false positive studies provoke an excessive number of unneeded heart catheterizations. And while the test is low-risk, it's not no-risk. Coronary CT angiography involves radiation exposure. With the first commercial devices, the radiation dosage was equivalent to five to seven cardiac catheterization procedures. More recently, in response to criticism, manufacturers have introduced advanced scanners that substantially reduce radiation dosage, but many first-generation scanners still exist. Finally, keep in mind that when coronary CT angiography suggests a blockage that might require treatment, you will still need a standard cardiac catheterization and angiogram to confirm the findings.

The bottom line: be wary if your physician advises you to have coronary CT angiography. Ask questions. Will you require a cardiac catheterization in addition? Will test results influence your medical therapy? How will the test lead to better health? Get a second opinion before you enter the scanner.

Radiation Exposure and Cardiac Testing		
TEST	RADIATION DOSE (MILLISIEVERTS)	NUMBER OF CHEST X-RAYS FOR EQUIVALENT RADIATION DOSE
Chest X-ray (single view)	0.05	1
Calcium scanning	1–2	20–40
Cardiac catheterization	2–16	40–320x
Coronary CT angiogram	2–20	40–400
Nuclear medicine stress test	8–30	160–600
Yearly background radiation from radon and cosmic rays	3–3.5	60–70

RADIATION AND HEART TESTS:
GETTING THE BIGGEST BANG FOR YOUR RADS

Radiation exposure can cause cancer. This means that medical imaging studies performed to improve your health may increase your risk for cancer down the road. Over the last thirty years, the average radiation exposure for American adults has doubled, largely as a result of a sixfold increase in radiation from medical imaging. Americans get the most medical radiation in the world, with imaging of the heart accounting for about one-third of the exposure.

In the cardiovascular field, nuclear stress tests and cardiac CT scans are the largest sources of radiation. Each of these tests can involve a radiation dose equivalent to that of several hundred chest X-rays, generally at least double the dose of a cardiac catheterization. Depending upon a hospital's equipment and protocols, radiation exposure from cardiac scans can vary by a factor of ten or more. These tests should not be used indiscriminately. We take particular issue with the common practice of annual checkups that include repeated stress tests or CT scans. In general, there is little justification for such serial testing and its attendant radiation exposure.

How much do cardiac imaging studies increase cancer risk? Radiation damages the DNA in the body's cells. Sometimes that damage can trigger a mutation that results in cancer. The best recent studies suggest that a CT coronary angiogram performed in forty-year-olds will eventually cause cancer in one in 270 women (most likely breast cancer) and one in 600 men. The lifetime risk of imaging-associated cancer is also increased in younger patients. Our advice is simple: there is no radiation dose that is completely safe, so we should think twice every time we order one of these tests.

Recognizing the risks, the FDA is considering a broad range of initiatives to regulate radiation-based medical testing:

- Setting standard radiation doses for common tests
- Requiring manufacturers to disclose radiation doses associated with each medical image
- Establishing a "radiation medical record" for each patient to keep track of cumulative radiation exposure (we already do this for doctors, nurses, and technicians who administer the tests, so why not do it for patients, too?)

But you don't have to wait for the FDA. Keep track of your cumulative radiation exposure with a log of all of the X-ray-based tests that you have had; give your doctor a copy each time a new test is ordered. When a doctor suggests a test involving radiation, make sure it is truly necessary, and ask how its results will influence your treatment or health. Ask whether the test has been optimized to limit your radiation exposure. Be particularly wary if you have had the test previously; make sure that your doctor has a good rationale for repeating this scan.

RX: TESTS FOR YOUR HEART

Everybody needs to check these:
    Blood pressure: at least every two years
    Lipid panel: at least every five years
    BMI and weight: at least annually

Ask six questions before advanced or invasive heart testing:
    What condition are we looking for?
    What is the likelihood that I have the condition?
    What is the ability of the test to detect the condition if I have it?
    What is the chance that a positive test is correct?
    What are the risks of the test?
    What are the benefits of the test (change in therapy, improved health)?

Don't have annual stress tests or cardiac CT scans

Keep track of your radiation exposure

FIXING THE BROKEN HEART

CHAPTER 11

MEDICINES FOR THE HEART: THE BIG SIX

THE BIG PICTURE

"Why do I have to take so many medicines?" John Simpson asked us. John has been our patient for over a decade, and he asks this every time we see him. He is not alone: we hear this complaint over and over from our patients, and their confusion often stems from misconceptions and biases about the drugs used to treat heart disease.

Some patients are really complaining about the cost of medications, which can be daunting, particularly for those without prescription drug insurance coverage. Others perceive taking medication as a kind of weakness. Many believe (usually mistakenly) that if they dieted and exercised more effectively, they would not need to take cholesterol-lowering therapy. Taking medicines reminds people that they are sick, and some patients don't like the constant reminder of a serious illness.

One of the most frequent conflicts between doctors and patients is the willingness of some patients to blame their symptoms on the drugs they take, rather than on their underlying disease. It's easy to be influenced by rumor and hearsay: "I heard that statin drugs can damage your liver." "My uncle had a terrible reaction to that drug and I don't want to take it." Other patients have inordinate fears about drug safety. In the wake of highly publicized drug recalls, these concerns are not irrational, but they become problematic when patients confuse risky drugs with therapies we have used safely for decades. Prominent cases of misconduct by drug makers have fueled patient fears about the safety of medications, leading to a strong reluctance on the part of many patients to accept drug therapy.

If you are a heart patient, you will need to take medicines. In fact, modern drug therapy represents one of our greatest triumphs in the battle with heart disease. While some key medicines, such as aspirin, have been around for centuries, most heart medicines were developed in the last few decades. With appropriate use, these medicines have helped millions, extending both the quantity and quality of life by preventing heart attacks and strokes. The key is "appropriate use." Many patients don't get the medicines that they need, or receive prescriptions that are inappropriate. If you or a family member is a heart patient, you almost certainly take one of the medicines we call the "Big Six." You must understand what these medicines do and how to use them safely. Your health depends upon it.

The "Big Six" Heart Medicines		
MEDICINE	PRIMARY USES	NOTES
Statins	Lower LDL cholesterol	
Aspirin	Prevent blood clots	Platelet inhibitor
Clopidogrel	Prevent blood clots	"Super" platelet inhibitor
Warfarin	Prevent blood clots	Blocks proteins that cause blood clots
Beta-blockers	Treat heart attack Treat heart failure Lower blood pressure	Decrease heart rate and force of contraction, decreasing heart's work
ACE inhibitors	Treat heart failure Lower blood pressure	Relax (dilate) arteries

The challenge of choosing drugs wisely for patients represents one of the most vexing aspects of modern medical care. Over the last three decades, we have seen an explosion of drugs to treat heart patients. This news is both good and bad. The good news is that we have more effective medicines available to treat the most complex and challenging cardiovascular conditions. The bad news is that physicians need to educate themselves about these new drugs to fully understand their optimal use, potential side effects, safety issues, and interactions with other drugs. For the busy practitioner, gathering and remembering all of this information is daunting; many physicians fall short. Intellectually lazy physicians rely too heavily on information provided by drug makers, usually conveyed by ebullient, articulate, and well-groomed representatives. This process, known as drug "detailing," recalls the experience of talking to a used car salesman; the company representative strives to leave the physician with an unrealistically favorable opinion about the efficacy and safety of the drugs that he or she sells. Since drug companies don't deploy their salespeople to detail generic drugs, which are inexpensive and available from many different manufacturers, practitioners hear exclusively about newer and more expensive drugs, which may or may not be more effective and safer than older drugs.

What can an informed patient do? Knowledge is always the best antidote to fear and doubt. By helping you to understand key principles underlying the rational use of medications, we will equip you to ask the right questions when a medicine is prescribed. Focusing on the most important cardiovascular drugs—medicines you will certainly encounter—we will explain their actions, highlight their side effects, and point out potential for interactions with other drugs.

HOW DO MEDICINES WORK?

There are six critical points underlying the safe and effective use of medications:

♥ *Absorption*

♥ *Elimination*

♥ *Mechanism of action*

♥ *Adverse effects*

♥ *Dosage*

♥ *Drug interactions*

By considering each of these issues, you and your doctor can ensure that you make the best choices from the hundreds of available cardiovascular drugs.

Absorption

Cardiovascular drugs commonly enter the body in one of three ways: injection (intravenous, subcutaneous, or intramuscular), transcutaneous administration (giving the drug via a patch placed on the skin), and oral administration (as a pill or elixir).

Each approach has advantages and disadvantages that influence the drug's safety or efficacy. For example, the route of administration will often have a major impact on the time required before the medicine exerts its effects. IV administration usually provides an instantaneous onset of action, whereas oral administration may take considerable time before the first effects are noted. Some, but not all, very important drugs are available by several different routes of administration. For example, an essential drug used to treat heart rhythm disturbances, amiodarone, can be given intravenously or orally depending on the urgency and specific problem being treated. On the other hand, aspirin is available only as an oral preparation.

Elimination

Drugs must be removed from the body. The most common routes of elimination depend upon the kidneys (excretion in the urine) and the liver (metabolism of the drug, followed by elimination in urine or feces).

Why must you take some medicines every eight hours and other medicines only once per day? This relates to how quickly the drug is eliminated from your body, which involves a concept called the *half-life* of the drug. The half-life is the time it takes for the effects of the drug (often measured by blood levels) to decline to one-half of the highest achieved level. The longer the half-life, the greater the interval between doses.

To prolong the half-life of a drug, pharmaceutical companies often develop long-acting formulations. These longer-acting preparations are generally as effective as their short-acting cousins, and they are far more convenient. All other factors being equal, most patients prefer the convenience of a drug that can be given once per day. If you are taking pills every six or eight hours, perhaps you can simplify your life. Ask your doctor if a longer-acting preparation is available for you.

Mechanism of Action

How does the drug produce the desired effects? Some drugs interfere with naturally occurring bodily processes that can contribute to cardiovascular disease. For example, blood thinners (anticoagulants) affect the body's clotting system, preventing blood clots from forming in places that might harm the patient. Other drugs boost a naturally occurring protective substance. For example, some drugs are designed to raise HDL ("good") cholesterol, believed to protect against heart disease. Understanding how medicines work—their mechanism of action—is important because it helps us to determine which drugs are likely to benefit which patients. A patient with a genetic tendency to form blood clots may benefit from an anticoagulant. A patient predisposed to coronary heart disease by a low HDL level might be a good candidate for an HDL-raising drug.

Adverse Effects

All drugs have side effects. Reading a medicine's package insert can be terrifying. The list of possible side effects can range from blue skin (amiodarone) to severe muscle damage (statins) to kidney failure (ACE inhibitors). Fortunately, most serious side effects are rare. When patients experience something they deem abnormal, they often search the Internet to see if their symptoms could relate to a medicine they are taking. For common complaints, such as headache and gastrointestinal distress, it is difficult to determine whether the drug is at fault. Don't simply stop taking a medicine if you experience this sort of problem; pay attention the next time that you take it and see if the symptom recurs. If it does, alert your doctor, as it may be time to try a different drug.

Drugs produce adverse effects in a variety of ways. An *on-target* adverse effect is a problem caused by the same mechanism of action responsible for the drug's principal benefit. For example, an anticoagulant, even when given in the correct dosage, may produce abnormal bleeding. An *off-target* adverse effect occurs when a drug interferes with a bodily process that is not related to the drug's mechanism of benefit. A classic example relates to the hugely popular class of blood-pressure-lowering drugs known as ACE inhibitors. In about 5 percent of patients, these drugs cause a dry but annoying and persistent cough because the drugs interfere with an enzyme system known as bradykinin. ACE inhibitors don't need to affect bradykinin to lower blood pressure, so the cough is an off-target effect.

Every time a doctor prescribes a medicine, he or she should ask you about drug allergies. *Allergic reactions,* another important category of adverse effects, are unpredictable side effects triggered by mechanisms similar to those responsible for common allergies such as asthma or hay fever. Allergic reactions to drugs can be mild, such as a skin rash, but they also can be severe or even life-threatening. The most feared allergic reaction, anaphylaxis, includes hives and swelling of the tongue and throat; this can lead to obstruction of breathing or death. *If you have had an anaphylactic reaction to a drug, you must inform every physician involved in your care.* Many patients who have had an anaphylactic reaction wear a bracelet warning medical caregivers of this danger.

Patients often confuse adverse drug reactions with allergic reactions. Patients will tell us they are allergic to a particular medicine, but on further questioning, it turns out that what they are experiencing is a common on-target effect, not a true allergy. If a drug has caused a reaction, do a little detective work with your doctors to determine whether this is an allergy or a standard side effect. If it is an allergy, you may need to avoid all drugs in that class, while simple side effects are often managed easily by reducing the medicine's dose.

Dosage

Safe use of drugs requires determining the proper dosage, not always an easy task. For most drugs, higher dosages produce greater benefits, but may also increase adverse effects. A general principle of good medical practice is to use the lowest dosage that is effective. Doctors select the lowest effective dose through a strategy called *titration*: we start with a low dose and assess the response. For example, we might prescribe a blood-pressure-lowering drug at a starting dose. After a few days or weeks, the patient returns and we measure the blood pressure. If the pressure is still too high, we increase the dose. With certain types of drugs, including statins for cholesterol, this process may take several visits.

Dosage titration produces an added benefit. If you experience an ad-

ARTHRITIS, PAIN RELIEF, AND THE RISK TO YOUR HEART

Every pharmacy and supermarket has an aisle filled with pain relievers, many of them targeted to ease the joint pain of arthritis. Before your knee pain convinces you to buy that oversized bottle containing 1,000 tablets, you need to consider your heart. While popular analgesics reduce joint pain, there are concerns about their cardiovascular side effects.

Since 2004, when Vioxx was withdrawn from the market, physicians, patients, and government agencies have questioned the cardiovascular safety of non-steroidal anti-inflammatory drugs (NSAIDs). Common NSAIDs include naproxen (Aleve, Naprosyn), ibuprofen (Motrin, Advil), diclofenac (Voltaren), and celecoxib (Celebrex). As a class, these agents have been associated with increased blood clotting, increased blood pressure, worsening kidney function, and retention of salt and water. Whether these changes increase the risks of heart attack, heart failure, and stroke remains uncertain. But many experts believe that those with a history of preexisting cardiovascular disease probably face the greatest risk with NSAIDs.

Different NSAIDs have different risk profiles. Observational studies (weak strength of evidence) suggest that naproxen may have the lowest cardiovascular risk and diclofenac the highest, with other drugs intermediate in risk. In addition, some of these medications (ibuprofen and naproxen) may interfere with the action of aspirin, reducing its ability to discourage clot formation. If you are a heart patient and you suffer from joint or muscle pain, we advice that you try other strategies—physical therapy, weight loss, heat and cold therapy—before taking NSAIDs. If these don't work, try acetaminophen (Tylenol). While the next step is often naproxen, you should take the lowest dosage that relieves your symptoms for the shortest period of time. This stepwise approach to treating arthritis pain may help to minimize the risk to your heart.

verse effect, the doctor can reduce the dose of the drug to a previous dosage that was tolerated. Be patient with your physician during drug titration. The lack of effectiveness at low dosage doesn't mean the drug won't eventually work. Give it time.

A common and occasionally lethal problem is failure to adjust a drug's dosage if the patient has kidney failure and the drug is eliminated by the kidneys. Thousands of kidney patients die or are injured every year when they receive medicines that should be used only in much smaller dosages in the presence of kidney failure. Similarly, patients with chronic liver disease quickly develop toxic levels of drugs metabolized by the liver if their physician fails to adjust the dosage downward. If you have liver or kidney problems, remind your doctor every time you receive a new prescription.

Drug Interactions

The problem of drug interactions represents one of the most treacherous areas of modern medicine. Today, it is the rare patient who takes only one medicine. In fact, it is not unusual for a patient to be taking five or more medications, many administered by different physicians. A patient's cardiologist prescribes three medications, the family physician two more, and the gastroenterologist adds yet another drug. Then the patient visits the emergency department with back pain and receives another medication. No single physician supervises the overall medication list, and many do not know what their colleagues have prescribed. The risk of drug interactions increases dramatically as the number of prescriptions increases.

This is where you need to take charge. It is critically important that you keep a list of all of your active prescription and non-prescription drugs. Present this list at every doctor's appointment. Your doctor will appreciate the help, and you will protect yourself from the dangers of drug interactions.

How do drugs interact to cause harm? The most common problem is one drug's interference in the metabolism of another. This is particularly common for drugs that are metabolized by the liver, where a group of enzymes known as cytochrome P450 are responsible for metabolizing many drugs. Some drugs cause overactivity of these liver enzymes, thereby increasing the rate of elimination of other drugs; this reduces the blood concentration and effectiveness of medicines.

A particularly dramatic example of this sort of drug interaction occurred on a college campus during a meningitis outbreak. Doctors prescribed the antibiotic rifampin to students who had been exposed to classmates with meningitis, to prevent them from developing this life-threatening illness. Within a few weeks, there was a campus-wide outbreak of unwanted pregnancy. What happened? Rifampin caused overactivity of the liver P450 enzymes that metabolize (break down) oral contraceptives, but young women were not told that it might reduce the effectiveness of their birth control pills.

Dietary supplements and over-the-counter medications can also cause drug interactions. A notorious example is the dietary supplement St. John's wort. A widely used over-the-counter remedy for depression—although deemed ineffective by the National Institutes of Health—St. John's wort increases activity of the liver P450 enzymes, significantly altering the metabolism of many important drugs, including medications administered for heart-related conditions. Heart patients should not use St. John's wort.

These examples illustrate just a few of the many ways that drugs can interact. They point out why it is so important that you, your physician, and your pharmacist carefully scrutinize every drug that you take, looking for common drug interactions.

WHERE CAN YOU GET GOOD INFORMATION?

Given the complex nature of drugs and the constant introduction of new medicines, how can you stay informed? Many sources of information exist, but not all of them are reliable. Every drug has an FDA-approved product insert, which is a complete description of the information known about the medication. Product inserts are written in scientific language and are intended for medical audiences, but some scientifically inclined patients may choose to read product inserts for their own edification. A compendium of product inserts, known as the *Physician's Desk Reference* (PDR), is available to all physicians. You can buy a copy of the PDR, but it makes for dense and difficult reading.

Many patients turn to the Web for information about medicines. Product inserts are generally available online as PDF files, and this is a good place to start. Many websites contain drug information, but unfortunately, they vary widely in quality and reliability. Be careful. One source of information should always be avoided: websites produced by the drug makers. These sites abound. If fact, if you type the brand name of a drug into a search engine, you will usually find a website administered by the drug manufacturer at the top of the list. Such websites are designed to promote use of the drug and are unreliable sources of information.

Get information from your doctor. When a physician prescribes a new drug for you, discuss the reasons she decided to use that particular medication. Don't hesitate to ask your doctor how long the drug has been marketed and how much is known about its long-term effects. Thoughtful practitioners consider newly introduced drugs (usually defined as medications approved within the past two years) to be riskier than those with a longer track record, because rare side effects may not show up until a drug is used for a longer duration in a larger and more diverse population. Of course, in some cases, it is entirely appropriate to administer a new drug because it has distinct advantages for an individual patient. Don't be afraid to take a new drug, but also don't hesitate to ask your doctor why she is prescribing this medication.

In recent years, the FDA has begun requiring drug makers to provide medication guides for drugs it believes will be used more safely if consumers have more information about them. Medication guides provide patients with a clear, easy to understand summary of the risks and benefits of each drug, along with guidance for safe use. If you receive a drug with a medication guide, read it carefully.

STATINS: RANKED NUMBER ONE

If we were evaluating heart medicines the way sportswriters rank college basketball teams, statins would come in at number one. With annual sales topping $26 billion, statins are the best-selling cardiovascular drugs in the world and have extended the lives of millions of patients. We provide a comprehensive discussion of statins in Chapter 3. Here we'll just give you an overview.

Statins are a relatively recent addition to our medicine cabinet, dating to the late 1980s. When diet and lifestyle interventions fail to bring LDL cholesterol levels down, we turn to statins to reduce cholesterol levels. About 80 percent of the body's cholesterol is produced by the liver, and the statins reduce LDL cholesterol by tricking the liver into removing more cholesterol from the blood.

Today we have seven different statin medications available in the United States. They tend to lower LDL cholesterol levels by 20 to 50 percent, depending upon the choice of drug and the dose. While atorvastatin (Lipitor) and rosuvastatin (Crestor) are the most powerful statins, this does not necessarily mean that they are the best. A patient who requires only a modest reduction in LDL cholesterol can be treated with an inexpensive generic agent such as simvastatin (Zocor). Unfortunately, many doctors prescribe a particular statin because they are familiar with the dosage or know the drug company representative. If your doctor prescribes a statin for you, ask if it is the best fit for you and whether it is available as a generic.

Why are doctors so enthusiastic about statins? The answer goes well beyond their cholesterol-lowering ability. We embrace statins because they prevent heart attacks and strokes and save lives. If you have had a heart attack or stroke, you should definitely be on a statin. If you have high LDL cholesterol unresponsive to diet and lifestyle changes, you should be on a statin. Doctors don't argue much about these two statements. But the noise level escalates rapidly when cardiologists debate the use of statins in people with normal LDL levels.

The controversy stems in part from a recent study known as the Jupiter Trial, in which statins were tested in nearly 18,000 people with normal LDL levels. Media reports characterized these subjects as "healthy," but they weren't healthy by all measures. They had increased inflammation in their bodies, which was measured by a blood test for C-reactive protein. Among these people, who had normal LDL but increased inflammation, statins reduced the risks of heart attack and stroke and the need for coronary artery bypass surgery or stenting.

Some doctors have proposed, perhaps only half in jest, just putting statins in the drinking water. Of course, we can't endorse this idea. Statins are medicines, and they should be used to treat people with cardiovascular disease and people at particular risk for cardiovascular disease. Based upon the Jupiter Trial, we do prescribe statins in patients with borderline elevations in LDL values and high levels of inflammation. Interestingly, in addition to lowering LDL, statins reduce inflammation, supporting the rationale for prescribing statins for these patients.

Like any medicine, statins have side effects. While many doctors worry about the possibility of liver damage, there has never been a case of serious liver damage attributable solely to a statin. If you take a statin, you do not need routine blood tests to check your liver. But if you develop severe muscle pain, particularly if accompanied by tea-colored urine, call your doctor immediately. In rare cases, statins cause severe muscle damage (rhabdomyolysis) requiring hospitalization. When muscle pain is mild and not associated with this condition, changing the dosing schedule or to a different statin can relieve symptoms. Don't give up on statins because of mild muscle discomfort.

As the most popular heart medicines in the world, statins are often the subject of rumor and innuendo. Statins have been linked to all kinds of illnesses, ranging from diabetes and kidney disease to a variety of cancers. Here is the truth: Statins are associated with a small increase in the risk of diabetes, but the cardiovascular benefits outweigh the risk. Statins do not cause kidney failure. Statins do not cause cancer, and some studies even suggest that statins might prevent development of certain types of cancer. Finally, contrary to other rumors, statins do work in women.

Used appropriately, statins save lives. If your doctor prescribes a statin, take this as good news—we have a medicine that will help to prevent you from having a heart attack and make you live longer.

ASPIRIN: WHO NEEDS IT?

In about 400 BCE, Hippocrates first described the use of the bark of the willow tree to relieve headache and reduce fever. Willow bark contains salicylic acid, a close chemical cousin to modern aspirin. More than twenty centuries later, in 1897, German chemist Felix Hoffman synthesized a derivative, acetylsalicylic acid, which was named aspirin by Hoffman's employer, Bayer AG. Within a few years, aspirin had become one of the world's most successful medications. The cardiovascular benefits of aspirin were not described until the 1960s, when British pharmacologist Sir John Vance determined the mechanism responsible for aspirin's cardiovascular effects. Vance was awarded the Nobel Prize in 1982 for his pioneering work. Today, 50 million Americans take an aspirin a day. Unfortunately, for many of them this is a mistake.

How Does Aspirin Work?

Aspirin inhibits the effects of a powerful group of naturally occurring substances known as prostaglandins. One of these circulating factors, thromboxane A2, plays a key role in clotting. When an artery is injured, the body's first line of defense against excessive bleeding is the formation of a platelet plug or "white clot" that initially stops the blood loss. To effectively plug the hole, platelets—small cell fragments that circulate in the blood—must stick together, and thromboxane A2 is an important factor that makes platelets "sticky," causing them to clump at the site of blood vessel injury and stop the bleeding. Aspirin, by inhibiting the formation of thromboxane A2, reduces the ability of platelets to clump together and form white clots.

This effect of aspirin on platelets and blood clotting occurs at very low dosages, much less than those required for pain relief. The typical dosage used in heart patients is 81 mg (one baby aspirin) given once a day. The anti-clotting effects of aspirin are permanent and irreversible, lasting for the entire life span of the platelet (about one week), until new platelets are manufactured by the bone marrow.

The anti-platelet and anti-clotting effects of aspirin benefit certain heart patients by keeping arteries open. The underlying cause of coronary heart disease is atherosclerosis, the buildup of fatty plaques in the coronary arteries. This can reduce blood flow through arteries, leading to chest pain with exertion. However, the most catastrophic plaque-related events, such as heart attack and stroke, are caused by fracture or rupture of an atherosclerotic plaque, exposing substances within the plaque to flowing blood. Platelets flock to the raw surface of the ruptured plaque, initially producing a platelet-rich white clot. The white clot quickly progresses to become a larger "red clot" (a thrombus). The thrombus can completely block blood flow through the artery, leading to a heart attack or stroke. Aspirin prevents the initial platelet plug and enhances the body's own mechanism for dissolving platelet plugs, thereby offering protection from heart attacks and strokes.

Aspirin in the Heart Patient:
Heart Attacks and Secondary Prevention

In the 1960s and 1970s physicians began to use aspirin to prevent clotting in patients with heart disease. A series of randomized controlled trials demonstrated unequivocal benefits in heart patients. Aspirin's benefits were greatest in patients with the most severe disease and far less evident in lower-risk populations.

In 1988, a 17,000-patient Italian study showed that administration of aspirin to patients suffering from an acute heart attack reduced the risk of dying by 23 percent over the following six weeks. Other well-designed randomized controlled trials confirmed these findings. This led to the universal practice of administering an aspirin tablet immediately to any patient with a suspected heart attack. It is very important to take an *uncoated* aspirin during a heart attack. Most emergency departments also ask the patient to chew and swallow the tablet to facilitate rapid absorption. Do not use enteric-coated aspirin to treat a suspected heart attack; the coating is designed to delay release of aspirin until the tablet reaches the small intestine, which occurs several hours after ingestion. When a heart attack is beginning, you need aspirin in your blood immediately. Although enteric-coated aspirin may be easier on the stomach and appropriate for normal use, regular aspirin must be used to treat a suspected heart attack.

Solid evidence from high-quality studies supports the continuous use of aspirin in most patients with established coronary heart disease. Patients with preexisting coronary disease include those who have had prior bypass surgery, major blockages in coronary arteries on catheterization, coronary stents, or known blockages in the arteries of the legs or the carotid arteries. Collectively, individuals with known artery disease are termed *secondary prevention* patients because the goal of therapy is to prevent a recurrence or second event. A meta-analysis of sixteen major trials demonstrated that aspirin produced a 19 percent reduction in the risk of a serious new coronary event in secondary prevention patients. This study also found an 18 percent reduction in the risk of stroke. The message is clear: if you have coronary heart disease, you need to be on aspirin unless you have another condition that makes aspirin too risky, such as an active stomach ulcer. For most patients—except for those with coronary artery stents—81 mg per day is the right dose.

Aspirin in Primary Prevention

Individuals are considered *primary prevention* patients if they have risk factors for heart disease, such as high cholesterol or hypertension, but have not yet suffered an event such as heart attack or stroke. The use of aspirin in these patients is more controversial. A large meta-analysis of primary prevention patients showed that aspirin did not reduce the risk of death or stroke, but it did result in a 12 percent reduction in the risk of a serious event such as heart attack. This statistic sounds favorable, but there is a problem.

Among primary prevention patients, the absolute event rates were very low, with only about 1 in 200 people experiencing a cardiovascular event each year; this compares to an incidence of 1 in 15 for some high-risk secondary prevention patients. These numbers mean that you would need to treat more than 1,000 primary prevention patients for a year to prevent a single cardiovascular event.

If you are a primary prevention patient (no known heart disease, no history of stroke) you might ask, "Why not take aspirin anyway, even if the benefit is small? After all, we all know that aspirin is safe, right?" Not so fast. Aspirin, like all drugs, has risks. In the primary prevention meta-analysis, the risk of a hemorrhagic stroke (bleeding into the brain) was increased by 32 percent, although the actual number of events was very small, just 1 in 250 patients per year. In primary prevention patients, the risk of serious bleeding not involving the brain was also increased, by about 50 percent, with an absolute risk of about 1 in 1,000 annually.

We can combine all of these findings into a risk-benefit analysis for aspirin in primary prevention patients. For every 10,000 patients treated for one year, there would be 6 fewer major coronary events and 2 fewer strokes due to blood clots, but at the cost of 1 additional stroke due to bleeding into the brain and 3 other episodes of serious bleeding. Based upon these observations, aspirin is not for everyone; we reserve it for primary prevention patients with the highest risk of a coronary event, such as smokers or certain diabetics who have other risk factors such as high blood pressure.

Let's compare these figures with similar calculations for secondary prevention patients. In patients with preexisting coronary disease, for every 10,000 patients treated for one year, there would be about 100 fewer major coronary events, 46 fewer strokes of all types, and 29 fewer deaths. The number of serious bleeding episodes caused by aspirin in these secondary prevention patients is about 5 patients per 10,000. Obviously, the balance of benefit versus risk tilts strongly in favor of aspirin for patients who have already suffered a cardiovascular event. In fact, the higher the risk, the greater the benefit. For these patients, we do recommend a baby aspirin a day.

Is Aspirin Right for You?

WHEN SHOULD YOU TAKE A BABY ASPIRIN EACH DAY?

History of heart attack, coronary artery stent or angioplasty, or bypass surgery

Coronary artery disease demonstrated on cardiac catheterization

Angina

Blockages in other arteries of the body (femoral or carotid)

History of certain type of stroke (ischemic stroke)

History of transient ischemic attack (TIA, or mini-stroke)

Is aspirin right for you? If you are a primary prevention patient, the answer is usually no. But you should discuss the issue with your doctor before you buy (or throw out) the aspirin bottle. On the other hand, if you are a secondary prevention patient, someone who has already had a coronary event, the reduction in heart attack, stroke, and death dwarfs the slight increase in bleeding with aspirin.

One final note on aspirin: for secondary prevention, aspirin works equally well in women and in men. No matter what your sex, if you have arterial disease in the heart or in other parts of the body, aspirin can be a lifesaver.

CLOPIDOGREL: "SUPER-ASPIRIN"

Because aspirin has proven so useful in heart attack and secondary prevention patients, pharmaceutical companies sought to develop more effective anti-platelet therapies. The most important drug of the newer platelet blockers is clopidogrel (Plavix). Clopidogrel is a kind of super-aspirin that very effectively prevents platelet clumping, particularly when used in combination with aspirin. In 2011, clopidogrel was the second-largest-selling drug in the world, right behind the statin Lipitor (atorvastatin). As with aspirin, the effects of clopidogrel are long-lasting, taking five to seven days to disappear. Because clopidogrel is more effective than aspirin at preventing platelet clumping, clopidogrel is also more likely to cause both minor and major bleeding, so the decision to administer it must be individualized. For patients at low risk of blood clots, the downsides often exceed the benefits.

But for the highest-risk patients, clopidogrel has proven very effective in well-designed randomized controlled trials.

The CURE Trial of heart attack survivors randomized more than 12,000 heart attack patients to aspirin alone, or aspirin and clopidogrel. Administered for three to twelve months after a heart attack, the addition of clopidogrel reduced the combined risk of death, heart attack, and stroke by 20 percent compared with aspirin alone. Not surprisingly, there was also a 38 percent increase in the risk of bleeding, but most bleeding episodes were not life-threatening. Expressed as number needed to treat, for every 10,000 patients treated for up to one year after a heart attack, clopidogrel prevented approximately 200 major cardiovascular events (including forty deaths), while causing about 100 major bleeding episodes, 30 of which were life-threatening. Following publication of these data in 2002, adding clopidogrel to aspirin for twelve months after a heart attack became the standard of care. Clopidogrel has also been shown to benefit patients admitted to the hospital with severe or worsening angina, a disorder known as acute coronary syndrome.

Clopidogrel is also routinely administered to patients after coronary stenting. Stents are small wire mesh devices designed to prop open arteries and keep them open for the long term. Compared with balloon angioplasty, an older procedure that dilated arteries with tiny balloons, stents are more effective at preventing the renarrowing of arteries (restenosis). However, the wire mesh of a stent is a foreign material that activates platelets within the body, which can cause a clot to form within the stent in the days or weeks following the procedure. When a clot forms in a stent (stent thrombosis), the result can be catastrophic, because the clot often obstructs blood flow, leading to a heart attack. The problem of stent thrombosis was so challenging that stents were not feasible prior to the development of drugs such as clopidogrel. Today, dual anti-platelet therapy (aspirin plus clopidogrel) has dramatically reduced, but not eliminated, the problem of stent thrombosis.

Clopidogrel is administered to all patients after stent placement to prevent thrombosis. For patients receiving a bare metal stent, current guidelines suggest treating with clopidogrel for at least three months. Current guidelines recommend twelve months of therapy for patients receiving the newer drug-eluting stents. Because stent thrombosis can occur many months or even years after placement of a drug-eluting stent, some doctors treat these patients for even longer periods. Regardless of type of stent and when the patient stops taking clopidogrel, aspirin should be taken for life following stent placement. A few patients who stop aspirin suffer late stent thrombosis—sometimes years after initial placement. The administration of clopidogrel after stenting is so important that cardiologists are reluctant to place stents in patients not considered reliable enough to take clopidogrel as prescribed.

When and How Long to Take Clopidogrel	
CONDITION	DURATION OF THERAPY
Heart attack	12 months
Unstable angina requiring hospital admission	12 months
Coronary stent—bare metal	3 months
Coronary stent—drug-eluting	12 months

Before clopidogrel can block platelets, it must be chemically changed by the liver. We now recognize that many people are poor metabolizers of the drug—that is, they obtain less anti-platelet effect from clopidogrel because their livers don't readily convert the drug into its active form. Although a genetic test can determine if a patient is a poor metabolizer, it is not yet clear if this test can help us take better care of our patients. For now, we use the genetic test only in patients who have suffered stent thrombosis while taking clopidogrel. To circumvent the problem of poor drug metabolism, a newer drug with a similar mechanism of action has been approved (prasugrel or Effient), but it is controversial because it appears to have a higher incidence of bleeding than clopidogrel. A third drug, ticagrelor (Brilinta), was approved in 2011 and has a distinct advantage—it is short-acting, which makes it desirable for patients who may need to stop therapy for surgery or bleeding.

As with aspirin, the major complication of clopidogrel is bleeding. The drug exerts a much more powerful effect on platelets than does aspirin, so it is not surprising that clopidogrel also has a greater tendency to provoke bleeding. Bruising of the skin is a common complaint among patients taking clopidogrel, but more serious bleeding can occur. About 3 percent of patients experience moderate or severe bleeding on clopidogrel.

If you take clopidogrel and you need surgery, you and your doctors

DIRECT-TO-CONSUMER ADVERTISING

Nearly every American who watches television—from ESPN to the Food Channel—knows something about Plavix (clopidogrel). The reason for this is direct-to-consumer advertising. Only two countries in the world, the United States and New Zealand, permit direct-to-consumer advertising of medicines. This form of drug advertising was first allowed in 1997, and pharmaceutical companies soon learned that it could increase sales dramatically. Today, this is a multibillion-dollar industry, with advertisements for medicines featured in newspapers, magazines, television spots, and annoying Internet pop-ups. Of course, promotions focus on expensive brand-name drugs, steering consumers away from high-quality, low-cost generics. Many advertisements use deceptive practices, employing sounds and video images to divert consumers' attention when side effects are mentioned.

So-called disease awareness advertisements represent a particularly insidious type of direct-to-consumer advertising. These promotional campaigns feature actors describing a relatively common series of symptoms and are designed to convince patients that they have a particular disorder such as "restless leg syndrome." Patients are urged to "discuss your symptoms with your doctor"; if they do, they frequently leave the office with a new prescription to treat a condition that they may not even have. Critics have called this type of advertisement "disease mongering."

Our advice? Keep the remote control close at hand and mute the television during drug advertisements. Don't rely on television actors to guide your medical decisions.

need to craft a plan to ensure your safety. For elective surgery, we stop the clopidogrel five days before the operation. Emergency surgery represents a major problem because discontinuation of clopidogrel in a patient with a stent might result in acute stent thrombosis, but proceeding with surgery might cause serious hemorrhage during the operation. Each case must be decided individually through collaboration between the cardiologist, the surgeon, and you.

The cost of clopidogrel is substantial, averaging more than $3 a day, but this will soon change. The Plavix patent expired in 2012, and the prices of brand-name pharmaceuticals usually fall by 80 percent or more during the first two years the drugs are available as generics.

Several newer clopidogrel-like agents will also be approved within the next few years, but they will be costly and must first demonstrate superiority to clopidogrel to succeed in the marketplace. It therefore seems likely that clopidogrel is destined for a role as one of the mainstays of cardiovascular drug treatment for many years to come.

CLOPIDOGREL AND ANTI-ULCER MEDICINES: A SAFE COMBINATION?

With every medicine, we must worry about side effects and interactions with other drugs. These two issues raised their heads simultaneously in the case of clopidogrel, which can cause bleeding from the stomach, and the proton-pump inhibitors, a class of drugs that prevents stomach ulcers.

Clopidogrel is a powerful anti-platelet agent, and it causes bleeding from the gastrointestinal tract in 2 to 4 percent of people. Therefore, doctors thought it would be reasonable to prescribe clopidogrel with a medicine that protects the stomach from this bleeding. Most doctors chose to use proton-pump inhibitors (esomeprazole, omeprazole, lansoprazole, and others) for this purpose. But then reports surfaced suggesting that these medicines reduced the effectiveness of clopidogrel, leaving people at increased risk of heart attack. The FDA responded to these reports by urging doctors to avoid combining proton-pump inhibitors and clopidogrel.

Many doctors questioned the FDA's pronouncement. Fortunately, in October 2010, we got the evidence that we needed to address this concern. In a large randomized controlled study, proton-pump inhibitors reduced the risk of bleeding associated with clopidogrel without reducing its cardiac benefit. The answer on this one is in: if a patient requires clopidogrel and has a history of ulcers or gastrointestinal bleeding, it is safe to add the protection of a proton-pump inhibitor.

WARFARIN AND OTHER ANTICOAGULANTS: FROM RAT POISON TO LIFESAVING DRUG

The development of one of the world's most important blood thinners began with a veterinary mystery. In 1920, American and Canadian farmers noticed a strange new disease in their cattle. Afflicted animals bled easily, and many died after minor surgical procedures. Canadian veterinarians, in a brilliant series of observations, demonstrated that cattle with the bleeding tendency had ingested sweet clover, which contained a naturally occurring anticoagulant. Scientists at the University of Wisconsin isolated and purified warfarin, the active ingredient in sweet clover that caused the bleeding, and then they found the perfect use for it—they marketed it as rat poison. Rats that ingested bait laced with warfarin bled to death. As rat poison, the drug achieved instant popularity.

In 1954, warfarin was introduced into human medicine, marketed under the brand name Coumadin as an anticoagulant to treat and prevent blood clots. The drug received considerable public attention when it was administered to President Dwight Eisenhower after his heart attack in 1955. Over the next five decades, warfarin became a unique and indispensable drug for heart patients.

Warfarin's effects as an anticoagulant are produced by its ability to block vitamin K, an essential factor used by the liver to produce proteins that cause blood to clot. Unlike aspirin and clopidogrel, warfarin's actions do not involve blood platelets. Warfarin is a far more potent anti-clotting agent than aspirin or clopidogrel.

Warfarin is widely used to prevent formation of clots in patients with atrial fibrillation. These patients have a striking elevation in the risk of stroke, caused by formation of blood clots in the atrium (upper chamber of the heart); when a piece of a clot breaks loose, it can travel through the bloodstream to the brain, where it blocks an artery and causes a stroke. By preventing clot formation in the atrium, warfarin reduces the likelihood of stroke by more than 50 percent in patients with atrial fibrillation.

Other patients treated with warfarin include those with mechanical (metal and plastic) artificial heart valves and those who have formed blood clots in veins of the legs. In a patient with a mechanical heart valve, life-long warfarin use is required to prevent clots from forming on the valve and causing a devastating stroke or valve malfunction. In patients who develop clots in the legs (deep venous thrombosis), warfarin is used to help dissolve the clots, which can break free and cause a potentially fatal pulmonary embolus (blood clot in the lungs). Tennis star Serena Williams recently survived such a blood clot and required several months of warfarin therapy to prevent a recurrence.

Although an essential drug in modern medicine, warfarin is extremely challenging to use safely; it interacts with dozens of other medicines that either increase or decrease its anticoagulant effects. If you take warfarin, you must tell your doctor every medicine that you take, including all over-the-counter medicines and supplements. In addition, because warfarin acts on vitamin K, which is found in green leafy vegetables, your diet greatly influences the action of warfarin. This is not a problem for patients who maintain a steady diet with a stable mixture of foods that contain vitamin K, but abrupt changes in diet can result in too little or too much blood-thinning effect.

We obtain frequent blood tests to monitor the effects of warfarin. Some patients are "brittle," meaning that their dosage requirements are so unstable that they need weekly blood tests to monitor the anticoagulant effect. If too little warfarin is administered, a dangerous clot may develop. If too much is administered, serious bleeding may be provoked. In some cases, patients can do this sort of testing at home, much as diabetics check their blood sugar. Ask your doctor if home monitoring of warfarin is an option for you. In order to make initial dosing easier, scientists have developed a genetic test that is recommended by the FDA to improve estimates of the starting dose. However, many doctors consider it impractical. Currently we do not recommend routine use of this test.

Finally, fifty-five years after the introduction of warfarin, a new anticoagulant received FDA approval in 2010. The drug, dabigatran (Pradaxa), works via a different mechanism from warfarin and produces a more reliable anticoagulant effect using a single approved dosage. Dabigatran must be given twice per day but requires no blood tests to monitor its anticoagulant effect.

A large randomized controlled trial showed that dabigatran was at least as effective as warfarin at preventing stroke, with similar bleeding risks. Unfortunately, the developers of this drug have set a very high price for it, about $7 per day. Other chemical cousins of dabigatran are nearing FDA approval, so competition may drive down costs. If you are doing well on warfarin and don't require frequent testing, we advise you to stay on your current warfarin regimen. If, however, you are struggling with finding a stable dosage, dabigatran may be worth discussing with your physician.

BETA-BLOCKERS: OLD BUT GOOD

As you learned in Chapter 8, our bodies are genetically programmed to respond to stressful situations by producing a surge of adrenaline. Physicians have long recognized that this fight-or-flight response is not always beneficial, particularly for patients with heart disease. Accordingly, pharmaceutical companies sought to create drugs that would block the effects of adrenaline in the body, and they finally succeeded in the early 1960s

BRANDS VERSUS GENERICS: WHICH IS BETTER?

Patients frequently ask whether we recommend generic or brand-name drugs. Current federal law and FDA regulations require bioequivalence testing of generics—generic drugs must produce blood levels between 80 percent and 125 percent of the original brand-name product. Despite this requirement, generics do present potential problems.

Patients often complain that generics seem less effective than their branded equivalents. In addition, some well-documented quality problems have occurred with generic drugs. Critics point out that many generics are now produced overseas, sometimes in third-world countries where FDA oversight is problematic. On the other hand, generics are often priced at a tiny fraction of brand-name drugs, and many insurance companies require higher co-payments for branded products.

So when is a generic acceptable? For most commonly used drugs, a slight difference in blood levels is unlikely to impair effect; therefore, generics are fine. On the other hand, with certain critical drugs that have a narrow margin for safety, brand-name products are preferred. Examples in this category include digoxin (Lanoxin) and warfarin (Coumadin). But for the most part, don't be scared of generics.

---

with the development of propranolol (Inderal); the pioneer in this research, Scottish scientist Sir James W. Black, won the Nobel Prize in Medicine in 1988 for this extraordinary work. Since then, nearly twenty beta-blockers have been introduced, although only a few are commonly used today. Beta-blockers are indispensable in the treatment of four common cardiac conditions: angina, heart attack, congestive heart failure (CHF), and abnormal heart rhythms.

For angina, the mechanism of action is easy to understand. When you exercise, your heart rate increases, and the heart contracts more vigorously to pump more blood to the muscles. This increase in heart rate and force of contraction is no problem for healthy individuals. But in the presence of blockages in the coronary arteries, the increased demand on the heart exceeds the ability of the narrowed coronaries to respond. Angina occurs when the heart muscle does not receive enough coronary blood flow to meet its demands. By blocking the increase in heart rate and contraction, beta-blockers allow patients to exercise without developing chest pain.

When the heart muscle is damaged by a heart attack, it becomes particularly sensitive to the effects of adrenaline. In 1983, a Swedish random-ized controlled study demonstrated for the first time that treating patients for three months with a beta-blocker immediately after a heart attack re-duced mortality by an astonishing 36 percent. Furthermore, the incidence of a second heart attack during that period was also reduced by about one-third. Today, the use of beta-blockers after a heart attack is considered so important that federal authorities use the percentage of patients receiving a beta-blocker after a heart attack as a measure of hospital quality.

The use of beta-blockers in the treatment of heart failure has an ex-traordinary history. When beta-blockers were first introduced, physicians recognized the potential hazards of administering these drugs to patients with a weakened heart muscle and congestive heart failure. After all, if the heart has been weakened, then reducing heart rate and force of contraction would be expected to worsen CHF and might even be lethal. Early experience confirmed that some patients developed acute heart failure after starting a beta-blocker. The original product inserts for beta-blockers warned that these drugs could precipitate heart failure, and phy-sicians were cautioned against administering these drugs to patients with known CHF.

Despite the warnings, courageous physicians, once again in Scandi-navia, proposed that beta-blockers might actually help CHF rather than worsen it. Meta-analyses suggested that they were correct, but many Amer-ican physicians were still extremely skeptical. Then in 1999, a randomized controlled trial led by Swedish physicians showed that a long-acting version of metoprolol (Toprol XL) reduced mortality by an amazing 34 percent in patients with moderate to severe congestive heart failure. Hospitalization was also reduced. The study was stopped early because the benefit was so striking that it was deemed unethical to continue the trial. Patients treated with beta-blockers felt better (had fewer heart failure symptoms) by the end of this one-year study. Although several beta-blockers have been shown to produce similar benefits, carvedilol (Coreg) eventually became the most common agent used in heart failure patients. Generic carvedilol is inexpensive and has a long enough half-life to permit twice-daily admin-istration.

How do beta-blockers improve patient outcomes in heart failure? The most accepted explanation is that patients with CHF have excess adrena-line in their bloodstream. This is the body's response to a failing heart, an attempt to compensate for CHF by stimulating more vigorous contraction of the heart muscle. Unfortunately, this stimulation is not entirely beneficial. Muscle cells in the heart are overstimulated and gradually die, resulting in slow deterioration of the heart muscle, eventually leading to death of the patient. By blocking the overstimulation by adrenaline, beta-blockers prevent loss of muscle cells, and the heart gradually strengthens.

Beta-blockers are also widely used to treat certain heart rhythm disturbances, particularly atrial fibrillation. In this disorder, the upper chambers of the heart beat wildly, sending too many electrical impulses to the ventricles, the main pumping chambers. This results in a rapid and irregular heart rate, which is uncomfortable and compromises normal heart function. Beta-blockers prevent an excessive number of electrical impulses from getting through to the ventricles, thereby slowing the heart and allowing it to function more normally. Usually physicians try to reduce the resting heart rate in atrial fibrillation patients to eighty beats per minute or less.

Occasionally beta-blockers are used to prevent other heart rhythm disorders, including the most serious rhythm problems, ventricular tachycardia and ventricular fibrillation, both of which are life-threatening. Beta-blockers are also administered to patients who have had a dissecting aneurysm, a tearing of the aorta that can compromise blood flow to various organs or lead to death. By reducing the contractile force of the heart, beta-blockers stop the tearing and allow the aorta to heal.

Although originally introduced as anti-hypertensive agents, beta-blockers are now considered passé for treating high blood pressure—they offer less protection against the complications of hypertension, such as stroke, than do other anti-hypertensive drugs. However, physicians are often slow to change old habits, so beta-blockers are still widely used for treatment of hypertension. In the absence of congestive heart failure, angina, or recent heart attack, we do not recommend beta-blockers as first-line agents for hypertension. We particularly avoid the drug atenolol (Tenormin) for hypertension because studies suggest that it offers little protection from the complications of high blood pressure.

Giving beta-blockers in a fixed dosage to all patients is one of the more common mistakes made by practicing physicians. Beta-blocker dose must be adjusted to achieve the desired response, usually by monitoring the heart rate. In addition, some beta-blockers are cleared from the circulation by the kidneys or liver, and therefore must be used cautiously in patients with kidney or liver problems.

Like all medicines, beta-blockers can cause complications. They can lower heart rate excessively, resulting in dizziness or low blood pressure. By blocking adrenaline, beta-blockers often cause a generalized sense of

BETA-BLOCKERS AND THE FEAR OF PUBLIC SPEAKING

Beta-blockers have important, and often lifesaving, cardiovascular effects. But many people use beta-blockers for an entirely different reason—to manage their fear of public speaking. Because they block the fight-or-flight response, beta-blockers can prevent the pounding heart, sweaty palms, tremor, and general panic that can accompany public speaking. But remember, all medicines have side effects. Beta-blockers lower heart rate and blood pressure, and this can cause a fainting spell in a person who already has a slow heart rate or a low blood pressure. In addition, in asthmatics, beta-blockers can precipitate an asthma attack; many inhalers used by asthmatics to relieve wheezing are actually beta-agonists, the opposite of beta-blockers. Because beta-blockers are powerful medicines with potential side effects, we generally do not recommend using them for managing performance anxiety. But if you are at wits' end and feel that you must try beta-blockers for this purpose, follow this checklist:

- Check with your doctor.
- Use the lowest available dose.
- Do a dry run at home (you don't want to give a speech that is memorable only because you fainted in the middle).

fatigue or listlessness, dubbed the "beta-blocker blahs." Some beta-blockers cross into the brain, resulting in nightmares and, occasionally, depression. Constriction of the airways in the lung may cause wheezing in susceptible patients, although inappropriate fear of this adverse effect prevents some physicians from using beta-blockers in patients who might benefit. However, some patients with asthma or other chronic lung diseases simply cannot take beta-blockers. Although beta-blockers are used chronically to treat congestive heart failure (CHF), these drugs can precipitate acute heart failure, particularly when therapy is first initiated. Men may experience erectile dysfunction, but this improves rapidly if the drugs are withdrawn. Finally, some beta-blockers may slightly worsen glucose control in diabetics.

ACE INHIBITORS: HELPING THE HEART TO PUMP

Sometimes medicines come from the most unlikely places. Case in point: angiotensin-converting enzyme (ACE) inhibitors, which were originally developed from snake venom produced by pit viper species found in South America. Today ACE inhibitors represent one of the most important classes of medicines for heart patients. There are many drugs in this group, including lisinopril (Prinivil), captopril (Capoten), enalapril (Vasotec), and several others with virtually identical effects.

Introduced in the 1980s, most ACE inhibitors are now available as generics, often for pennies a day. ACE inhibitors prevent the body from producing a hormone called angiotensin, which causes arteries to constrict. Because ACE inhibitors allow arteries to relax, they lower blood pressure. Not surprisingly, ACE inhibitors were initially offered as blood-pressure-lowering drugs and are still widely used for this purpose.

Soon after these drugs were introduced, cardiologists learned that they could be used for several other heart problems. Congestive heart failure (CHF), a serious heart condition in which the heart's pumping ability is reduced, often occurs due to damage from a heart attack. Randomized clinical trials showed that patients with CHF lived longer when given long-term treatment with ACE inhibitors. ACE inhibitors also improved patients' symptoms, such as shortness of breath and fatigue, reducing the need for hospital admission.

For patients who have had a recent heart attack causing reduced heart function, ACE inhibitors actually prevent deterioration in heart function and the subsequent development of congestive heart failure. Like beta-blockers, administration of ACE inhibitors to patients with CHF or a recent large heart attack is so important that federal authorities grade the quality of hospitals based upon the percentage receiving an ACE inhibitor at the time of discharge.

In addition to improving outcomes in patients with CHF, ACE inhibitors are still widely used as anti-hypertensive agents. These drugs produce a moderate reduction in blood pressure when used alone, but a more striking reduction when combined with a low dosage of a diuretic. This combination is so effective in treating hypertension that many manufacturers make combination products that include both classes of drugs. One of the most common is known generically as lisinopril-HCT, a combination of the ACE inhibitor lisinopril and the diuretic hydrochlorothiazide. The syn-

MEDICINES AFTER A HEART ATTACK

If you have survived a heart attack, you have one overriding health goal: prevention of a second heart attack. Each time you have a heart attack, heart muscle dies. If you lose enough heart muscle, your heart cannot beat effectively, and you develop congestive heart failure. We have a wide variety of therapies to prevent heart attacks, including lifestyle and dietary changes, exercise, quitting smoking, stenting, bypass surgery, and, of course, medicines. We know which medicines improve prognosis after a heart attack. But, surprisingly, not all people get the right prescriptions. If you or a family member is leaving the hospital after a heart attack, check your medicines against this list:

- Aspirin
- Clopidogrel
- Beta-blocker
- Statin
- ACE inhibitor

After a heart attack, you should almost always be on at least three of these medicines. Make sure that you get the right medicines so that you can avoid a return trip to the coronary care unit.

ergy between ACE inhibitors and thiazide diuretics is particularly useful in treating hypertension.

Although these drugs have been used safely in millions of patients, ACE inhibitors can occasionally produce serious adverse effects. Reduced kidney function is the most common concern with ACE inhibitors, but this problem is almost always reversible if the drug is discontinued. The patients most vulnerable to kidney problems are individuals who already have impaired kidney function prior to starting therapy. Importantly, when ACE inhibitors are given long-term to patients who already have reduced kidney function, the rate of decline in kidney function actually slows. For that reason, thoughtful physicians use ACE inhibitors to treat patients with kidney disease, gradually adjusting the dosage while closely monitoring kidney function.

A second kidney-related issue is an increase in blood potassium levels; this is more common among those with preexisting kidney problems, emphasizing the need to monitor routine blood tests when starting an ACE inhibitor. Patients taking ACE inhibitors should usually not take potassium supplements.

A rare, but very serious, adverse reaction to ACE inhibitors is known as angioedema. This disorder is characterized by swelling of the lips or tongue, sometimes followed by obstruction of the airway; it can be fatal. Angioedema usually occurs during the first week of treatment with an ACE inhibitor. Fortunately, most cases run their course without treatment as long as the drug is promptly stopped, but patients with this condition should always seek medical attention. If you have had such a reaction in the past, you should wear a bracelet alerting physicians to your history with ACE inhibitors.

As we previously mentioned, cough is a common, although reversible, side effect of ACE inhibitors. It is not a serious reaction, but it is often so bothersome that patients request withdrawal of the drug. For unknown reasons, Asian patients have a higher incidence of ACE-inhibitor-induced cough. Dizziness when suddenly standing, also known as postural hypotension, can occur with any anti-hypertensive agent, including ACE inhibitors.

ANGIOTENSIN RECEPTOR BLOCKERS: NEW AND IMPROVED?

Recognizing limitations of ACE inhibitors, drug companies sought to develop new drugs with similar benefits but fewer side effects. This led to the angiotensin receptor blockers, or ARBs. Like ACE inhibitors, these medicines lower blood pressure and improve symptoms in heart failure patients.

Although ARBs are more expensive than ACE inhibitors, they are not superior. In clinical trials, both ACE inhibitors and ARBs confer substantial benefits to heart patients. With the exception of cough, the side effects of ARBs are similar to those of ACE inhibitors. Nevertheless, because of aggressive promotion by the manufacturers, ARBs have become the world's best-selling drugs for high blood pressure. Don't misunderstand—they are good medicines. But if an ACE inhibitor works for you and does not cause an irritating cough, it makes no sense to take an expensive ARB as a substitute.

MEDICINES FOR THE HEART

If you have coronary heart disease or risk factors for its development, odds are that you take at least one of the medicines discussed in this chapter. Collectively, these drugs have prevented millions of heart attacks and have saved countless lives. So taking heart medicines is not an admission of defeat on your part. But failing to understand your medicines—why you need them, their side effects, and their potential risks—puts you at risk. Keep your list of cardiac medicines in your wallet or purse at all times. Do you know what each medicine does? If not, make sure that you get an answer at your next doctor's appointment.

RX: MEDICINES FOR YOUR HEART

Keep a list of all your medicines, including over-the-counter medicines and supplements

Every time you receive a new prescription, ask:
   What does the medicine do?
   What are the common side effects?
   Does it interact with any medicines that I already take?

Save your money: ask about generics

If you have coronary heart disease, go over your medicines with your doctor. You should be on at least two of these medicines:
   A statin or cholesterol-lowering medicine
   Aspirin
   Clopidogrel
   A beta-blocker
   An ACE inhibitor

STENTS VERSUS SURGERY FOR CORONARY HEART DISEASE: TO A MAN WITH A HAMMER, EVERYTHING LOOKS LIKE A NAIL

THE BIG PICTURE

Your doctor has given you the news, and it is not what you wanted to hear. You have coronary artery disease (also called coronary heart disease). You have joined the ranks of the 16 million Americans with plaque buildup in the heart's arteries, limiting blood flow to the heart muscle. You are at risk for a heart attack. The questions start immediately: "What should I do now? What do I do if I think I am having a heart attack?"

For the person with coronary heart disease, knowing the right answers is lifesaving. Most patients simply accept the procedures and medicines their doctors recommend. We want you to trust your doctor, but we subscribe to Ronald Reagan's motto: "Trust but verify." Your therapy should be tailor-made for you, addressing your unique medical history. But in many cases, your choices are determined by where you live, the capabilities of the hospital you go to, or the type of doctor you see. We will give you the information that you need to ensure that your treatment is based upon your medical condition, not geography or your doctor's particular training and favorite procedure.

You can't get this information on your own. If you search the Internet for the term "coronary heart disease," you will find 17.3 million websites filled with confusing, contradictory and often incorrect information. You will encounter recommendations ranging from chelation therapy (worthless) to immediate stenting and angioplasty (usually not the first step for people with stable coronary artery disease). We will help you sift through this overload of contradictory information and help you find the answers that are right for you.

Understanding the treatment options for coronary artery disease is actually pretty straightforward. No disease in cardiology and cardiac surgery has been studied as intensively. The three broad treatments for coronary heart disease are medical therapy, stenting with balloon angioplasty, and bypass surgery. The key is to match the therapy to the patient to maximize benefit and minimize risk.

The first thing to understand is that medical therapy is the correct choice for *everybody* with coronary heart disease, even if you also receive a stent or have bypass surgery. Every person with coronary heart disease must follow a heart-healthy lifestyle—diet, exercise, no smoking, and so on—and must take certain medicines, usually starting with aspirin and a statin.

Medical therapy is not controversial, but it is frequently overlooked as people seize upon more immediate interventions to treat the blockages in coronary arteries. The direct approaches to the heart's arteries include stenting and balloon angioplasty, which clean out the insides of arteries, and bypass surgery, which lays down new blood vessels to reroute blood around blocked arteries. Because stenting and bypass surgery directly improve blood flow, they are grouped together under the label "revascularization." While the concept of fixing the heart's plumbing is appealing, these procedures are not appropriate for all patients with coronary heart disease. Like all medical procedures, they are invasive, exposing you to some risk.

So before you grant a cardiologist or cardiac surgeon free rein to work on your heart's arteries, you need a clear understanding of your options. The choice and timing of intervention are critically important. We will arm you with the information you need to make the right decisions, so that you don't wind up with the problems, headaches, and heartache experienced by our patient Jim Sutton.

JIM SUTTON AND THE FULL METAL JACKET

In the consultation room to discuss Jim Sutton's upcoming bypass surgery, we pulled up the images from his most recent cardiac catheterization on our computer, prepared to review the study with Jim and his wife, Susan. After the first few frames we could see that Jim's arteries were a surgeon's nightmare. Metallic stents outlined each of the three main arteries on Jim's heart, where they had been placed to treat blockages. With an internal lining of stainless steel stents, Jim's coronary arteries had what we call "a full metal jacket."

Jim's steel-lined arteries represented nearly a decade of work by his interventional cardiologist. Now sixty-seven years old, Jim first encountered his cardiologist when he was fifty-eight. At that time, Jim was a hardworking, successful senior executive at a telecom company—and a medical disaster in the making. Like the other high achievers at his firm, Jim took care of his job but paid little attention to his health. At five feet ten inches and 235 pounds, he was an overweight smoker who rarely exercised. Jim could not remember when he had his last checkup and did not know the key numbers that every adult should know—his blood pressure and blood cholesterol values.

Jim's visit to the cardiologist nine years earlier was spurred by chest tightness during his short morning walk from his parking spot to the office elevators. Although the chest tightness went away when Jim stopped walking, he recognized that he had classic angina, chest pain associated with exertion and relieved by rest.

That afternoon, Jim reluctantly canceled an important sales meeting and went to see his internist, who diagnosed coronary heart disease and referred Jim to a cardiologist in the same building. The cardiologist explained that Jim's pain was probably the result of one or more blockages in arteries of his heart. When Jim walked or exercised, his heart worked harder but did not get enough blood flow; this imbalance between blood supply and demand caused his chest pain.

Jim's course of treatment was determined by the cardiologist to whom he was referred. A well-known quotation from Mark Twain explains the medical procedures that Jim endured over the next nine years: "To a man with a hammer, everything looks like a nail." Jim's cardiologist was an interventional cardiologist, the type who specializes in procedures such as angioplasty and stenting to open blocked arteries. His hammer was the coronary artery stent.

The cardiologist immediately recommended a cardiac catheterization, also called a coronary angiogram, in which he would inject dye into the arteries of the heart and take X-ray pictures, enabling him to check for blockages. At the end of the consultation, after Jim and his wife agreed to the catheterization, the doctor said that he could probably use stents to fix any blockages that he found right then and there. That sounded pretty good to Jim and Susan.

The next day, barely twenty-four hours after his first bout of chest pain, Jim had his first cardiac catheterization. Lying on his back and feeling relaxed—almost happy, actually—as a result of the cocktail of sedatives that he received, Jim heard his doctor say that he had identified two blocked arteries and that he would prop them open with stents, relieving Jim's chest pain and preventing him from having a heart attack down the road. That sounded like a pretty good plan—one-stop shopping with diagnosis and treatment in a single sixty-minute session.

After a few hours' recovery, Jim left the hospital with two new metal stents in his coronary arteries and a prescription for Plavix to add to his Lipitor, aspirin, and beta-blocker. He felt like he had been given a new beginning on the journey to heart health. But Jim would soon learn that this new beginning did not lead down the road he expected.

Three months later, Jim noticed a return of that same chest tightness while walking his Chihuahua. He saw the cardiologist and learned that 20 to 30 percent of people with bare metal stents develop recurrent chest pain. The pain results from a condition called "in-stent restenosis," in which the stent becomes partially blocked by overgrowth of scar tissue. The good news was that the cardiologist could "fix" this problem with another catheterization and more stents. Later that week, Jim received three more stents.

Two years later, Jim had chest pain again. This time, the catheterization showed involvement of the heart's third artery, in addition to new plaque buildup in the two arteries that had already been treated. Four drug-eluting stents later, Jim was a new man—again. But the pattern continued. Over the next seven years, Jim had four more catheterizations and six more stents. By the time Jim consulted us, he had had fifteen stents and seven catheterizations.

Meanwhile, Jim was not doing too well on other fronts. Over the nine-year course, Jim remained overweight, exercised only occasionally, and, believe it or not, still smoked (although he had cut back from two packs to ten cigarettes per day). When his cardiologist finally conceded that a different sort of heart plumbing was needed, he referred Jim to us for bypass surgery. The angiogram we reviewed with Jim and Susan showed stents throughout his heart's arteries, and blockages both within the stents and in the remaining segments of unstented arteries.

Susan told us that Jim was crippled by his angina. He could barely make it up one flight of stairs before chest pain forced him to stop and rest. He could no longer play golf, and his beloved but unused golf clubs were a constant, painful reminder of his heart problem. He wanted us to "fix" his heart with bypass surgery.

We explained that we could do four bypasses, rerouting blood flow around the blockages by placing arteries and veins from other parts of his body on his heart. Although we anticipated successful surgery, Jim's collection of coronary artery stents would complicate the operation because we could not sew his bypasses into the regions of his arteries that were filled with stents. In addition, we told him, we could not "fix" his coronary heart disease. No treatment cures coronary heart disease. We emphasized that medical therapy is the cornerstone of treatment. Jim responded, "I already do medical therapy. I fill my prescriptions and take my pills religiously." Susan nodded in agreement. We told him that taking the medicines is good, but that a complete medical approach must include key lifestyle changes that Jim had not undertaken.

Jim's situation was not entirely of his own making. He had been talked into having stents when comprehensive medical therapy alone might have relieved his angina and prevented him from ever needing stents or surgery. Jim also had some bad luck, experiencing repeated bouts of stent failure as a result of in-stent restenosis. He was referred for surgery at a late stage, when bypass surgery is technically difficult because of the presence of so many stents. But if Jim had understood his disease and his options at the outset instead of being rushed to the cardiac cath lab for stents, he might not have spent nine years of his life on his cardiologist's "frequent flier" list.

The good news we shared with Jim is that it's never too late to correct course. We explained his condition and the steps that Jim could take to improve his prognosis. Two weeks later we did his bypass surgery, using mostly arteries (rather than veins) to bring additional blood flow to his heart. After surgery, we referred him to cardiac rehabilitation, where he quit smoking completely and started exercising.

Today, Jim looks good. Although he sports a scar on his chest courtesy of his heart surgeon, he is down to 180 pounds. He eats sensibly and exercises for forty-five minutes each day. He is even thinking about training for a 5K road race. And at work he takes the stairs instead of the elevator.

CORONARY HEART DISEASE:
THE FACTS ABOUT THE TREATMENTS

There are three basic treatments for coronary heart disease: medical therapy, balloon angioplasty with stenting, and bypass surgery. During his nine-year odyssey through the worlds of cardiology and cardiac surgery, Jim Sutton had all of them. Sometimes this combination of approaches is necessary. Former president Bill Clinton has also experienced each of the three therapies, although his order was different (bypass surgery, then medical therapy, and, most recently, stenting). The key to success is starting with a clear and sensible strategy tailored to the particular patient. In many cases, getting the right treatment at the outset minimizes the need for subsequent invasive treatments.

Medical Therapy

At this point, we do not have a cure for coronary heart disease. It would be ideal if we had a medicine that worked like Drano or Liquid-Plumr—one pill and the plaques would magically dissolve, leaving your arteries unobstructed. If and when we discover such a medicine, it will be the most important advance in heart care since the development of statins.

One of the key challenges is that coronary heart disease is a systemic problem—it extends well beyond the obstructing plaque in an artery. Coronary heart disease is a form of atherosclerosis, a diffuse process that can affect all of the arteries on the heart and other arteries throughout the body, including those that bring blood to the brain, kidneys, and legs. Local therapies like stenting and bypass surgery address only segments of individual arteries; contrary to public perception, they do not "fix" the system-wide problem. By contrast, medical therapy *does* have the ability to influence all of the body's arteries.

People with coronary heart disease need to take several medicines. We realize that it is a hassle to refill your medicine cupboard every month, but the medicines are not optional, and they are not interchangeable. Aspirin limits blood clotting, reducing the chance of a heart attack. Statins prevent progression of coronary heart disease and may even cause some plaque regression. Beta-blockers, nitrates (nitroglycerin), and calcium channel blockers improve blood flow and reduce the heart's work, decreasing chest pain. Additional medicines are often necessary to treat high blood pressure and diabetes, conditions frequently present in people with coronary artery disease.

As in Jim's case, medical therapy requires more than a regular trip to the pharmacy. A lifestyle that includes exercise, a sensible diet, weight control, and smoking cessation is as important as any prescription from your doctor. We actually write these instructions down on a prescription form and hand the slip to patients. Taking your medicine—both the pills from the pharmacy and the lifestyle instructions—is the foundation of treatment for coronary artery disease.

Bypass Surgery

In many people, medicines are combined with direct plumbing work on the heart's obstructed arteries. Coronary artery bypass graft (CABG) surgery was the first successful direct interventional treatment for coronary artery disease. Developed in 1968, the idea was simple: if an artery on the heart is like a pipe that is blocked, lay some new pipe that gives blood an alternative route around the blockage. There are a variety of veins and arteries in other parts of the body that can be transplanted to the heart to carry blood.

Studies from the 1970s and 1980s showed that bypass surgery worked. Although it required use of the heart-lung machine, bypass surgery relieved chest pain and extended life in people with the most advanced forms of coronary heart disease, especially those with heart damage from heart attacks and diabetes. It quickly became the most common procedure performed in people with coronary heart disease, peaking at nearly 500,000 operations per year in the United States.

Bypass surgery is highly invasive: it usually requires a median sternotomy incision, which goes straight down the middle of the chest through the breast bone. It generally takes about six weeks for this bone to heal completely. The odds are that you know several people who have had this sort of operation. If you flip through the television channels and happen to catch a glimpse of David Letterman, Bill Clinton, or Regis Philbin, you are looking at living proof that bypass surgery is safe and effective.

While the incision and the six-week healing period concern some patients, others worry more about the heart-lung machine. Using the heart-lung machine, surgeons can stop the heart and lungs for up to four or five hours, and people nearly always make an uneventful recovery. Some surgeons do perform bypass surgery on the beating heart ("off-pump"), though this is quite challenging. Read more about surgical techniques on page 506.

If you are going to have bypass surgery, ask your surgeon whether he or she will be using the heart-lung machine. If the surgeon says that the operation will be performed off-pump, ask how many such operations he or she has performed. Because this technique requires special skill, you want to ensure that you have an experienced surgeon.

DOES THE HEART-LUNG MACHINE MAKE YOU DUMB?

A 2000 *New England Journal of Medicine* paper from Duke University suggested that patients suffer cognitive decline as a result of the heart-lung machine. In that study, 261 patients had neurologic and cognitive testing before and after bypass surgery. Shortly after surgery, 53 percent of patients showed some loss of mental function; five years after surgery, this figure was 42 percent. The authors concluded that open heart surgery damages the brain. Patients became scared of developing a condition that some called "pump head."

The problem with the Duke study was that there was no control group—a group of similar patients who did not have bypass surgery but who underwent assessments of memory and other mental functions over time. Johns Hopkins researchers corrected this mistake, measuring mental function in 244 patients with coronary artery disease. Their study included some patients who had bypass surgery, some who had stenting with angioplasty, and some who had medical therapy alone. Over a six-year period, there was similar cognitive decline in each group, no matter what the heart therapy. Their conclusion was that older people with coronary heart disease also have atherosclerosis affecting the arteries in the brain. Progression of disease in the brain is the real cause of changes in mental function over time.

However, it is true that heart surgery has short-term cognitive effects. After hospitalization for any major surgery, people are often confused and a bit slow. This relates to administration of pain medicines, disruption of sleep-wake cycles, and general fatigue. These symptoms usually disappear within a couple of weeks. So don't be afraid that an operation on your heart will hurt your brain. In most people, treatment of the heart does not cause cognitive decline. The next time you can't find your keys, don't blame your cardiologist or heart surgeon.

The choice of arteries or veins for the bypasses is more important than whether or not the heart-lung machine is used. Arteries are better than veins, so every bypass operation should include use of at least one artery (preferably one or both of the internal mammary arteries) as a new "pipe" (see page 320). Therefore, in your preoperative consultation, make sure that your doctor plans on doing at least one bypass with an artery.

Today, bypass surgery remains the most frequent cardiac surgical procedure, relieving chest pain and prolonging life in nearly 250,000 Americans per year. However, it is the number two interventional therapy for coronary artery disease. Stenting and balloon angioplasty have surpassed bypass surgery and are now used in more than 1 million Americans per year.

Stenting and Angioplasty

Swiss cardiologist Andreas Gruentzig performed the first coronary artery angioplasty on September 20, 1977. In that procedure, he threaded a long, thin catheter with a deflated balloon at its tip through the femoral artery in the leg and into the heart of a thirty-seven-year-old man with chronic angina. Gruentzig actually manufactured the balloon in his kitchen sink! After positioning the tip of the catheter at the site of an obstructing plaque, he inflated the balloon. X-ray images confirmed that this simple maneuver crushed the plaque against the wall of the artery, creating a large channel for the flow of blood. The procedure was a success, and the patient's pain was relieved. In 2000 (twenty-three years later), the patient underwent cardiac catheterization, which demonstrated that the artery treated in 1977 remained open.

Gruentzig's success led to widespread application of balloon angioplasty in people with coronary artery disease. But as with many new medical technologies, initial results were spotty. Among the first fifty patients, success was achieved in only 64 percent; in addition, one in seven patients required emergency bypass surgery, and one in twenty had a heart attack caused by the procedure. Although the safety profile improved rapidly, the primary long-term limitation of balloon angioplasty quickly became apparent. As many as half of patients developed a recurrent blockage, called restenosis, within six months of the initial procedure.

Today, we know that you need to place a stent in the artery to keep it open and prevent restenosis. Coronary artery stents, ultra-thin metal tubes that are positioned inside arteries after an angioplasty balloon is used to dilate the area of obstruction, push the arterial walls outward to maintain the opening.

The first coronary artery stent was placed in Toulouse, France, in 1986. The FDA approved coronary artery stenting in 1994, and the combination of balloon angioplasty and stenting became standard. Stents cut the risk of restenosis to about 20–30 percent—better than balloon angioplasty alone, but still not perfect. Therefore, scientists investigated the causes of restenosis in stents, and found that blockage inside of stents is caused by activation of the body's normal healing mechanisms. Balloon angioplasty and stent deployment cause injury to the arterial wall, which leads to an inflammatory reaction. Cells migrate to the site, scar tissue forms, and the stent becomes partially blocked.

The search for ways to prevent this inflammation and scarring led to the idea of coating stents with medicines to inhibit cell growth and inflammation. If we could block this normal healing response by local release of medicines from the stents, maybe we could keep stents open longer. The first drug-eluting stents were approved for use in the United States in 2003, and large studies showed that they reduced restenosis rates by half, from about 20–30 percent to 10–15 percent. Although the long-term risk of heart attack was not reduced by drug-eluting stents, they did limit the need for subsequent procedures on the same artery. The development of drug-eluting coronary artery stents was hailed as one of the greatest advances in interventional cardiology.

Then came some concerning news. In 2006, investigators studying drug-eluting stents reported a higher incidence of a serious condition called stent thrombosis, which occurs when a blood clot forms inside a stent, shutting off blood flow to the artery. This can be catastrophic, causing heart attacks in most patients and death in about half. While stent thrombosis had been observed early after implantation of the original, non-medicated stents (bare metal stents), people with drug-eluting stents seemed to still be at risk months and even years after the procedure.

Alarmed by these reports, doctors temporarily returned to using bare metal stents. Meanwhile, cardiologists and the FDA considered the problem of clotting after placement of drug-eluting stents. It turned out that the same chemicals that keep the drug-eluting stents open also slow the body's normal response to stent implantation, which should include covering the inside of the stent with a person's own cells. With no protective layer of cells, blood remains in contact with the metallic surface of the stent for several months. And when blood comes into contact with foreign surfaces or materials, it clots. This is a natural response that prevents us from bleeding to death when we are injured.

Cardiologists did not want to abandon drug-eluting stents and their superior durability. They decided that the best strategy was to prescribe additional medicines that prevent blood clotting during the slow healing phase after placement of a drug-eluting stent. This was great news for the manufacturers of clopidogrel.

Today, people who receive coronary artery stents are treated with aspirin and clopidogrel to inhibit blood clotting. Nearly all stent patients should take aspirin for life. Clopidogrel is required for at least one month (and preferably three months) after placement of a bare metal stent. For those receiving a drug-eluting stent, the FDA recommends that people continue clopidogrel for at least one year, though some cardiologists recommend they continue it forever. We treat all stent patients with aspirin and clopidogrel for one year, and then continue aspirin indefinitely. (For a more detailed discussion of clopidogrel, see Chapter 11.)

CLOPIDOGREL: DON'T DELAY AND DON'T STOP

Formation of a blood clot in a stent—stent thrombosis—is the most feared complication of coronary artery stenting. While some complications occur unpredictably, this one is usually preceded by a mistake: 88 percent of people who experience stent thrombosis failed to take their aspirin and clopidogrel as instructed. A recent study showed that one in six patients delays filling the clopidogrel prescription. And of those who delay, 14 percent *never* get their prescriptions filled. These patients have double the risk of heart attack or death, particularly in the first thirty days after the stenting procedure.

One reason that people fail to fill their prescriptions is that nobody explained the medicines to them. At hospital discharge, most patients can't list their medicines or explain their purposes. Don't be part of that majority. Before you leave the hospital, make sure that a nurse or doctor takes the time to explain what each of your prescriptions does. Then place the clopidogrel prescription on top of your stack and get it filled first.

If you take a combination of aspirin and clopidogrel, the risk of catastrophic stent thrombosis is low for both drug-eluting stents and bare metal stents. Overall, somewhere between 0.5 and 2.0 percent of people develop a blood clot in a stent. But these two medicines represent a double-edged sword, as they also cause bleeding in some patients. Clopidogrel should be avoided in people with ulcers, those who have a history of brain hemorrhage, and those at particular risk for trauma—for example, elderly people who are unsteady on their feet. The choice of stent must be tailored to the patient, and you should be part of this discussion.

If your cardiologist recommends a coronary artery stent, there are a few additional things you should consider before deciding that the latest drug-eluting stent is right for you. Long-term treatment with brand-name clopidogrel (Plavix) has been expensive. If it is not covered by your insurance, you can expect to pay $1,000 to $1,500 a year for this important medicine, so make sure that you can afford it. Fortunately, clopidogrel became available as a generic in 2012, and the price is falling rapidly.

Next, think about your general health. Are you likely to need any sort of surgery or a major medical procedure in the next year? Because clopidogrel inhibits blood clotting, it must be stopped in patients who are having surgery, particularly some types of eye and brain surgery, where a little bit of bleeding can create a huge problem. If you anticipate having surgery in the next twelve months, consider requesting a bare metal stent because it is safer to temporarily stop clopidogrel with this type of stent.

WHEN YOU SHOULD CONSIDER A BARE METAL STENT INSTEAD OF A DRUG-ELUTING STENT

Do you have bleeding problems (ulcers, gastrointestinal bleeding, history of stroke with bleeding)?

Are you at risk for trauma (unsteady on your feet, dangerous occupation such as police officer, firefighter, or active military)?

Are you going to require surgery within the next 12 months?

Is clopidogrel a problem (it is too expensive, you are unwilling to take it for 12 months)?

MAKING THE RIGHT CHOICE: WHICH THERAPY IS RIGHT FOR YOU?

Now that you understand the medical, stenting, and surgical options, it is time to figure out which one is right for you. The first key factor is

YOU NEED SURGERY BUT YOU HAVE A CORONARY ARTERY STENT

Patients with stents must take aspirin and clopidogrel. For bare metal stents, at least 1–3 months of clopidogrel are necessary; in patients with drug-eluting stents, the duration of clopidogrel treatment should be at least a year. But what if you develop a gallbladder problem or suffer a hip fracture and require surgery? What is the risk of temporarily stopping clopidogrel? It depends how long it has been since the stent was placed. When clopidogrel is stopped for elective surgery within six weeks of implantation of a drug-eluting stent, 42 percent of patients experience a cardiovascular event. The risk falls with time, reaching about 12 percent by one year. Scottish investigators who studied this problem noted that 20 percent of the stent patients who stopped clopidogrel to have surgery actually had cosmetic procedures. The messages here are:

- Do not plan elective surgery within six weeks of stent implantation.
- Delay cosmetic surgery, preferably for at least a year; don't let vanity get in the way of heart health.

It is essential that you continue aspirin after stopping clopidogrel for surgery. If you stop both drugs, the risk of stent thrombosis rises to unacceptable levels.

your symptoms. Among the 16 million people in the United States with coronary heart disease, the most common presentation is chronic, stable angina. This usually manifests itself the way it did in Jim Sutton—predictable and reproducible chest pain or tightness that comes on with exertion and goes away with rest.

The more alarming presentation is the sudden onset of chest pain that is more severe or does not go away. This dramatic pain usually is caused by acute formation of a blood clot in an artery on the heart. These symptoms are termed acute coronary syndrome and, unlike chronic stable angina, require urgent attention. If you develop sudden chest pain that does not go away or is worse than your normal exertional chest pain, chew an aspirin and call 911. When you get to the hospital, use the information in this chapter to ensure that you get the right treatment.

Chronic Stable Angina: You Have Time to Choose

Stents Versus Medicine

Although chronic stable angina is common, there is considerable debate concerning the best initial therapy for patients with this condition. Should they be treated with medicines, or should they be shuttled straight to the cardiac catheterization laboratory for immediate stenting and balloon angioplasty, like Jim Sutton?

The idea of performing a cardiac catheterization, identifying the blockages, and propping them open with stents seems attractive. It satisfies our natural desire for a quick fix, and results in a nice-looking angiogram that makes your cardiologist proud. But remember that atherosclerosis is a widespread, systemic problem. Local treatment of selected narrowings does not cure the disease.

The April 2007 issue of the *New England Journal of Medicine* contained a carefully designed study that compared medical therapy to stenting as initial treatment for patients with chronic stable angina. In this study, called the Courage Trial, 2,287 patients were randomly assigned to one of two initial treatments: 1,149 received optimal (aggressive) medical therapy, while 1,138 had both optimal medical therapy and angioplasty with stenting. After five years, there was no difference between treatment groups in the percentage of people who suffered a heart attack or died. Symptoms improved dramatically with both treatments: 74 percent of stent patients and 72 percent of medicine patients were free of angina. One-third of medicine patients did experience "crossover," meaning that they eventually required stenting in addition to medicines to relieve their symptoms. But the key point is that patients in both groups did equally well over the long term, no matter what their initial therapy.

The conclusion from the Courage Trial was that an initial strategy of medical therapy is the right choice for most people with chronic stable angina. The majority of patients can be rendered pain-free with medicines alone. If chest pain recurs in spite of the best medical therapy, the patient can then undergo elective stenting. But there is no penalty for trying medicines first. And, as we noted previously, everybody who receives a stent should continue with optimal medical therapy as well.

Critics—mostly interventional cardiologists—argued that stenting provided more rapid relief of angina and improved quality of life more quickly than medical therapy did. This is true, although both quality of life and reduction in chest pain were equal by three years. Others noted that in the real world it is hard to achieve the excellent medical treatment enjoyed by patients in the Courage Trial. One editorialist wrote that ensuring that people receive the best medical therapy requires "a Herculean effort, unlike that typically seen in routine clinical practice."

The problem is not that we can't deliver good medical care on a routine basis; it is that we don't do it. Today fewer than half of patients who receive stents get the best medical therapy. This is unacceptable. If doctors prescribe the correct medicines and lifestyle interventions and take the time to formulate a strategy and explain it to our patients, we can provide excellent care. If you or a family member receives a stent, urge your doctor to plot out the right medical course and discuss it with you.

Again, we recommend a strategy of "trust but verify" when it comes to your doctor's recommendations. Below is a list below of the medicines used in the Courage Trial. If you have chronic stable angina—whether you have received a stent or not—bring this list to your doctor and discuss what you should be taking. You are probably not receiving a medicine in every one of these categories, and that is okay. But you should be on at least three, and possibly four or five, of these medicines. Make sure that you are getting the right treatment. And, of course, couple these medicines with a heart-healthy, tobacco-free lifestyle.

MEDICINES FOR CHRONIC STABLE ANGINA

Aspirin

Statin medication

Other anti-lipid or anti-cholesterol agent

Beta-blocker

ACE inhibitor

Calcium channel blocker

Nitrate (nitroglycerin or similar agent)

The Courage Trial was a landmark study of treatments for chronic stable angina. Nevertheless, the allure of a quick fix with rapid stenting remains a strong temptation for many patients and cardiologists. Like Jim Sutton, too many people are subjected to stenting as first-line therapy, when medicines alone might have been extremely effective. And stenting is expensive. If doctors followed the recommendations from the Courage Trial and tried medical therapy first, our health care system would save $5 billion a year.

CHELATION THERAPY FOR HEART DISEASE: A "WALLET BIOPSY"

We sometimes refer to procedures that make money for doctors but provide no benefit to patients as "wallet biopsies." Chelation therapy for coronary heart disease falls into this category. Chelation therapy involves giving patients intravenous infusions of chemicals that bind to calcium in blood and tissues and cause the calcium to be excreted from the body in the urine. Because calcium is present in atherosclerotic plaques, proponents contend that removal of calcium with chemicals will make plaques shrink or dissolve, reducing obstruction to blood flow and eliminating chest pain. Other supporters claim that chelation therapy also improves blood vessel function. Scientific studies find no evidence supporting either of these alleged mechanisms for treatment of coronary heart disease.

There is only one hard fact that we know about chelation therapy: a typical six-month course costs $3,000 to $5,000. It is estimated that every year more than half a million Americans undergo chelation therapy to try to treat coronary heart disease. Are they getting their money's worth? The answer is a resounding no. The few well-conducted clinical studies of chelation therapy demonstrate absolutely no benefit to this treatment.

In medicine, we frequently discuss the risk-benefit ratio of therapies and procedures. Chelation therapy has no benefit for patients with coronary heart disease, but it does pose risks. At least thirty people have died as a direct result of chelation therapy. Another risk is that some patients put off or forgo proven and effective therapy in favor of chelation therapy, leaving themselves at risk for heart attack and death from their untreated coronary heart disease. The American Medical Association, the American Heart Association, and the FDA agree that chelation therapy is an unproven and unsafe therapy for heart disease. In our opinion, chelation therapy is even worse than just a wallet biopsy; it is a dangerous and potentially life-threatening choice for patients with coronary heart disease.

Stents Versus Surgery

In addition to representing the most common indication for coronary artery stenting, chronic stable angina is the condition that most frequently gets people to the heart surgeon. As we discussed, improvements in stenting and angioplasty have cut into the cardiac surgeons' business. The turf war between cardiac surgeons and cardiologists has generated considerable controversy and confusion. As with the stents-versus-medicine debate, the answers are in the data.

LOCATION, LOCATION, LOCATION

Many factors determine the therapy a person receives for coronary artery disease. You would think that a person's medical condition—the anatomy of the heart's arteries, overall heart function, and presence of other diseases such as diabetes—would be the primary considerations, but this is not always the case. Where a person lives can be one of the most important determinants of therapy. In the United States, there are 2.6 stenting procedures performed for every bypass operation. However, if you live in Davenport or Burlington, Iowa, the ratio of stents to bypasses is more than ten to one. In contrast, in Santa Maria, California, or Fayetteville, North Carolina, bypass surgery is performed twice as often as it is in other parts of the country. Even within different regions of New York State, stenting rates vary by a factor of two.

Is it possible that patients with heart disease are that different across the regions and states? We don't think so. The difference lies in the types of doctors that patients see and in their approaches. For example, regions with more interventional cardiologists tend to report higher rates of stenting. There is particular concern when it comes to areas served by special "heart hospitals," which tend to be physician-owned, creating the possibility of a financial incentive to perform procedures. A recent study confirms that when a brand-new heart hospital opens in a neighborhood, the number of heart-related procedures goes up two- to threefold. In contrast, when an existing hospital adds a heart program, there is no such increase in procedures. Use our guidance to ensure that your therapy is based on your heart's condition, not on your neighborhood or zip code!

Though relatively invasive, bypass surgery is the right answer for certain patients with chronic stable angina. When compared to stenting and angioplasty, coronary artery bypass grafting is associated with longer life spans in people with the most severe and complex coronary artery disease. This includes people with blockages in all three of the heart's major arteries, and certain people with blockage of the critically important left main coronary artery, which supplies blood to 70 percent of the heart muscle.

Among patients with extensive coronary artery disease, those with heart damage and those with diabetes derive a particular advantage from surgery when compared to stenting.

The largest contemporary study comparing bypass surgery to stenting is the Syntax Trial, which enrolled 1,800 patients from seventeen different countries and was widely reported by the media. Patients with severe coronary heart disease were split into two groups, with half of the patients having bypass surgery and half receiving stents. At the end of one year, the rates of heart attack and death were similar with the two therapies. However, patients undergoing stenting were about twice as likely to require further procedures on the heart's arteries, while patients having bypass surgery were more likely to suffer a stroke.

Reading the same report, surgeons and cardiologists both claimed victory. Each group said that their procedure was better. A closer examination of the data shows that both procedures are good, and provides guidance for their use. Patients with the most severe and diffuse coronary heart disease did better with surgery. Those with more localized or discrete blockages were generally best served by an initial strategy of stenting. A new scoring system called the Syntax Score, which reflects the severity and complexity of coronary heart disease and helps to guide therapy, allows doctors to be more objective as they recommend the best medical approach for each patient.

Perhaps the most important result of the Syntax Trial is the concept of a "heart team" to review each patient's case and determine the best therapy. The heart team includes a cardiologist and a cardiac surgeon; we want to add one more member—you, the patient. Instead of being assigned a treatment by the cardiologist or the cardiac surgeon, make sure that you discuss the risks and benefits with both of them, and make your choice together.

This concept of evidence-based, personalized decision making by a heart team is spreading. It may eventually replace the more common scenario of the patient laying sedated on the table in the cath lab, hearing his cardiologist say, "I can fix your blockages right now or the surgeon can crack your chest tomorrow." Under those circumstances, the expedient option seems most attractive, but it is not always best. Make sure that you have a team on your side before making big decisions about your heart.

Acute Coronary Syndromes:
Emergency, but Still Some Time to Choose

Patients with chronic stable angina have lots of time to convene a heart team and choose a therapy. The situation is dramatically different for the person with an acute coronary syndrome with sudden onset of severe chest pain caused by a newly formed blood clot in a coronary artery. In these patients, rapid diagnosis and treatment are often lifesaving. But even then, the informed patient can use his or her knowledge to ensure the best possible care.

Blood clots form in the heart's arteries when the thin cap covering a vulnerable plaque is disrupted. When this cap erodes or ruptures, the underlying components of the plaque are exposed to blood, causing activation of platelets and blood clotting. Vulnerable plaques are often not at a location with a severe blockage that restricts blood flow. Rather, these cholesterol-rich plaques are different from the hard, fibrous plaques that narrow arteries and are treated by stenting or bypass surgery. We cannot yet reliably identify the vulnerable plaques that are going to rupture.

Your first action if you develop sudden, severe chest pain is to take a non-coated 325 mg aspirin and chew it; chewing it gets the medicine into your bloodstream more quickly than simply swallowing the pill. If the chest pain lasts more than five minutes, call 911. Don't worry about potential embarrassment if it turns out to be a false alarm—each year, more than 6 million Americans visit emergency departments because of chest pain, and only about 25 percent of them actually have an acute cardiac condition. If the problem is not your heart, you will go home within a day feeling reassured. If the issue *is* your heart, you will get the treatment you need to prevent a heart attack.

Within five to ten minutes of your arrival in the emergency department, you should have an electrocardiogram. Some ambulance crews do this simple test before you get to the hospital. The EKG gives your doctors critically important information. If one part of the EKG tracing, called the ST segment, is elevated, or raised, this is a sign that an artery on the heart is completely blocked by a clot. This means that you are having a heart attack, or myocardial infarction. This type of heart attack is called an ST-elevation myocardial infarction, or STEMI. STEMI is a medical emergency. Irreversible heart damage begins within thirty minutes of blood clot formation.

If your EKG shows that you are having an STEMI heart attack, there is only one goal—get the artery open. The more quickly the artery is opened, the smaller the heart attack, the better the heart function, and the lower the risk of death. There are two ways to try to open the artery—stenting with angioplasty, or administration of clot-busting drugs, which are also called thrombolytics.

Stenting is better than clot-busting drugs for STEMI. The problem is that stenting is not always available. Although there are more than 5,000 acute care hospitals in the United States, only 25 percent of them have the equipment and doctors to open blocked arteries with stents. However, 80 percent of Americans live within a one-hour drive of a hospital that does stenting. But even if you are taken to a hospital with stenting capability, if you arrive after hours or on a weekend, the treatment may not be immediately available.

We know that you can't schedule your heart attack. But if you are a heart patient or have a family member with heart disease, ask your cardiologist which nearby hospital performs stenting. Get this information in advance so that if you develop sudden chest pain, you can ask to be taken to that hospital. Unfortunately, current rules may not allow the ambulance to take you to the hospital of your choice, so some patients will be transported to the nearest hospital. Often, a helicopter or fast ambulance is available to transfer you to a hospital that performs acute stenting for heart attacks.

In medicine, we love to record numbers and analyze data. When stenting is used to open a completely blocked artery in a patient having an STEMI, the key number that we track is the door-to-balloon time. This is the interval from the time that you hit the hospital doors to the moment that a balloon is inflated in the artery to open it up. The shorter the door-to-balloon time, the better your prognosis. The American College of Cardiology recommends that the door-to-balloon time be less than ninety minutes. In the recent past, this was achieved in only about half of patients. However, new studies demonstrate that when hospitals focus on improving their processes, they can reach the ninety-minute goal in ninety percent of patients, resulting in better outcomes.

When we examine the numbers, we find that certain groups of patients have a notoriously long door-to-balloon time. These include the elderly, minorities, and women. Sometimes the issue is that their symptoms are vague. Other times the picture is complicated by additional medical problems. If you or a family member has an acute heart issue and falls into one of these groups, be proactive and encourage rapid action by your medical team.

What if stenting is not available for a patient having an STEMI? While the idea of immediately transferring a patient to a hospital with stenting capabilities sounds attractive, this may take too long to be practical in some cases. Transfer should be considered only if it introduces a delay of less than sixty minutes. This is no time to be stuck in traffic. Clot-busting drugs are the next-best choice and should be administered within thirty minutes of hospital arrival.

About one-third of patients with sudden chest pain and acute coronary syndromes have a completely blocked artery causing an STEMI. The other two-thirds have a disrupted plaque and a clot, but the artery is not completely obstructed. Because there is still some blood flow to the heart muscle, the situation is less dire. Some of these patients still suffer a heart attack, but it is usually a smaller heart attack without the classic

EKG changes of an STEMI. We have a clever name for this kind of heart attack—we call it a non-STEMI, or NSTEMI.

Still other patients with acute chest pain and a partially obstructed artery do not have heart attacks at all. They have unstable angina, which usually presents as chest pain that is new or more severe (greater frequency, occurring at rest) than their normal chest pain. Unstable angina and NSTEMI are very similar, and we approach them the same way.

The goal of treatment here is to prevent further clot formation, which could trigger a large heart attack. There is some controversy about whether people with NSTEMI or unstable angina benefit more from an invasive strategy or from simple medical therapy. An early invasive strategy means taking these patients to the cardiac catheterization lab, taking pictures of their coronary arteries, and then treating the blocked arteries with stents or bypass surgery, as appropriate. A more conservative strategy involves administration of medicines to stop progression of the blood clot (aspirin, clopidogrel, and blood thinners) and to reduce the heart's work (beta-blockers, nitrates, and others). Patients treated conservatively undergo catheterization only if they have persistent chest pain or if an exercise stress test demonstrates that segments of heart muscle have inadequate blood flow.

Which is the best strategy? As with everything in medicine, the choice of therapy depends upon the patient's situation. Certain patients with NSTEMI or unstable angina should be treated with early cardiac catheterization, generally within twenty-four hours of presentation to the hospital. These are the patients who are at greatest risk and therefore stand to gain the most from an invasive procedure.

FACTORS SUGGESTING EARLY CATHETERIZATION FOR UNSTABLE ANGINA OR NSTEMI

Chest pain that is unrelenting or occurs at rest

Decreased blood pressure

Changes in ST segment of EKG

Blood test detects troponin, a component of cardiac muscle, in blood, meaning that heart muscle cells have been damaged

Previous stenting or bypass surgery

Known coronary heart disease based on previous cardiac catheterization

Reduced heart function on echocardiogram

If a patient has chest pain and has one or more of the features on this list, it is reasonable to discuss cardiac catheterization. On the other hand, if the chest pain eases with time and medications, the EKG and blood tests improve, and the person has none of the other findings in the table, it may be reasonable to avoid urgent catheterization and follow-up closely with a cardiologist.

DO CORONARY ARTERY STENTS *PREVENT* HEART ATTACKS?

Surprisingly, they don't. But why not? If an artery on the heart is tightly narrowed by a cholesterol-filled plaque and we prop it open with a stent, shouldn't that prevent a future heart attack? Although this assumption seems logical, the biology of heart attacks produces a different answer.

Plaques that cause heart attacks often differ from the plaques that cause chronic chest pain. Heart attacks occur when the surface of a plaque suddenly ruptures or erodes, leading to formation of a blood clot at the site that completely blocks the artery. These heart-attack-causing plaques frequently *do not* result in tight narrowings of arteries. They only declare themselves when they rupture and a blood clot forms at their surface. So when we place stents to open up tightly narrowed arteries, we do not stent the segments of the arteries that could be responsible for future heart attacks. We have not yet developed the capability to identify in advance which plaques will cause heart attacks, so we can't use prophylactic stents to keep them from occurring. Medicines, however, including statins and aspirin, do reduce the risk of heart attack in patients with coronary heart disease.

Although stents do not prevent heart attacks or prolong life in those with chronic chest pain, they are extremely important for someone who is having a heart attack. For this patient, who is losing heart muscle cells every minute as a result of a blocked artery, placing a stent to open the artery limits the damage and is often lifesaving.

Coronary artery stents represent a huge advance in our ability to treat heart disease. But as with any medical device, we should use them only when the patient benefits. We must avoid what some doctors refer to as the "oculo-stenotic stenting reflex"—a term that refers to the interventional cardiologist who sees ("oculo") a blockage ("stenotic") and places a stent simply because it is possible.

SPEAK UP

There is never a good time to develop coronary heart disease or to have a heart attack. Prevention comes first. However, this is the best time in the history of medicine to receive treatment for these problems. Diagnosis and therapy have never been better. If coronary heart disease does develop, we have three types of effective treatment that can improve prognosis dramatically. Medical treatment, including a heart-healthy lifestyle, is the foundation. Interventional strategies, whether catheter-based or surgical, relieve symptoms, prevent heart attacks, and prolong life—when used in the right patients.

Don't leave the choice of therapy to the first heart specialist that you meet. This is a decision for the heart team. With your newfound knowledge, you are a key member of the team. Speak up!

RX: CORONARY HEART DISEASE

Medical treatment is the right choice for everybody:
  Medicines: statin, aspirin, beta-blocker, and others
  Lifestyle—diet, exercise, no smoking

Know your stent:
  If you have chronic stable angina, ask whether a trial of medical therapy should be tried before stenting and angioplasty
  Drug-eluting stents require at least 12 months of clopidogrel. This is a problem if:
  • You have bleeding issues and can't take blood thinners
  • You will require surgery in the next 12 months
  • You don't like taking medicines
  • You can't afford clopidogrel

Find out which nearby hospitals perform stenting procedures, just in case of emergency

When bypass surgery may be the right answer:
  Complex disease of all three heart arteries or the left main coronary artery
  Diabetes
  Reduced heart function

A CHANCE TO CUT IS A CHANCE TO CURE: WHAT YOU NEED TO KNOW *BEFORE* HEART SURGERY

THE BIG PICTURE

Doctors often use the phrase "routine heart surgery." But while heart surgery is routine for an experienced surgical team, it is anything but routine for the patient and family experiencing the surgery. Heart surgery is a big deal. It can be lifesaving, but it is also life-changing. And, of course, there are risks involved, sometimes small, but occasionally large. We are going to show you how to control the experience and lower the risks. Understanding the processes involved—from choosing the right heart surgeon to recognizing and combating postoperative depression—is critical to ensuring the best possible outcome of heart surgery.

Facing open heart surgery, patients and their families are frequently overwhelmed. They don't know which questions to ask or how to prepare for the operation. And things happen quickly. Patients are often shuttled straight from the cardiologist to the surgeon and then to the operating room, all within a few days' time. This rush to the operating room is necessary in urgent situations, but most heart surgery is elective, meaning that the patient has time to do research, ask questions, and construct an appropriate surgical plan.

The first step in preparing for heart surgery is to educate yourself. Before you buy a new car or choose a laptop, you take the time to get the facts—you check the Internet, read *Consumer Reports,* and even test the products. While you can't take your heart surgeon for a test drive, you can gather information to ensure that you are in the right place and getting the right procedure. In fact, as of September 2010, you can even check out your hospital's heart surgery results in *Consumer Reports,* just as you do your car or laptop.

Choosing the best heart surgeon and receiving a technically excellent operation are critical, but they represent only the first phases of the heart surgery experience. The typical heart operation usually lasts about four hours. The recovery takes weeks or months, its duration and success depending in part on how you manage it. That's right: *you* will take charge of your recovery. There are some secrets to ensuring a speedy, successful recovery, and the first is to understand what is going to happen to you, including the elements of a normal recovery and the danger signs that signal problems. Early recognition of subtle changes can prevent serious infections, prolonged depression, and a host of other complications.

You need to approach heart surgery with both a solid understanding of the process and a well-designed plan for success. You must take an active role from the very beginning.

FRANK WALLACH AND THE BACK OF THE YELLOW PAGES

No physician wants to meet Frank Wallach. For years his familiar face has graced the back of the Yellow Pages, accompanied by the promise that he and his team of lawyers will help if you have been injured in an auto accident or have suffered as a result of medical malpractice. As we returned to the office after a full day in the operating room, it was an unwelcome shock to see his name on the long list of people who had called during the afternoon.

When we returned his call, the voice on the other end of the line sounded familiar—Frank also does television commercials touting his courtroom skills. His first words were, "Don't worry, I'm not going to sue you. I'm calling about my heart."

Frank called us on a Wednesday. He explained that his cardiologist had been following his heart murmur for five years. An echocardiogram (ultrasound of the heart) on Monday had showed a leaking mitral valve.

The cardiologist walked him down the hall to meet a heart surgeon, and he was now scheduled for heart surgery on Friday, just two days away. Could he come in for a second opinion? With great relief, we answered, "Of course."

Accompanied by his wife, Penny, Frank came in the next morning for a repeat echocardiogram, and then to talk with us. On a scale from 0 (no leak) to 4 (severe leak), his leak was a 3. His heart size and function were normal. He had no symptoms and had been playing golf—carrying his own bag—the entire summer. We concluded that he didn't need surgery at this time. Frank was pleased with our recommendation.

For the next five years, Frank did well, returning for an annual echocardiogram each July. During his sixth-year follow-up, we noticed subtle changes in both Frank and his echocardiogram. Penny said that Frank seemed a little short of breath at times, particularly after climbing a flight of stairs. Frank reported that he had started using a golf cart. His echocardiogram showed that his leak was now severe, a 4 out of 4. We recommended surgery, but we emphasized that the surgery was elective, meaning that Frank and Penny could take their time with scheduling.

They went home to do some thinking and some research. The following week, Frank called to schedule surgery. Being an expert litigator, he also had a carefully prepared list of questions that every heart surgery patient should ask *before* surgery: Could he have minimally invasive surgery instead of a standard, down-the-middle-of-the-chest sternotomy? Should he donate his own blood preoperatively? What were the risks of infection and depression after surgery? Should he enroll in a cardiac rehabilitation program once he was discharged from the hospital? Would he be able to climb stairs? How long until he felt completely normal?

After we answered Frank's questions, he and Penny set their expectations and formulated a plan for a speedy recovery. Frank had his minimally invasive surgery and was home four days later. His recovery was smooth initially, but ten days after discharge, Penny called to say that Frank's progress was slowing down. He had stopped taking his pain medicines—he was afraid of becoming addicted and convinced that he could "tough it out." As a result, he was sleeping poorly and had limited his exercise because of discomfort. We told him that the pain medicines were necessary and that he would not become dependent on them. Frank heeded our advice and was soon back on track.

Although Frank initially resisted going to cardiac rehab, Penny put her foot down, and he began a rehab program two weeks after returning home.

Meeting other patients in the rehab program sped his recovery and lifted his spirits.

The next few weeks were marked by steady progress. Frank was back on the golf course in eight weeks. His golf game was intact, and the murmur from his leaking heart valve was gone.

GETTING THE NEWS AND TAKING YOUR TIME

As in Frank's case, a cardiologist usually drops the bomb by telling the patient that heart surgery is needed. When you hear this news, take a moment and let yourself experience whatever emotions rise to the surface. Then take a deep breath and begin the steps to take control of the process and put yourself on the road to surgical success. Unless you are in an emergency situation—experiencing chest pain, acutely short of breath—you have time to gather information to help you make smart choices.

There are three questions that you should ask your cardiologist right off the bat:

1. *What in my heart is broken?*

2. *Will fixing my heart make me live longer?*

3. *Will fixing my heart make me feel better?*

Pose these questions to your cardiologist and to each of the surgeons that you interview. You should have heart surgery only if something is broken and fixing it will benefit you. Though this sounds pretty simple, it is often overlooked. Sometimes a component of the heart is "broken"—like Frank's valve the first time we saw him—but fixing it will confer no benefit. Resist the impulse to fix the heart merely because it appears to be broken. Plenty of people have non-threatening cardiac abnormalities that can be managed without surgery. You should have heart surgery only if it will make you live longer or feel better.

After receiving answers to these three questions, it's time to meet the surgeons. Yes, we said surgeons, with an *s.* Your cardiologist will recommend a particular heart surgeon, somebody that he or she knows and trusts. The odds are high that this is a good recommendation. But you should still take some time to learn about this surgeon and consider getting a second opinion. To ensure that you are getting the best team that you can, you need to understand how to assess heart surgeons and their hospitals.

CHOOSING YOUR SURGEON AND HOSPITAL

This is one of the most important choices of your life. But how can you judge the quality of your surgeon and hospital?

The traditional method of determining quality is to assess the number of procedures that a surgeon or a hospital performs. The basic idea is that heart surgery is like golf or tennis; if you practice your swing for hours on end, you should become pretty good. In fact, there are theoretical reasons that practice makes perfect in heart surgery.

BENEFITS OF HIGH SURGICAL VOLUME

Surgeon skill increased

Technical errors reduced

Anesthesiologist more skilled

Postoperative care streamlined

Team function improved

Management of complications more effective

With these factors in mind, patients and families frequently ask the surgeon, "How many of these operations have you done?" This is a good question to ask. But it is not the *only* question.

There is a relationship between surgical volume and outcomes in heart surgery, but it is not as simple as you might think. Coronary artery bypass grafting (CABG for short) is the most common type of heart surgery and the most frequently performed complex operation in the world. In general, hospitals and surgeons that do large numbers of CABG procedures have a lower mortality than those that do smaller numbers. For example, the risk of dying from bypass surgery is 2.6 percent in hospitals that do fewer than 100 operations per year, versus 1.7 percent in hospitals that do more than 450 cases per year. This sounds like a small difference, but it means that mortality is increased by 49 percent at low-volume hospitals. This is an important difference.

Nevertheless, you can't apply the rule that high surgical volume equals good surgical outcomes indiscriminately. Some low-volume centers have excellent outcomes, and a few high-volume hospitals deliver below average results. Analyzing the data more closely, we see that nearly all centers do well with low-risk patients. However, elderly, complex patients with multiple medical problems—diabetes, kidney failure, poor heart function—tend to do better with busy surgeons in high-volume hospitals. If you fall into one of these high-risk categories, it is worth your while to go to a higher volume surgeon and hospital. If you are a low-risk CABG patient, a smaller program is probably fine.

It's good to find out the number of CABG procedures that the surgeon performs annually. But you need more specific information about the surgeon and the hospital before signing the surgical consent form. For this particular surgeon at this particular hospital, what are the actual outcomes? What percentage of patients die as a result of the surgery or suffer major complications (stroke, heart attack, infection)? The surgeon should be able to give you his or her numbers. With an expert surgical team and a low-risk patient, each of these complications should occur in less than 1 percent of patients.

The preceding discussion relates to CABG surgery, the most common type of heart surgery. This is a procedure performed by nearly all heart surgeons, and you have many options when choosing a doctor and a hospital. Other cardiac conditions require surgeons who specialize in particular operations. If you need heart valve surgery, repair of an aneurysm, treatment of an abnormal heart rhythm, or surgery for a disease of the heart muscle (cardiomyopathy), you should seek out a specialist. Find the right doctor with a combination of three strategies: (1) ask your cardiologist for a specific referral to a surgeon with this specialty, (2) go to the websites of large, well-known medical centers, and (3) search for information about your condition on the Internet. For most specialty conditions, a handful of surgeons and programs will keep popping up. These are usually your best choices. When you meet the surgeons from these programs, ask the same questions about surgical volume and outcome that we have outlined for CABG surgery.

CONSUMER REPORTS TACKLES HEART SURGERY

Today you can get valid information about heart surgery results online. The idea of publicly reporting heart surgery outcomes has been around for more than twenty years. In 1989, New York State began to report results of coronary artery bypass grafting in its hospitals. Pennsylvania has a similar program, reporting the risk of death after CABG. In September 2010, *Consumer Reports* added heart surgery to the list of services and products that it evaluates, with 221 of the 1,100 U.S. hospitals performing heart surgery agreeing to release their results. The hospitals are rated based upon four outcomes—mortality, complications, use of appropriate medicines, and technique for performing the surgical procedure—and receive one, two, or three stars, with three stars being best.

Should you check to see if your heart surgery program was evaluated? Yes. But you need to know a few things before you decide how to use the information provided by *Consumer Reports*.

First of all, the rankings apply only to CABG surgery; if you are having another kind of heart surgery (such as heart valve surgery), the results don't apply. The ratings rank entire hospitals and therefore may not represent outcomes for your individual surgeon, as there may be as many as ten different heart surgeons at a single hospital. And at this point, results are provided for a small number of programs. So if your hospital is not listed, it should not be taken as a negative or as a sign that it is trying to hide its results. Still, if you are going to have CABG surgery, check out your hospital on *Consumer Reports*. If results are provided, use them as a starting point to discuss outcomes with your surgeon. But remember that your job is to go deeper than the staff of *Consumer Reports,* getting more specific information from your doctor.

MEETING THE SURGEON: BASIC QUESTIONS

You don't have to be a skilled litigator like Frank Wallach to know the important questions to ask your surgeon. And the surgeon should not behave like a hostile witness. In fact, if your surgeon is a good communicator, he or she will supply answers to your questions before you even ask. However, if important issues such as risk of infection, blood transfusions, pain control, and operative approach are not discussed at your initial meeting, it is perfectly reasonable for you to say, "I have a few questions that I was hoping you could answer. I really appreciate your taking the time to listen

MEDICAL TOURISM: HEART SURGERY ABROAD

Sometimes it is necessary to travel to a major medical center for your cardiac treatment. There is a long history of people traveling for specialized health care. Thousands of years ago, pilgrims from all over the Mediterranean journeyed to Epidauria, thought to be the home of the healing god Askleios. In the eighteenth century, Europeans traveled hundreds of miles to experience the healing waters of spas. Today, people often travel across the country for cardiac care, particularly if they require complex heart surgery or desire a minimally invasive approach. This approach—traveling for excellent outcomes or special approaches—makes sense.

But people are willing to travel even greater distances to save money on their heart surgery. Each year, approximately 750,000 Americans leave the country to get a variety of medical services and procedures at cut-rate prices. By going to Thailand, Costa Rica, India, or a host of other destinations, patients can save 20 to 80 percent on coronary artery bypass or heart valve surgery. Websites advertise "highly qualified and experienced English-speaking surgeons" and promise that having surgery abroad is convenient and safe. This sort of medical experience, which is coordinated by a travel agent instead of your cardiologist, is termed "medical tourism."

We cannot endorse the concept of medical tourism for lifesaving heart surgery. It is one thing to travel within the country to a recognized center of excellence to receive treatment from a surgical team with a well-known track record. It is another situation entirely to sign up for heart surgery online or through a travel agent, with no means of verifying the quality of the medical providers. If money is a problem, most hospitals have programs in place to assist those who cannot pay, whether for lack of insurance or even trouble handling the co-pays.

to them." No reasonable surgeon would be put off by this request. If you encounter a surgeon who is so busy or arrogant that he or she won't answer your questions, get a new surgeon.

While each operation has its own technical details, certain questions pertain to all types of heart surgery. As we emphasized earlier, you should begin by finding out how many procedures like yours the surgeon performs, and the surgeon's overall results, including risk of death and complications. You want an experienced surgeon who has excellent results that can be backed up with numbers. If a surgeon is eager to do your operation because he has always wanted to tackle a case like yours but never has, leave him with his enthusiastic yearning and move on to a surgeon who already has a track record.

Once you find this surgeon, it is time to dig a little deeper into the hospital experience and the operative plan. We are frequently asked about infections, blood transfusions, neurologic issues, and pain control. Let us give you some background on these topics so that you can have a productive discussion with your surgeon.

INFECTION

A hospital-acquired infection can derail your recovery and destroy the results of an excellent operation. Each year in the United States, there are 1.7 million health-care-associated infections, causing 100,000 deaths. Serious infections after heart surgery occur in 1 to 3 percent of patients. For the most part, these infections can be prevented by thorough antiseptic technique. In this regard, simple hand washing is very important—more on this in a moment.

Any postoperative infection is bad, but infection by MRSA (methicillin-resistant *Staphylococcus aureus*) is particularly dangerous and difficult to treat. Many hospitals have programs in place to prevent MRSA and other infections. Although hospital-acquired MRSA infections have decreased substantially in recent years, they have not completely disappeared. Infections tend to occur in clusters, sometimes signaling a systemic problem in a hospital. Ask your surgeon about the risk of infection and find out if your hospital and surgeon are in the middle of an infection cluster; if they are, you need to look elsewhere.

BLOOD TRANSFUSION

A second important point that you need to address when you meet the surgeon is blood transfusion. Twenty percent of all blood transfusions in the United States are given as a result of heart surgery. Will you need a blood transfusion at the time of heart surgery? Should you donate your own blood so that you can get it back after surgery? To answer these questions, we need to provide a bit of background on the risks and benefits of blood transfusions.

DON'T FORGET TO WASH YOUR HANDS!

This is a message that you need to pass on to family, visitors, and, most important, your doctors and nurses. Transmission of bacteria from the hands of health care workers is the main source of cross-infection in hospitals. Scientific studies prove that these infections can be prevented by hand washing. Yet appropriate hand washing is performed only 48 percent of the time by hospital personnel. Nurses do better than doctors on this score. Hand washing is particularly lax on weekends.

The problem is that bacteria are everywhere in hospitals, and unwashed hands will deposit them on you. One study found that 25 percent of hospital computer keyboards are culture-positive for MRSA. So be proactive. Anybody coming in to your hospital room should wash hands both on entrance and on exit—even a nurse or doctor who is going to wear gloves. Standard soap and water and newer antiseptic foams are both acceptable options. Your job is to make sure that the hand washing occurs. In one English study, patients were instructed to ask health care workers, "Did you wash your hands?" before they had direct contact. Patients were reluctant to remind their physicians—only 35 percent of patients were willing to pose the question to their doctors. But this program increased hand washing by 50 percent. Don't be timid—make sure that *everybody* who enters your room washes their hands. You want their concern. You want their medical help. But you don't want their bacteria.

When you get a blood transfusion, you are actually receiving a transplant from another person. The transplant is not a solid organ and it is not permanent, as red blood cells survive only three to four months in the circulation. But people are still wary of blood transfusions; one-third of the population believes that blood transfusions are unsafe. The biggest concern is that receiving another person's blood could lead to illness and infection.

The truth is that today transfusions are quite safe—but, as with any medical therapy, the risks and benefits must be weighed. The risks associated with blood transfusion fall into three broad categories: infection, immunologic reaction, and clerical error. A complication that we should add to this list is anxiety; many patients become very anxious when told that they need a blood transfusion. We will allay that anxiety.

As the table shows, serious complications are rare. Every unit of blood is carefully screened for transmittable diseases. If a person is anemic (has a low red blood cell count), reduced oxygen delivery to the tissues can cause serious organ damage, and a blood transfusion can be lifesaving and speed recovery as well.

With that background, let's tackle the question of whether you will need a blood transfusion with your heart surgery. The answer depends upon your personal profile and the operation you are having. About one-third of patients having open heart surgery require a transfusion, but certain patients are more likely to need blood than others. Those at greatest risk include people who are anemic before surgery, smaller people (particularly small women), older individuals, those who require complex reoperations or emergency surgery, and people with kidney disease. In addition, if you take aspirin or clopidogrel up to the time of surgery, your risk of needing a transfusion increases; this is why these medicines, which interfere with platelet function and blood clotting, should be stopped five days before heart surgery. If you fall into one or more of these groups, the odds are increased that you will need blood at the time of heart surgery.

What can you do to avoid receiving a blood transfusion? If your preoperative blood tests show that you are anemic, your anemia should be investigated before elective heart surgery. Blood loss through the gastrointestinal tract (stomach ulcers, colon problems, hemorrhoids) is relatively common and should be treated. A diet low in iron may also contribute. If you are mildly anemic (hemoglobin less than 12 mg/dl), add an iron supplement (and a high-fiber diet or a stool softener to prevent iron-induced constipation) a few weeks before surgery. This may increase your red blood cell count enough to avoid transfusion.

Many people are interested in donating their own blood before surgery, the idea being that they would receive this blood and thereby avoid exposure to blood from others. Donating and receiving your own blood, a practice called autologous blood donation, has fallen out of favor with heart surgeons. A patient with serious cardiovascular disease may not be able to tolerate preoperative blood donation. In addition, the blood must be donated weeks before surgery. This means that the blood is old by the time the person gets it back. Blood has a limited shelf life, and the longer it sits outside the body, the less effective the transfusion. Large studies show no medical advantage to autologous blood donation.

If your doctor tells you after surgery that you need a blood transfusion, ask a few questions before agreeing. How will it help you? If the transfusion will raise your blood pressure, increase blood flow to the kidneys or heart, or make you feel stronger and less short of breath, it will speed your recovery. Also find out your hemoglobin level. If it is 10 mg/dl or greater, blood transfusion is usually not needed.

While it is not necessary for you to know your blood type, you do need to pay attention to the process as you receive a blood transfusion. Before the bag of blood is hung on your IV pole, there should be a two-person check-in to ensure that you are receiving the correct unit of blood. The two people checking the blood will repeat your name and hospital identification number out loud, making sure that the information on your hospital bracelet matches that on the label of the unit of blood. Make it a three-person check-in—listen to them and make sure that they state your name, not your roommate's.

NEUROLOGIC INJURY

Recently, a university anthropology professor called us to delay his aortic valve replacement for six months so that he would have time to complete a grant application before the operation. Although his application for funding was not due for twelve months, his reasoning was that he would no longer be intellectually sharp after heart surgery and he wanted to write the best possible application before his mental powers declined.

We had two problems with this strategy. First, review of his echocardiogram and his history showed that he had severe and symptomatic aortic valve stenosis. This meant that there was a real risk that he might die during the surgical delay. The second issue was misinformation: heart surgery rarely causes permanent cognitive decline.

When we sat down to discuss our recommendation for early surgery, we explained that there is a small risk of stroke at the time of heart surgery—this is generally about 1 percent. That is the primary neurologic issue with heart surgery, and it is an uncommon occurrence. Early after heart surgery, as after any surgery, lingering effects of anesthesia make people tired, and short-term memory is temporarily impaired. These effects may last for a few weeks, but they virtually always disappear. People can expect heart surgery to fix their hearts without harming their brains.

PAIN CONTROL

"How much will it hurt? How will you control my pain?" These are perfectly valid questions. Although only one-third of patients will need a blood transfusion with heart surgery, 100 percent will require pain relief. We are surprised by the number of people who do *not* ask questions about pain control. You should definitely raise the issue of pain management with your surgeon, and expect a well-thought-out response to your questions. You need an answer that goes beyond "Don't worry, we'll take care of the pain" or "Pain is unavoidable after surgery."

Some discomfort will occur, but it does not have to be extreme. Your medical team can and should take a variety of measures to limit your pain. If your incision is on the side of the chest, the surgeon can inject a long-acting local anesthetic into the incision before you wake up; this sort of nerve block, similar to what a dentist employs, is extremely effective. In addition, the anesthesiologist or surgeon should make sure that you receive intravenous pain medicines *before* you awaken. These might include both a narcotic and, if you do not have coronary artery disease, a non-narcotic, Motrin-like compound called ketorolac (Toradol). If you have experienced nausea with pain medicines in the past, tell your doctors before surgery so that they can create a pain management strategy that works for you.

Ask the surgeon if pain medicines will be given around the clock (every four to six hours) or if you have to ask for pain medicines. It is generally preferable to take them regularly instead of waiting for pain to hit you and then requesting the medicine. Many hospitals use patient-controlled analgesia (PCA), where the patient presses a button and pain medicine is automatically administered by a pump through an IV in the arm. If you like this idea of cutting out the middleman and taking charge of your own analgesics, tell the doctor that you would like to try this option. Remember, a well-executed plan for pain control will speed your recovery, shorten your hospital stay, and make your entire experience a whole lot better.

You will leave the hospital with several prescriptions, including one for a pain reliever. Don't make the same mistake as Frank Wallach—take the pain medicine. It will make it easier to exercise and will help ensure that you sleep well, two crucial elements of a good recovery. Expect to use narcotic pain relievers for up to one month. After that, Tylenol or Motrin will help, although you should discuss Motrin with your doctor if you are on aspirin or warfarin (Coumadin), as each of these medicines impairs blood clotting.

TECHNICAL DETAILS OF THE SURGERY

Although you don't ask your car mechanic exactly what he is going to do when he looks under the hood of your car, it is okay to ask your heart surgeon how he is going to fix your "engine" when he opens your chest. There are several technical questions that are well worth asking before the surgery. These questions vary with the type of operation.

Coronary Artery Bypass Grafting

A surgeon can employ many different techniques to do your bypass surgery. Some approaches will serve you better than others. It turns out that many of the techniques that are best for you and your heart—in particular, the use of arteries rather than veins for your bypasses—require greater effort and more time on the surgeon's part. This means that you need to be prepared to lobby for the best possible operation.

The first technical question for your heart surgeon is, "What are you going to use for my bypasses?" If you have a blockage in an artery on the heart, the surgeon uses an artery or vein from a different part of the body to reroute the flow of blood around the blockage. Your mission is to ensure that the surgeon plans to use at least one of your internal mammary arteries as a bypass. The left internal mammary artery, a long artery running down the inside of the chest wall behind the ribs, is easily detached from the chest wall, leaving the upper part connected to the large subclavian artery. The lower end of the artery can be sewn onto a coronary artery on the heart, bringing extra blood flow to the heart muscle. This bypass is extremely durable; it is still functioning in about 90 percent of people twelve years after surgery. When this artery is used during a bypass operation, the patient is more likely to live longer than when all of the bypasses are accomplished with veins from the legs. For relatively young patients (under seventy) who are not diabetic or obese, the right internal mammary artery can be used as well.

Because most people having CABG surgery require three or more bypasses, your surgeon will need to supplement your internal mammary arteries with other arteries and veins. Bypasses can be completed with veins from the legs (saphenous vein), arteries from the arm (the radial artery), and even an artery that courses along the stomach (the gastroepiploic artery). In general, the younger the patient, the greater the number of arteries that should be used for bypass surgery, as arteries stay open longer than veins and give better long-term results.

Blood Vessels Used in Coronary Artery Bypass Grafting

BLOOD VESSEL USED	PROBABILITY IT IS STILL OPEN AT 10 YEARS
Internal mammary artery	> 90 percent
Radial artery (from arm)	70–80 percent
Saphenous vein (from leg)	50–60 percent
Gastroepiploic artery (from stomach)	50–60 percent

It's your heart. Don't be afraid to ask the surgeon for his or her plan. If the surgeon does not mention that one or more arteries will be used, ask why not.

In addition to understanding your new plumbing, it is a good idea to ask if using a less invasive approach is an option for you, and whether or not the surgeon will use the heart-lung machine during the operation. A minimally invasive approach may be possible in the rare person who requires just one bypass. If your only blocked artery is the left anterior descending coronary artery, the surgeon can perform the operation through a small incision between the ribs on the left side of the chest. However, the majority of patients need several bypasses, and this almost always requires a sternotomy—an incision through the breast bone—as the surgeon must be able to bypass arteries on the right and left sides and front and back of the heart.

So the odds are that you are going to get a sternotomy for your CABG. Don't worry—it almost always heals just fine. David Letterman, Bill Clinton, Robin Williams, Arnold Schwarzenegger, Barbara Walters, and Regis Philbin are just a few examples of people who have had a sternotomy for heart surgery. They all healed well and returned to active lives. You will do the same.

Each of these celebrities also spent a couple of hours on the heart-lung machine, a collection of tubes and pumps that temporarily takes over the action of the heart and lungs. Heart surgery involves sewing together blood vessels that are the diameter of thick shoestrings, so most surgeons prefer to work on a motionless and blood-free field. This is what is provided by temporarily rerouting the circulation through the heart-lung machine, which surgeons call "the pump."

WILL YOU STOP MY HEART? WILL IT START AGAIN?

Most heart surgery requires stopping the heart and lungs for a period of one to three hours. The heart-lung machine makes this possible. Credit for the first successful use of the heart-lung machine goes to Philadelphia surgeon John Gibbon. On May 6, 1953, Gibbon placed an eighteen-year-old woman on the heart-lung machine, made an incision in her heart, and in twenty-six minutes repaired a hole between the heart's upper chambers.

Today, use of the heart-lung machine (also called cardiopulmonary bypass) is routine. Venous blood is removed from the body by a tube placed in the right atrium of the heart. This blood is routed to the heart-lung machine, where oxygen and nutrients are added and carbon dioxide is removed. The blood is then pumped through a tube into the aorta, the body's largest artery, which supports the circulation. Meanwhile, the heart is stopped by injecting a cold, potassium-rich solution into its arteries. This special medicine, called cardioplegia, preserves the heart during the time that the surgeon works on it. When the surgeon is finished, he allows normal blood flow to wash out the cardioplegia. He than shocks the heart with paddles—just like on television—and the heart starts to beat. So, yes, your heart will usually be stopped during surgery. But don't worry about this feature of the operation. We have progressed quite a bit in the decades since Dr. Gibbon's first attempts. We can always start the heart again when we are finished fixing it.

Although the heart-lung machine has enabled safe and effective heart surgery in millions of patients, it is possible to do bypass surgery without it. This is called off-pump coronary artery bypass (OPCAB) grafting. With this approach, special instruments are used to stabilize the area in which the surgeon is working as bypasses are sewn to arteries on the beating heart. The initial thinking was that avoiding the heart-lung machine would improve the safety of CABG surgery, but recent large studies demonstrate that this offers no benefit for most patients. And, not surprisingly, most surgeons are able to perform better bypass surgery on a still and bloodless heart.

Nevertheless, some surgeons do achieve excellent results when performing OPCAB. OPCAB requires a lot of practice and extra surgical skill. Ask your surgeon if he or she is planning to do your procedure on-pump or off-pump. If the answer is on-pump, you are getting the standard approach. If the answer is off-pump, ask your surgeon if he or she is experienced with this technique.

A CHECKLIST BEFORE INCISION

We are all familiar with the fact that airplane pilots go through an extensive preflight check list before takeoff. Now surgeons do the same thing, and you get to participate. A 2009 study reported in the *New England Journal of Medicine* demonstrated that use of a surgical safety checklist cuts the risk of death by 50 percent and hospital complications by 35 percent. This really shook up the medical establishment, as we thought we were doing pretty well without this step. The checklist includes identification of the patient, discussion of the planned operation (which heart valve, how many bypasses), confirmation that the necessary equipment is available, review of important medical information, and answers to any questions you may have. Recently, one of our patients stared in bewilderment as we went through our checklist after he was rolled into the operating room. "Do you really wait until now to figure all of this stuff out?" he asked us. We assured him that this was just a final check before doing something very important. It is worth an extra three minutes to ensure that we have everything exactly right.

Heart Valve Surgery

While nearly all heart surgeons are comfortable with CABG surgery, surgeons vary considerably in their experience and ability when it comes to fixing heart valves. The heart has four valves—aortic, mitral, tricuspid, and pulmonic. Of these, the aortic and mitral valves most frequently require surgery, usually because they are leaky (regurgitant) or narrowed (stenotic).

Aortic Valve Surgery

Aortic stenosis is the most common heart valve problem that leads to surgery. The aortic valve acts like a gateway between the heart and the rest of the body. When the left ventricle squeezes or contracts to send blood out to the body, every drop of blood must pass through the aortic valve. A normal aortic valve is about the size of a half dollar. If the valve is narrowed—say, to the size of a dime or smaller—the heart has to work harder, and serious problems arise. Left untreated, severe aortic stenosis is almost uniformly fatal. If you have been told that you have aortic stenosis and you have any symptoms—shortness of breath, chest pain, or fainting—you need surgery. And you may need it soon, within two or three months.

If you have aortic stenosis, the primary decision to make is which type of new valve you want. The stenotic aortic valve cannot be repaired; it must be replaced. Patients frequently tell us that their surgeon told them what kind of valve they will receive. This is the wrong way to make the decision. It is not the surgeon's job to tell you which valve you should get. Rather, it is your job to ask the right questions and then work with the surgeon to make a choice together.

So what are the options? There are two basic categories of heart valve replacements—tissue valves and mechanical valves. Tissue valves are made from the tissue of pigs, cows, or humans. While it might seem logical that the best valve for a person would be a human valve, implantation of a human valve (also called a homograft) is technically challenging, takes longer, and offers no advantage when compared to valves from pigs or cows. Valves from pigs are actual aortic valves from pig hearts, while valves made from cow tissue are constructed from pieces of cow pericardium, the tough, leather-like sack that surrounds and protects the heart.

Both cow valves and pig valves are excellent. The key benefit of tissue valves is that they do not require that you take blood thinners. But the trade-off is durability: tissue valves can wear out. This does not appear to result from an immunologic response. Rather, the valves are subject to the wear and tear associated with 100,000 heartbeats per day. Over the course of ten to twenty years, most tissue valves wear out. Your age becomes a factor here. If you are sixty-five or older, a tissue valve is likely to last your entire life. If you are in your forties or fifties and you receive a tissue valve, it will likely wear out during your lifetime, necessitating a second operation to place a new valve.

How can a younger person avoid a second operation? Choose a mechanical valve. Mechanical valves, also called metal valves, are made of carbon and metal surrounded by a cloth sewing ring—this is the part that is attached to the heart. These valves virtually never wear out. But they do require that the recipient take a blood thinner every day for the rest of his or her life. As we discussed at greater length in Chapter 11, warfarin (Coumadin) is the most common blood thinner. It is effective, but it has its dangers. Each year, 1 percent of people on Coumadin experience a bleeding problem that requires medical attention. Sometimes the issue is minor, such as a nosebleed that will not stop. Occasionally the problem is major, such as bleeding into the brain resulting in irreversible neurologic injury.

In addition to this medical requirement, there are lifestyle differences between tissue and mechanical valves, too. While tissue valves may require replacement down the road, you can pretty much ignore them in the meantime (except for a yearly echocardiogram and taking antibiotics before dental work or medical procedures). Mechanical valves, on the other hand, give constant reminders of their presence. They make a clicking noise with each heartbeat. Years after receiving a mechanical valve, one patient told us that the clicking still bothered him—but it was preferable to the alternative of no clicking!

People with mechanical valves require a monthly check (sometimes more often) of their warfarin (Coumadin) level with a blood test called the INR, either at a lab or by checking it themselves. If you are contemplating a mechanical valve, ask your doctor about measuring your INR at home. It turns out that people who manage their own INR values do a better job than harried doctors and nurses who are trying to follow dozens of patients at once.

One common question is whether you can have an MRI after receiving a mechanical heart valve. The answer is yes. Heart surgery does not interfere with MRI scans. As long as you do not have a permanent pacemaker, you can have an MRI after any type of heart surgery.

So how do you choose your new aortic valve? Most studies show that neither option is better or worse. You should settle on the valve that sounds best to you. If you really don't want to be on a blood thinner, or if you have a bleeding problem or a lifestyle that places you at risk for physical harm (police officer, firefighter, soldier, martial arts enthusiast, etc.), choose a tissue valve. If you are relatively young and your primary motivation is to avoid a future procedure, go with a mechanical valve—as long as you are willing and able to take warfarin every day.

No matter which type of valve you choose, ask your surgeon whether a minimally invasive approach to aortic valve replacement will work for you. Most people who require isolated aortic valve surgery can get a three-to-four-inch incision instead of a ten-inch incision. The minimally invasive approach for aortic valve replacement is most frequently an incision in the middle of the chest (partial sternotomy), but it is sometimes possible to fix the aortic valve via an incision off to the right side. Ask your surgeon about your options.

Mitral Valve Surgery

After the aortic valve, the mitral valve is the second most common heart valve that requires surgical treatment. When the mitral valve is narrowed or stenotic, usually as a result of a childhood bout of rheumatic fever, valve replacement is usually necessary. In that case, the choice of valve (tissue versus mechanical) follows the same decision process as aortic valve replacement. The difference between the mitral and aortic valves becomes important when a person has the more common problem of a leaking, or regurgitant, mitral valve, like Frank Wallach had.

In most cases, leaking mitral valves should be repaired rather than replaced, but many are not. Here is where you need to act as your own advocate to ensure that you get the best treatment. Compared with people who have mitral valve replacement, those who receive repair generally live longer and are less likely to suffer reduced heart function, blood clots, strokes, and cardiac infections. In addition, taking warfarin is not necessary after valve repair.

The most common cause of a leaking mitral valve is mitral valve prolapse, which means that the valve is a somewhat loose or floppy. While 2 percent of all people have mitral valve prolapse, only a few progress to the sort of severe leak that requires surgery. But if you do have mitral valve prolapse and a severe leak, you need to find a surgeon who satisfies three criteria: he or she should have a 90 percent or greater rate of successful repair, should have an extremely low rate of death from surgery (less than 1 percent), and should be proficient in operating with less invasive approaches. If your surgeon can't provide these sorts of numbers, you need to move on to one who can.

It is worth exploring the possibility of a less invasive approach for mitral valve repair. Many patients who require isolated mitral valve surgery are candidates for valve repair via a small incision in the right chest. These procedures entail a two-to-four-inch incision and may or may not employ a surgical robot. In this approach, the artery and vein in the leg (femoral artery and vein) are used to hook the person up to the heart-lung machine. Blood is pumped from the heart-lung machine into the artery of the leg, sending blood up toward the brain (opposite to the normal direction of blood flow). If there is any plaque present in the femoral artery or the aorta, the stream of blood could dislodge a piece of calcium and carry it to the brain, where it would cause a stroke. CT scanning before surgery is used to identify people who face this risk with minimally invasive surgery; these patients receive a standard sternotomy, which is safer for them.

Criteria for Minimally Invasive Approach to Mitral Valve Repair	
YES	**NO**
Mitral valve appears repairable	Calcified or irreparable mitral valve
Good heart function	Disease of aortic valve
	Need for bypass surgery
	Small leg vessels (less than 7 mm in diameter)
	Atherosclerosis or calcium in leg arteries or aorta
	Previous heart surgery
	Poor heart function

Patient selection is the key to making less-invasive surgery safe and effective. You and your surgeon should consider it only if it is right for you. Advantages to less invasive surgery include a better cosmetic result, less blood loss, and faster recovery. We occasionally encounter patients who focus only on the size of the incision. Don't forget why you are seeing a heart surgeon. If the surgeon says that a less invasive approach is also *less safe,* don't push it. This is not plastic surgery, where the result is judged by the beauty of the incision.

VIGILANCE IN THE HOSPITAL

Immediately after heart surgery, you will be taken to the intensive care unit, the best place for us to monitor you closely. While you are in the ICU, your heart rate, blood pressure, respiratory rate, urine output, blood tests, chest X-ray, and a variety of other data points will be assessed continuously in order to ensure that there are no problems during the critical first few postoperative hours. Nurses, respiratory technicians, special doctors called intensivists, and your surgeon will receive minute-to-minute reports on

PREPARING FOR SURGERY

In most cases, heart surgery is not an emergency. This gives you time to prepare, and we have some advice on that topic, including steps you can take to increase the success of your surgery. Your doctor may ask you to stop certain medicines that cause bleeding at least five days before surgery; these include ibuprofen (Motrin, Advil), naproxen (Aleve), and similar pain relievers. Tylenol is okay. Also stop taking over-the-counter supplements, as some of these interfere with blood clotting.

Stop smoking. Active smokers have a 30 percent risk of lung-related complications from heart surgery. If you quit, you can cut this risk in half. In addition, smokers spend twice as long on the breathing machine. Nobody likes having that breathing tube down their throat. Do yourself a big favor and quit smoking, ideally at least two months before surgery, and you will minimize this unpleasant experience.

Modest alcohol consumption—a glass of wine or a bottle of beer the night before surgery—will not affect your surgery. But if you have more than two drinks per day on a regular basis or drink heavily from time to time (binge drinking), be honest and tell your doctor. Knowing this information will enable your doctor to prevent you from going through alcohol withdrawal after surgery, which can cause serious complications and even death.

If you are overweight and your heart condition allows it (mitral valve disease, stable coronary artery disease), get your doctor's permission and continue to exercise modestly before surgery. This may help you lose a few pounds, which will reduce your surgical risk and speed your recovery.

Preparing emotionally is also helpful. Specialized websites, including Heart-Valve-Surgery.com, enable you to communicate with former patients, who can provide reassurance and valuable information. Finally, put together your personal support team before surgery. Emotional support from friends and family hastens recovery.

your progress. You may remember bits and pieces of the ICU experience, but for most patients the time spent there is a blur.

If everything goes as planned, within twenty-four hours your doctor will proclaim that you are on track and you will leave the ICU. You will transition quickly and dramatically from someone with a tube or monitoring line in every orifice to a person with a peripheral IV and a bit of oxygen supplied through a nasal cannula. On the regular nursing floor, you will be cared for by a single nurse (who has several other patients), a nursing technician, and a team of doctors (who make rounds on many patients). They will help you make steady progress, steering you toward hospital discharge in about a week.

That's the plan. But sometimes things go wrong. About half of heart surgery patients will have some sort of bump in the road on the way to recovery. The most common event is atrial fibrillation, a temporary irregular heart rhythm that will be picked up by your heart monitor; this is rarely serious and is easily treated.

Other complications can be insidious and harder to recognize. Rapidly moving from patient to patient, your nurses and doctors may miss important signs. This is where you and your family and friends come in. Frequently the patient or family is the first to recognize that something is not quite right. Look for the warning signs listed below and speak up. Your vigilance may speed a recovery or save a life.

Warning Signs to Watch For

SYMPTOM OR SIGN	POSSIBLE CAUSES
Loss of energy	Low blood pressure, low blood sugar, anemia, depression, overmedication
Confusion	Low blood pressure, low blood sugar, anemia, overmedication, depression, stroke
New difficulty speaking or finding words	Stroke
New weakness of an arm or leg	Stroke
Increasing paleness	Bleeding, anemia, low blood pressure
Pain in abdomen	Intestinal problems, constipation
Little or no urine production over an 8-hour period	Low blood pressure, kidney problems

You should also be on the lookout for signs and symptoms of depression, which is common among people with cardiovascular disease. One-third of patients develop symptoms of depression after CABG or heart valve surgery. Patients at particular risk include those with preoperative depression and older women. If you have suffered from depression, let your doctors know before surgery so that they can take measures to help you prevent postoperative depression.

Depressed cardiac surgery patients have longer hospital stays, more hospital readmissions, slower recoveries, more pain, and reduced quality of life. For reasons that are not completely understood, they are also more prone to suffer heart attacks and to die within the first year of surgery. Possible mediators of these negative outcomes associated with depression include lower compliance with medical care, poor health habits (smoking, unfavorable diet, lack of exercise) and effects on blood clotting, inflammation, and heart rate.

The primary challenge with depression is diagnosis. Your medical team will regularly check your standard medical tests, including blood tests, chest X-ray, and EKG. But the diagnosis of depression requires more than a glance at a computer screen and a five-minute visit on rounds. Once again, this is where the patient and family come in.

DEPRESSION AFTER HEART SURGERY: SIGNS AND SYMPTOMS

Loss of energy, fatigue

Feelings of hopelessness or worthlessness

Loss of interest in activities formerly enjoyed

Loss of appetite

Inability to concentrate

Recurrent thoughts of death/suicide

Depression tends to occur within the first three months of surgery. If you develop these signs, either in the hospital or in the first few weeks after going home, alert your doctor. Most depressions pass with time. But if the depression is particularly severe or persistent, treatment is imperative. Whether by short-term use of an antidepressant medicine or a few visits to a mental health professional, successful intervention will speed recovery and improve outcomes. So don't ignore depression after heart surgery. It is common. It is dangerous. But it is treatable.

SHOULD I ENROLL IN CARDIAC REHAB?

Yes.

You have just committed to a huge investment in your health. You made it through open heart surgery. You spent several days away from home in the hospital. Now you are looking at another month or two to complete your recovery. Do it the right way. Enroll in a cardiac rehab program near your home. It may be at a health club, hospital, or family health center. The site does not matter. Follow the Nike motto: "Just do it!"

You may not realize it, but you have actually already started cardiac rehabilitation. Phase I cardiac rehab includes the walking, stair climbing, and educational activities that you completed in the hospital.

Phase II cardiac rehab begins one to three weeks after surgery. As Frank Wallach quickly learned, this is far more than a supervised exercise program. It also covers diet, risk factor modification, optimization of medicines, and lifestyle counseling. Instructors and other participants provide emotional and psychological support. Patients realize that they are not alone, and hearing others' stories is both comforting and empowering. This feature of the rehab is particularly beneficial for those who are suffering from depression or who have been deeply affected by the sense of mortality that often accompanies the heart surgery experience. And make it a family affair: patients are more likely to adopt beneficial and long-lasting changes if their spouses or significant others accompany them to the rehab sessions.

Patients who participate in cardiac rehab after heart surgery have increased exercise tolerance, better lipid levels, less chest pain and shortness of breath, and a more rapid return to independence. With these advantages, it is hard to accept the numbers: only 10 to 20 percent of Americans and 35 percent of Europeans participate in cardiac rehab after heart surgery. The elderly and women are particularly underserved.

One reason for this low enrollment is that many people think that they are "fixed" after heart surgery and that no further effort is necessary. Of course, this is not accurate. Heart surgery is the beginning of a second chance. Seize that opportunity! Others fear that a rehab program will be expensive. Don't worry about the expense. Medicare and most insurance companies cover cardiac rehab; it is actually cost-effective, as it improves your health, reducing future expenditures and returning you to productivity more rapidly.

You need a physician's referral for cardiac rehab. Don't leave the hospital without one.

A ROAD MAP TO RECOVERY

During the two to three months after your operation, you will gradually return to normal, resuming all of your customary activities. But what is the right pace of recovery? Which activities are appropriate, and when can you engage in them? How soon after surgery can you climb stairs, drive, or have sex? Is there a special diet you should follow? How can you tell if your recovery is on track? Let us answer these and other common questions. The answers will help you ensure that you stay on the road to recovery.

Exercise

You should exercise daily. Plan to walk every day. Over the first two to four weeks, build up to twenty to thirty minutes of walking per day. You can climb stairs immediately. Stop any activity if you feel shortness of breath, chest pain, faintness, or dizziness; call your doctor if these symptoms do not subside within twenty minutes. When sitting, elevate your legs on an ottoman or stool. If you have had a sternotomy, avoid lifting weights more than ten pounds for six weeks; this is the time it takes for the bone to heal. If your incision is on the side of the chest, avoid lifting with that arm for four weeks.

Heavy exercise can begin three months after surgery. Joggers and weight lifters face no restrictions after three months. Thereafter, ensure that daily exercise remains an important part of your life; it will not interfere with any of the repair work done on your heart.

Diet

No matter what your operation, avoid heavily salted foods for two to four weeks. People tend to gain three to ten pounds of fluid weight during the course of heart surgery. Most of this disappears before hospital discharge, but limiting salt when you get home will help you to shed any remaining excess fluid and prevent water retention early after surgery. It is common to have a poor appetite and a diminished sense of taste in the first few weeks after surgery. These will pass within a couple of months. Meanwhile, make sure that you take in an adequate number of calories to ensure healing. Many find it easiest to eat small, frequent meals. Milk shakes and high-energy liquid supplements may help. Once your recovery is complete, follow a heart-healthy, Mediterranean-style diet to preserve the effects of your operation.

Sex

You may resume sexual activity as soon as you feel able. This is generally two or more weeks after hospital discharge. Apprehension in the beginning is common, but don't worry. With your newly efficient heart, things will be fine. Men who take Viagra or other medications for erectile dysfunction can resume this medication in almost all cases, but check with your doctor first.

Caring for Your Incision

You can take a shower; you probably already took one in the hospital. Wash your incision daily with soap and water. Do not use creams or oils on the incision. Do not soak in a bathtub for the first two weeks after returning home. Avoid tanning in the area of the incision for at least twelve months, as sun exposure can cause permanent dark pigmentation of your incision.

Driving

If your incision was a sternotomy, we recommend that you avoid driving for six weeks from the date of surgery. However, you may ride as a passenger. If your incision was on the side of the chest, you may start driving seven to ten days after surgery. Of course, avoid driving while you are taking prescription pain medicines.

Pain Control

Take your pain medicines. When you leave the hospital, you will be given a prescription for a narcotic pain reliever. Use it. Even if you had a minimally invasive surgical approach, you still had a major operation. Limiting your discomfort will enable you to breathe more deeply and exercise regularly.

This will speed your recovery and reduce your risk of complications like pneumonia and blood clots in the veins of the legs. To ensure a good night's rest, consider taking a pain pill before you go to sleep for the first two to four weeks. Remember that narcotics can be constipating; include fruits and fiber in your diet, and, if constipation develops, ask your doctor about a gentle laxative.

Return to Work

After a sternotomy incision, it is wise to take six to eight weeks off work, particularly if your work involves strenuous physical activity. People with desk jobs will often do one or two hours of light work beginning as soon as three or four weeks after surgery. But your main job after heart surgery is to take care of yourself. Before returning to work, make sure that your recovery is on track.

Monitoring Your Recovery

Buy a notebook and record the following information every day for the first month after surgery:

DAILY CHECKLIST: FIRST MONTH AFTER RETURNING HOME

Record weight (same time each day)

Check legs for swelling

Record temperature

Check incision (dry, weeping, or red; clicking with movement)

Note walking duration

Record use of incentive spirometer (5 uses per day)

Danger Signs

Your recovery will be gradual, and you may not feel better every single day. Modest variability in how you feel from day to day is normal and is not a cause for concern. However, certain signs or symptoms should prompt medical attention—either immediately or within twenty-four hours.

Warning Signs and Symptoms	
GO TO EMERGENCY ROOM OR CALL 911	**CALL LOCAL DOCTOR**
Chest pain—similar to preop pain or new in onset	Fever greater than 100°F or 38°C twice within 24 hours
Fainting spell	Extreme fatigue
Heart rate faster than 150 beats per minute or newly irregular heartbeat	Persistent bleeding or oozing from incisions
Shortness of breath not relieved by rest	Sharp pain when taking a deep breath
Sudden weakness in arms or legs or difficulty speaking	Weight gain of more than 2 pounds within 24 hours
	Worsening shortness of breath
	Worsening ankle swelling or leg pain
	Incision becomes red, painful, or weepy or clicks with movement

(Adapted from Society of Thoracic Surgeons)

Continued vigilance at home will both prevent complications and identify problems early, enabling rapid treatment that gets the recovery back on track.

Finally, let's address the toughest question of all: "When will I feel completely normal?" The answer varies from person to person. At the earliest, a young person who had minimally invasive surgery might feel completely normal in four to six weeks. After a sternotomy, it will take three months for most patients to get back to normal. After that, most people will actually feel *better* than they did before surgery—many people notice increased energy and endurance.

There is life after heart surgery, and it is usually of excellent quality. More than 75 percent of people report substantially increased quality of life after heart surgery. By following our prescriptions, you will place yourself squarely in this majority.

RX: SUCCESS WITH HEART SURGERY

Do your research:
  Don't rush into heart surgery
  Get a second opinion

Meet the surgeon and ask questions:
  What are the surgeon's results?
  Bypass surgery—will the left internal mammary artery be used?
  Valve surgery—is repair possible?
  Is a minimally invasive approach an option?

Prepare for surgery:
  Put together your support team
  Quit smoking
  Lose weight if you are overweight

In the hospital:
  Be vigilant for early signs of complications: confusion, major change in energy level
  Watch for signs of depression

At home:
  Enroll in cardiac rehab
  Keep a daily checklist to chart your recovery

CHAPTER 14

YOU'VE GOT THE BEAT: KEEPING YOUR HEART IN RHYTHM

THE BIG PICTURE

If you had a dollar for every time your heart will beat over the course of your lifetime, you would be hanging out with Bill Gates, Warren Buffett, and their billionaire friends. Your finances would look pretty good even if you received only a penny for each heartbeat. The average life expectancy in the United States is seventy-eight years, which translates into about 3.3 billion heartbeats. Alas, we are not in a position to provide this kind of money. But we can give you something of greater value—a plan to ensure that your heart reaches this number of beats.

A healthy conduction system is the key to your heartbeat. Think of the conduction system as the electrical component of the heart, regulating the plumbing associated with heart muscle contraction and blood flow. The conduction system consists of groups of cells that act like a generator and wires, initiating and carrying electrical impulses through the heart muscle. These coordinated impulses tell the heart muscle what to do, establishing your heart rate and rhythm. Many of us can't dance, but when it comes to the heart, we all have rhythm.

As with the arteries, valves, and muscle of the heart, things sometimes go wrong with the conduction system. This is actually very common, and there is an entire field within cardiology—electrophysiology—that focuses only on the conduction system. When the conduction system is not working, the heart rhythm changes, and we call this an arrhythmia. Although the heart muscle itself may be undamaged, arrhythmias can cause serious problems with heart function. Just as an orchestra needs a conductor, your heart muscle requires the direction of a normal conduction system.

Over the course of your lifetime, the odds are about one in three that you will develop a heart rhythm abnormality. There are many different types of arrhythmias. People may suffer from heart rhythms that are too fast (tachycardias) or too slow (bradycardias). Some abnormal heart rhythms are of no concern—the relatively slow heart rate of an athlete is technically a bradycardia, but in this situation it is actually a sign of health. Other arrhythmias cause problems, ranging from mild shortness of breath to life-threatening strokes.

You are already familiar with some of the more common manifestations of heart rhythm issues. Like almost everybody, you probably have occasional palpitations, which feel like extra or skipped beats. These are usually harmless. Fainting spells are also common, but these sometimes signal serious underlying heart rhythm abnormalities. Fortunately, simple clues can help identify which fainting spells are dangerous. You need to be able to recognize these signs.

The most common serious heart rhythm abnormality is atrial fibrillation, which will eventually affect 25 percent of us. The primary danger of atrial fibrillation is stroke; people with atrial fibrillation face a fivefold increase in the risk of stroke. Yet most of these strokes can be prevented. Unfortunately, medicines for stroke prevention are underprescribed. If you have atrial fibrillation, you need the correct prescription.

Treatment of abnormal heart rhythms covers a spectrum ranging from simple pills to the implantation of complex electrical devices. You probably know somebody who has a pacemaker, a technological marvel indispensable for many people with abnormally slow heart rates. Elton John, Bob Dole, and Dick Cheney all have them. You don't need to understand the engineering necessary to produce a pacemaker. But if you or a family member is facing pacemaker surgery, you should know that there are many different types of pacemakers, and that up to 10 percent of people feel *worse* after receiving a pacemaker because they receive the wrong type, or because the pacemaker they received is programmed incorrectly. We will explain how to avoid this problem, and the preventive maintenance required if you have a pacemaker.

Don't take your heart rhythm for granted. We will help you to recognize warning signs of arrhythmia, explaining when you must step in and join your doctor in active management.

CATHERINE HENRY LOSES HER RHYTHM

The first time that we saw Catherine Henry, we were struck by her unusual poise and balance, apparent even in the way she reached for her bag to extract her medical records for our review. It came as no surprise that she had been a ballet dancer and instructor for forty years.

At the age of seventy, Catherine was retired from ballet but still very active in life. One of her favorite weekly events was the Friday evening concert on the green at a local outdoor shopping mall, where she and her husband enjoyed dancing to big band music. They danced together so well that crowds gathered to watch them. They clearly had rhythm.

Catherine's heart rhythm problems began one Friday while she was dancing on the green. She suffered a fainting spell and collapsed. She recovered within minutes and attributed her spell to summer heat and dehydration. But later that week, it happened again. This time she felt faint while lying down. She went to see her doctor, who measured her vital signs, listened to her heart, and recorded an EKG. After reviewing these tests, he pronounced her "fine" and suggested that she take it easy for a couple of weeks.

Fortunately, Catherine discussed these events with her neighbor, a family practice physician. He was not convinced that she was okay, and suggested that Catherine see us for a second opinion. For us, Catherine's story set off warning bells. A fainting spell that occurs when a person is resting signals a heart rhythm problem. We sent her home with an event recorder—a special EKG that records heart rhythm when a person presses a button. Two days later, Catherine felt faint again. She pressed the button to record her rhythm. When we reviewed the recording, we found that Catherine's symptoms occurred when her heart rate plummeted from eighty beats per minute (normal) to twenty-five beats per minute (much too slow).

The treatment for this was a pacemaker to correct her slow heart rhythm. We set Catherine up with our colleague Jennifer Shaw, an electrophysiologist. Dr. Shaw implanted a pacemaker, set to kick in and take control of her heart every time the heart rate dipped below fifty beats per minute. Catherine had no more fainting spells.

Catherine had her pacemaker checked every six months, frequently using simple equipment that enabled Dr. Shaw to assess the pacemaker over the phone. Five years later, at age seventy-five, Catherine was still dancing on Friday evenings. From the outside, her rhythm looked good. But her next over-the-phone pacemaker examination revealed a new problem—an irregular heartbeat called atrial fibrillation.

After reviewing the data, Dr. Shaw called Catherine to schedule an in-person appointment. When she arrived at the office, Catherine said, "I thought the pacemaker fixed my heart rhythm. I don't feel anything. I'm fine." Dr. Shaw explained that pacemakers cannot correct all heart rhythm problems and that some heart rhythm abnormalities cause no symptoms. She emphasized that the primary threat associated with Catherine's atrial fibrillation was stroke, and prescribed warfarin, a blood thinner, to reduce this risk.

Catherine did well on warfarin for two years. Then she switched doctors because of insurance issues. The new doctor stopped her warfarin, pointing out that it increases the risk of bleeding, particularly in older women, who are prone to falls.

The next time we saw Catherine was in the neurology ICU. Without warfarin to thin her blood, the atrial fibrillation had caused a blood clot to form in Catherine's heart. A piece broke off, traveling to her brain and causing a stroke. The result was that Catherine's left arm and leg were paralyzed. Her dancing days were over, at least for a while.

Catherine left the hospital a week later. After six months of grueling rehab, she learned to walk again. Eighteen months after her stroke, she was finally able to resume dancing. Catherine was one of the lucky ones. She recovered from her stroke. But with the proper knowledge, she might have been able to discuss treatment options with her new doctor, stay on warfarin, and avoid a devastating stroke. We will give you the facts that Catherine needed, information that will ensure that you and your family get the right treatments for your rhythm and keep dancing through life.

CONDUCTING THE ORCHESTRA: YOUR HEART'S CONDUCTION SYSTEM

In order to recognize the signs of heart rhythm problems and understand their treatments, you need a little background on the normal conduction system. Your heart has its own internal pacemaker, called the sinus node, which is a group of specialized cells in the right atrium, one of the heart's upper chambers. Acting like a spark plug, the sinus node generates an electrical impulse about once every second. This impulse travels quickly down specialized conduction tissues that are almost like the wires that carry impulses from your iPod to your earbuds. As it traverses the heart's upper chambers (the atria), the impulse causes the muscle cells to contract. This contraction moves blood through the upper part of the heart toward the ventricles, the lower chambers.

Contraction of the upper chambers of the heart makes up the first half of your heartbeat, and it occurs in less than half a second. After the atria are activated, the impulse reaches a second group of cells, the atrioventricular (AV) node. The AV node serves as an electrical way station. It delays the impulse for about a tenth of a second and then sends it down to the ventricles, which are the heart's primary pumping chambers. This delay at the AV node is necessary to give the ventricles time to fill with blood before they squeeze.

Both the right ventricle, which pumps blood to the lungs, and the left ventricle, which sends blood to the rest of the body, contract simultaneously at the precise moment that they are filled with blood. Any alteration in this timing reduces cardiac efficiency, which can cause a decrease in blood flow to the body.

As the ventricles contract, the sinus node is already preparing to initiate the next heartbeat. This intricate, precisely timed set of steps is repeated over and over. It happened twice while you read the last sentence. Your conduction system even adjusts to your activity level. During exercise, signals from your body cause the sinus node to pick up the pace, speeding up your heart to meet the demands of your muscles. When you are sleeping, your energy needs are diminished, and your heart slows. Your sinus node is in charge, and its dedicated cells take care of your body's cardiovascular requirements.

But, as with any complex apparatus, your conduction system is vulnerable to breakdown. Problems can occur at any level. The sinus node may fail to fire, leaving the muscle without the proper signal to initiate a heartbeat. The delay at the AV node can become too long, dangerously slowing the heart rate. The impulse may move through the two ventricles at different speeds, causing uncoordinated contraction. In some people, other cells take over the heart rhythm entirely, resulting in dangerously fast or disorganized heart rhythms that reduce blood flow to the body.

Some of these heart rhythm changes are threatening, while others cause no problems. The challenge is to distinguish the dangerous from the harmless. Let's start by clarifying the issues involved with palpitations, the most common heart rhythm complaint.

PALPITATIONS: USUALLY HARMLESS

Skipped beats, missed beats, pounding, or fluttering in the chest—these momentary sensations, marked by acute awareness of your heartbeat, are termed palpitations. Everybody gets them from time to time. The question is, when do they signal a dangerous arrhythmia or other heart problem?

While palpitations certainly feel abnormal, about one-quarter of the time they actually represent normal beats originating at the sinus node. In these cases, a person simply has an unusually strong sensation of a normal heartbeat. The rest of the time, palpitations signal a misfire of the conduction system. Usually they are harmless extra or early beats that originated in the atria or ventricles rather than at the sinus node. Such premature beats occur occasionally in everybody and are not dangerous.

Although doctors frequently ignore the patient who complains of a pounding heart or extra or skipped beats, these common symptoms occasionally represent underlying medical issues that require evaluation and treatment. The trick is knowing when to see a doctor if you are bothered by palpitations.

Palpitations: When to Get Medical Help	
SYMPTOM	RESPONSE
Chest pain	Call 911
Shortness of breath	Call 911
Heart racing for more than 20 minutes	Call 911
Fainting spell	Call 911
New, frequent palpitations	Call your doctor for an appointment

Chest pain, shortness of breath, a prolonged increase in heart rate, and fainting associated with palpitations all require urgent evaluation—this means calling 911, not waiting to see if the problem goes away. With these symptoms, the chance of a sustained abnormal heart rhythm is high. Rapid medical attention is necessary to identify the heart rhythm on EKG and then to treat it.

In the absence of these symptoms, frequent palpitations are rarely medically dangerous, but they can be uncomfortable. If palpitations bother you, we can help you feel better. The first step is to identify those triggers that cause your palpitations. Common triggers include strong emotions such as anxiety or fear, exercise, fever, and medicines containing stimulants, such as asthma inhalers and cold medicines with pseudoephedrine (like Sudafed). Some people are very sensitive to the effects of caffeine contained in coffee, tea, and even chocolate. If one or more of these factors causes your palpitations, simple avoidance of the stimulus may cure you. When stress is the precipitating factor, deep breathing, yoga, and meditation are frequently effective.

If you can't identify your triggers or your palpitations persist, your doctor will probably ask you to wear a Holter monitor, an EKG that measures your heartbeats over a period of twenty-four to seventy-two hours, to assess the relationship between your symptoms and your heart rhythm. In most people, Holter monitor results are reassuring, documenting extra beats but revealing no serious problems. This reassuring information itself often reduces symptoms. If your evaluation shows nothing dangerous but your symptoms continue, a low dose of a beta-blocker medicine is often a good, safe option.

Palpitations are common, but they are rarely a sign of serious heart problems. If they are associated with bothersome symptoms or interfere with your life, they should be investigated. Simple, noninvasive testing provides reassurance in most cases, and occasionally enables early diagnosis and treatment of a real problem.

FOR THE FAINT OF HEART:
WHEN FAINTING SPELLS SIGNAL HEART DISEASE

Fainting spells—also called syncope—usually have nothing to do with the heart. But when fainting spells originate in the heart, as in the case of Catherine Henry, important clues point to the diagnosis. And treatment can be lifesaving.

Forty percent of people will suffer a fainting spell at some point. The loss of consciousness is usually brief—thirty seconds or less—and full recovery takes only a few minutes. These features distinguish fainting spells from strokes, which are not associated with rapid recovery, and seizures, which often involve rhythmic movements of arms or legs followed by a confused state that lasts thirty minutes or longer.

Before we tell you when a fainting spell should make you worry, let us describe the standard scenario, which represents no threat to your heart. The most common fainting spells are termed "reflex syncope" or "vasovagal syncope." These are fainting spells triggered by a specific factor. Common emotional triggers include distress, anxiety, and fear. Pain, needles, the sight of blood, and prolonged standing can also precipitate a fainting spell. Situational triggers include coughing, sneezing, urinating, exercising, eating a large meal, and even laughing. The unifying theme with these benign episodes is that there is a trigger.

In these situations, the trigger causes temporary dysfunction of the nervous system, and inappropriate nerve signals reach the cardiovascular system. The result is a decrease in heart rate and relaxation of blood vessels, causing blood to pool in a person's legs. Together, these cause blood pressure to fall. Blood flow to the brain is briefly decreased, and the person loses consciousness. Just before fainting, people often become pale, sweaty, and nauseated and feel light-headed or dizzy.

This sort of fainting spell—associated with a particular situation or trigger, preceded by symptoms, and brief in duration—does not require medical evaluation. If you feel a fainting spell about to occur, lie down and raise your legs, or if you're sitting, put your head between your knees—these maneuvers increase blood flow to the brain and may prevent loss of consciousness.

So, when *is* a fainting spell a sign of a heart problem? Ten to 15 percent of fainting spells signal underlying cardiac issues, the most common being an abnormal heart rhythm. The abnormality may be marked by a very slow heart rate, as with Catherine Henry, or a rapid heart rate that does not give the heart enough time to eject blood. Structural heart problems, including heart valve disease, heart muscle disorders, and even tumors of the heart, can also cause fainting spells.

CLUES TO A CARDIAC CAUSE OF FAINTING

Chest pain

Shortness of breath

Palpitations before fainting

Fainting when lying down or during exercise

No obvious trigger

Personal history of heart disease

Family history of sudden cardiac death

Age over 60

If a fainting episode is associated with any of these features, medical evaluation is mandatory. Call 911 if you have a fainting spell accompanied by chest pain or shortness of breath. In the other instances, call your doctor for an appointment.

To evaluate a fainting spell, your doctor should perform a few simple, noninvasive tests. An extensive and expensive evaluation—CT scan, MRI, cardiac catheterization—is unnecessary for most patients in the initial evaluation of a fainting spell. What is required is some old-fashioned medical detective work, which requires your input. Help your doctor by trying to remember the exact circumstances. Was there a trigger? Did you feel sweaty or light-headed before fainting?

The doctor will listen to your heart, trying to detect murmurs that might represent heart valve issues. She will measure your heart rate and blood pressure when you are lying flat and then standing. If standing causes your heart rate to increase and your blood pressure to fall, the fainting spell was likely caused by either dehydration or incorrect signals from your nervous system to your cardiovascular system; serious cardiac problems are unlikely. The doctor will also obtain an EKG, and if you are in the emergency room, you will be placed on a heart monitor during your stay.

If your story, physical examination, or EKG suggests an abnormal heart rhythm or other cardiac cause, you will either be admitted to the hospital or sent home with a Holter monitor. Most patients should also have an echocardiogram, which is an ultrasound of the heart that demonstrates its pumping action and allows examination of the heart valves. This will help determine if you have heart valve disease. If your heart function appears normal on the echocardiogram, a dangerous heart rhythm abnormality is unlikely. Results of these simple tests guide definitive treatment, which can range from beginning a medicine to implanting a pacemaker, as in Catherine Henry's case.

TECHNOLOGY STEPS IN
PACEMAKERS FOR HEART RHYTHM

The development of the pacemaker is one of the great medical advances of the twentieth century. And in the twenty-first century, these devices are becoming smaller, better, and smarter. A modern pacemaker has two components—a generator that is placed under the skin beneath the collar bone, and wire leads that travel through veins until they end inside the heart.

The generator is the "heart" of the pacemaker. The size of a pocket watch, the generator includes a battery and a computer with complex circuitry. The wire leads that connect the generator to the heart transmit electrical signals in both directions, enabling the computer to sense the heart's natural electrical activity and to respond by sending impulses down the leads to stimulate heartbeats. The computer also records and stores data on heart rhythm, which your doctor can use to assess function of both the pacemaker and your own conduction system.

Nearly all pacemaker systems rely on a conducting wire (lead) placed in the right ventricle; they may also incorporate leads in the right atrium and the left ventricle. A combination of leads enables coordinated pacing of multiple cardiac chambers at once, which more closely approximates the normal conduction initiated by the sinus node.

Today there are dozens of different types of pacemakers and leads. Many pacemakers are even rate-responsive, meaning that they increase or decrease heart rate according to activity level. When you receive a pacemaker, it is programmed to integrate with your heart as efficiently as possible. By holding a computerized wand over your pacemaker, a technician can program the heart rate, the chambers paced, and the pacemaker's response to your heart's intrinsic rhythm. It is usually best to set the device to pace only when your heart needs the help. Limiting the extent of pacing is best for heart function and extends the pacemaker's battery life. Many people with pacemakers are not paced 100 percent of the time.

Each year, more than 200,000 Americans receive a pacemaker. But many do not know why they have it. Most believe the myth that pacemakers fix all heart rhythm abnormalities; as Catherine Henry learned, this is untrue.

Bradycardias, or slow heart rates, are the primary reason for pacemaker implantation. Abnormally slow heart rates—fifty beats per minute or less—become more common as people age. The most frequent cause is

A POWER OUTAGE LEADS TO THE FIRST PACEMAKER

For more than a century, doctors have recognized that electrical signals regulate the heart. With this understanding, they correctly reasoned that delivering small electrical impulses to the heart could stimulate it to beat. By the early 1950s, bulky external pacemakers plugged into wall sockets were used to maintain heart function in people whose natural conduction systems had failed, but these were not the sort of device that allowed the patient to resume normal life. Pioneering Minneapolis heart surgeon C. Walton Lillehei thought that we could do better. He enlisted the help of a medically oriented engineer named Earl Bakken. Bakken got to work in earnest after a profoundly disturbing visit to Northwestern Hospital in Minneapolis. That day, a storm caused a hospital-wide power outage, and a patient died because his external pacemaker had no power.

Bakken attacked the project with renewed vigor, and in 1957 he produced the first self-contained, wearable pacemaker unit. This invention laid the foundation for Bakken to form Medtronic, the world's largest medical device and pacemaker manufacturer. A patient named Arne Larson received the first totally implantable pacemaker in 1958; this was a major surgical procedure that required direct access to the surface of the heart. Over the course of his life, Larson became something of a human laboratory for new pacemaker technologies. By the time of his death in 2001, at age eighty-six, he had received a total of twenty-six pacemakers. Thanks to the work of Bakken and others, Larson's last pacemaker was computer-driven and long-lasting with leads located inside, rather than outside, the heart—all dramatic improvements over his first device forty-three years earlier.

dysfunction of the sinus node, the heart's internal pacemaker. Problems with the AV node can also lead to a pacemaker; if the electrical impulse is blocked (instead of delayed) at this way station, a pacemaker can ensure timely arrival of the electrical signal at the ventricles. Finally, some people have a normal resting heart rate but fail to experience an increase in heart rate when they exercise; this can cause fatigue with only minimal exertion. If this happens, a pacemaker can markedly improve exercise capacity.

Most people who receive a pacemaker have both an abnormally slow heart rate and symptoms caused by the slow heart rate, such as fatigue, decreased exercise tolerance, shortness of breath, and fainting spells. In these circumstances, pacemakers relieve symptoms and improve quality of life. But a slow heart rate in a person who feels fine is not usually a reason to place a pacemaker. Lance Armstrong has a resting heart rate of thirty to forty beats per minute—but he clearly does not need a pacemaker. On the other hand, if an otherwise healthy seventy-two-year-old man has a heart rate of forty-five beats per minute and gets short of breath when he climbs one flight of stairs, a pacemaker will usually make him feel better.

If your doctor says that you need a pacemaker, make sure that you understand the reason, and ask the following questions: "What is my heart rate? Will a pacemaker make me feel better?" The answers will help determine if a pacemaker is right for you.

Your next step is to ensure that you have the right doctor. Many different types of doctors place pacemakers, but you want an electrophysiologist, a cardiologist who specializes in heart rhythm disorders. Electrophysiologists can place a pacemaker in less than two hours with a very low risk of complications and will know how to program your pacemaker so that you feel better, not worse.

That's right—if you get the wrong kind of pacemaker or if it is programmed unfavorably, you may feel *worse* than you did before you received it. We call this "pacemaker syndrome."

SYMPTOMS OF PACEMAKER SYNDROME

Dizziness or fainting spells

Shortness of breath

Fatigue

Weakness

Swelling of the ankles

Pounding or sense of fullness in the neck with each heartbeat

You should feel fine within a couple of weeks after receiving a pacemaker. If you don't feel better, or feel even worse, you may have pacemaker syndrome. The problem is easily remedied. Explain your symptoms to your electrophysiologist, who can reprogram your pacemaker or place additional leads to achieve more normal, synchronous activation of your heart and a better quality of life for you.

Once you have a properly functioning pacemaker, the maintenance program is simpler than that for your car. You will see your electrophysiologist for a follow-up visit at three to six months. After that, you will be able to use remote electronic surveillance to send information from your pacemaker to the doctor's office over the telephone or the Internet. This ensures that your pacemaker is working properly without requiring an office visit. You typically need to go for an office visit only once a year.

Unfortunately, you cannot charge pacemaker batteries the way you charge your cell phone each night. After five to six years your pacemaker battery will wear out and you will need a new one. This is not a big deal. In a simple outpatient procedure, the doctor will numb the skin over the pacemaker and make an incision to reach the pacemaker generator. At that point, the doctor will give you a whole new pacemaker so that you can benefit from new technologies developed since you received your original pacemaker. (The leads that go into your heart are not replaced.) After this quick upgrade, you are good to go for another five years or more.

SPECIAL PACEMAKERS FOR THE FAILING HEART: CARDIAC RESYNCHRONIZATION THERAPY

Until recently, pacemaker implantation was used only to correct a slow heart rate. Building on the work of pioneers such as Earl Bakken, we now have pacing systems that address more than heart rate; these pacemakers actually improve the function of hearts that have been weakened by heart attacks and other conditions. They do this by optimizing the sequence of contraction of the heart muscle to get the maximum force possible out of each beat.

The need for this sort of pacemaker is growing. Today, we are better than ever at helping people to survive heart attacks. But heart attack survivors often have severe heart damage, and doctors are challenged as we try to ensure their longevity and quality of life. Many heart attack victims have so much cardiac damage that they suffer from a constellation of symptoms called congestive heart failure: fatigue, shortness of breath, fluid retention, swelling of the ankles, and limited exercise ability. The first line of treatment for people with heart failure is medical therapy. We have medicines that remove fluid (diuretics) and drugs that make it easier for the heart to pump blood by reducing the downstream resistance (ACE inhibitors). These treatments tend to work for a while, but they often lose effectiveness over time.

The ideal solution would be a means of growing new, functioning heart muscle cells to replace those that were damaged or killed by the heart attack. That is undoubtedly part of our future. In the meantime, pacemaker therapy is a key component of our approach to patients with severe heart damage. About one-third of heart failure patients have conduction system problems that cause an inefficient and abnormal pattern of contraction of the muscle cells that still work. This is where specialized pacemakers come into play: they resynchronize the heartbeat, getting the biggest bang for the buck from each impulse that originates at the sinus node.

The use of pacemakers to coordinate contraction in this way is termed cardiac resynchronization therapy, or biventricular pacing. With this approach, pacemaker leads are placed in the right ventricle and in a vein near the left ventricle. The pacemaker generator has special software that resynchronizes the ventricles' contraction, ensuring that each ventricle ejects its blood at the same time to maximize the heart's output.

Doctors are not perfect when it comes to predicting which heart failure patients will benefit from this kind of pacing. We identify the most likely candidates by examining their EKGs. Two-thirds of heart failure patients who receive the pacing system respond favorably. Successful pacing therapy for heart failure can have dramatic benefits, including a 25 percent increase in the chance of being alive three years down the road, a 40 percent reduction in the need for hospitalization, increased exercise capacity, and improved quality of life.

These pacing systems are more expensive than standard systems, costing $20,000 to $30,000 each (about double the cost of a standard pacemaker). This may be one of the main reasons that they are underutilized. But if you or a family member has suffered a heart attack and has serious limitations from heart failure symptoms, ask your cardiologist about a biventricular pacemaker. Patients with the most heart damage and the worst symptoms derive the greatest benefit. This sort of pacemaker therapy can turn your life around.

DEFIBRILLATORS AND CPR: CHARGE THE PADDLES

If you have ever watched a medical show on television, you are familiar with this scene. A patient collapses suddenly. Somebody begins chest compressions while a nurse or doctor yells, "Get the paddles." After a few moments of chaotic activity, defibrillator paddles are placed on the victim's chest. The doctor shouts, "Clear!" and then pushes a button to send an electric shock through the victim's chest. The body jumps. The camera shifts to the EKG, which now displays a normal heart rhythm. The patient is saved.

This scene is one of the few accurate vignettes in the medical dramas that fill television. It depicts the most dramatic example of a heart rhythm disturbance. The electric shock is used to restart the heart when a person suffers sudden cardiac death. In real life, however, 400,000 Americans die from this cause each year. If sudden cardiac death occurs outside the hospital, the good outcomes written into television scripts are uncommon. Three-quarters of victims receive no therapy at all—no CPR and no defibrillation. Only 5 percent survive. But the combination of quick action, CPR, automatic external defibrillators, and internal defibrillators can improve these numbers.

First, let's get back to heart rhythm. Sudden cardiac death is different from a heart attack. When a person experiences a heart attack, the blood supply to a part of the heart is blocked, and heart muscle cells begin to die; this is usually a local problem, affecting only part of the heart muscle. With sudden cardiac death, a person develops a heart rhythm abnormality that disrupts the entire heart's ability to pump blood. Blood flow to the body ceases, and without intervention, death occurs within minutes.

The heart rhythms that cause sudden cardiac death are almost always either ventricular fibrillation or ventricular tachycardia. As the names imply, these heart rhythms originate in the heart's lower chambers, the ventricles. In 80 percent of cases, coronary artery disease or a weakened heart muscle is the underlying condition that leads to the electrical problem. These abnormal heart rhythms can occur in a patient with a history of a heart attack, somebody who is actually having a heart attack, or a person who has undiagnosed coronary heart disease that has been silent until he or she collapses. In 50 percent of people, the sudden arrhythmia and collapse are the first signs of a heart problem.

Because this scenario is so common—both on television and in real life—every one of us should know how to follow the script that will save a life. In this case, television got it right: CPR and the defibrillator paddles are the keys to survival.

CPR: A CHANGE IN ORDER—FROM ABC TO CAB

The first documentation that CPR saves lives appeared in a 1960 medical journal. Every few years, the American Heart Association reevaluates CPR protocols and makes recommendations for improvement. The 2010 guidelines for CPR include a change in the order of steps, from ABC to CAB. In this acronym, A stands for airway, B for breathing, and C for circulation. The new order emphasizes the importance of chest compressions to restore blood circulation.

These are the steps to take when an adult collapses:

1. *Recognize the arrest*
   a. Person is unresponsive
   b. No breathing or only gasping

2. *Call 911*

3. *Begin CPR*
   a. Chest compressions first
   b. Rescue breathing if you are willing and able to do so (most important in drowning victims and children)
   c. Minimize interruptions to compressions

4. *Use an automatic external defibrillator if available and you have help, but minimize interruption of chest compressions*

High-Quality Chest Compressions Are the Key

The rules for chest compressions are "push hard" and "push fast." With one hand on top of the other, each compression should push the center of the chest in at least 2 inches (5 cm). The rate of compressions is 100 per minute. Between compressions, allow the chest to recoil completely. To keep you from going too fast or too slow, some suggest that you deliver compressions to the beat of the 1970s song "Stayin' Alive," which is actually about 100 beats per minute. You can see the technique (without the disco music) at www.learncpr.org.

Let's dispel a myth that limits bystanders' willingness to perform CPR at a cardiac arrest: *you do not have to perform mouth-to-mouth resuscitation to save somebody's life.* Don't let the idea of rescue breaths stop you from performing CPR. Studies demonstrate that in most adult victims of cardiac arrest (with the exception of drowning victims), compression-only CPR is as effective as traditional CPR that alternates compressions and rescue breathing. Focus on the compressions. Remember, the new order is *compressions, airway, breathing*. If your CPR delivery keeps you at the C, you still may save a life.

In most cardiac arrest scenarios, the heart rhythm disturbance causes the medical problem. That is why in television dramas they always yell, "Get the paddles!" Chest compressions and CPR support circulation and buy time, but they do not actually correct the heart rhythm. To do that usually requires a defibrillator. Because of the importance of defibrillation, automatic external defibrillators were invented and are now available in many public places, including airports, federal buildings, sports stadiums, fitness centers, and schools. In fact, one of the best places to suffer sudden cardiac death is a casino. Casinos all have these defibrillators, and as a result, the chance of surviving a dangerous arrhythmia in a casino is 50 to 75 percent.

If there is a defibrillator immediately at hand and somebody can get it, you can work with a second person to use the defibrillator to try to restore normal sinus rhythm. While you deliver chest compressions, your partner can review the simple instructions inside the defibrillator and prepare to shock the victim. But if you are alone and do not know how to use a defibrillator, stick with chest compressions and CPR; this is not the right time to learn.

Again, when performing CPR, remember to minimize interruptions to chest compressions. There are only three reasons to stop compressions: if the person revives; to use the defibrillator, which should take no more than a few seconds; and if help arrives.

Speed is critical when a person collapses with an abnormal heart rhythm. Without resuscitation, the victim will die within ten minutes. The average time for an ambulance to respond is eight to fifteen minutes. If you can fill that gap and maintain circulation for just eight to fifteen minutes, you can save a life. Classes on CPR and basic life support are offered at most community centers and YMCAs. Make sure that your family and friends know these techniques as well—it is not a bad idea to be surrounded by people who can save *your* life if you get into trouble.

IMPLANTABLE DEFIBRILLATORS

The most significant medical advance in treating sudden cardiac death has been the development of the implantable cardioverter-defibrillator (ICD). Like standard pacemakers, these devices include a generator/computer and leads that travel through veins to the inside of the heart. In fact, the ICD can function like a pacemaker if it needs to. But unlike a standard pacemaker, it can also treat the heart rhythms that cause sudden cardiac death. If the patient develops a threatening heart rhythm, the ICD can correct it either with a special pacing protocol or by delivering a shock directly to the heart—no external paddles required.

People with heart failure and heart damage who receive special pacemakers to resynchronize heart rhythm and improve heart function are often candidates for an ICD. For these people, an ICD is an insurance policy, reducing the risk of sudden death. The person with an ICD can resume most normal activities, but there are a few rules. ICDs will shock abnormally fast heart rates (greater than 180 to 200 beats per minute). Most people never get their heart rate this high, even with heavy exertion. But if you are very athletic, discuss your activity level with your doctor, as your ICD may need to be programmed to accommodate a higher-than-average heart rate before triggering a shock. People who have ICDs can drive a car; however, if you have experienced sudden cardiac death or a shock, do not drive for six months in order to make sure that the abnormal rhythm does not recur. You certainly don't want to be on the receiving end of a shock while you are traveling down the highway at sixty-five miles per hour.

ATRIAL FIBRILLATION

Atrial fibrillation is the most common sustained heart rhythm abnormality. Today, nearly 3 million Americans have atrial fibrillation, and this number is expected to double over the next four decades. You may not have this problem now, but there is a one in four chance that you will develop atrial fibrillation at some point in your life. The older you are, the greater your chance of getting it. Atrial fibrillation is uncommon in those under age forty but affects one in ten people over the age of eighty.

Causes of Atrial Fibrillation

Surprisingly few people with atrial fibrillation take the time to understand what is going on with their heart rhythm. The basics are not that complicated, so we will take just a moment to explain the "hostile takeover" of your heart rhythm that causes atrial fibrillation.

MY PACEMAKER OR DEFIBRILLATOR WAS RECALLED: WHAT SHOULD I DO?

Reading in the *New York Times* that your pacemaker or defibrillator is defective and the subject of a recall or safety advisory understandably provokes great anxiety. The first thing to understand is that the words *recall* and *advisory* have different meanings when they come from the FDA than when they come from Toyota or Ford. A medical device safety advisory or alert is issued by the FDA when a device may pose considerable health risk. An advisory is coupled with a recall if the device is defective in some way. Most important, a recall or advisory concerning a pacemaker or defibrillator does not necessarily mean that the device must be removed and a new one implanted.

The FDA divides recalls into three classes according to the level of danger posed by the medical device:

Class I: There is a reasonable chance of the product causing serious harm or death.

Class II: The product may cause temporary or reversible health consequences, but there is only a remote possibility of serious harm.

Class III: The product is not likely to cause health problems.

These distinctions are important. Obviously, we are far more likely to consider replacing a device with a Class I recall (chance of serious harm or death) than a Class III recall (serious consequences unlikely).

If you hear that a pacemaker or defibrillator or one of its components (often a wire lead) is recalled, follow these steps:

1. Don't panic.

2. Determine if you have the pacemaker or defibrillator in question. A recall of one type of defibrillator or pacemaker is not a recall of all devices. After your device was placed, you received a card that included the manufacturer, product, model number, and serial number. Determine whether your information matches the recalled device.

3. If your device is included in the recall, note whether it is a Class I, II, or III recall.

4. Call your doctor to schedule an appointment.

5. Ask whether it is riskier to get a new device implanted or to live with the device you have. Sometimes a simple programming change or software update takes care of the problem.

Pacemakers and defibrillators are complex medical technologies and are not 100 percent free of design, manufacturing, and performance flaws. With periodic checkups by telephone or in person, your doctor can ensure that your device is functioning properly. Don't let this preventive maintenance slide. If it has been more than six months, it is time for a checkup.

INTERFERENCE: PACEMAKERS AND DEFIBRILLATORS VERSUS CELL PHONES AND MRI SCANS

People with pacemakers and defibrillators must be careful to avoid electromagnetic interference that can cause device malfunction. Fortunately, you need to know only a few simple things to stay safe in this regard. If you have a pacemaker or defibrillator, you cannot have an MRI scan. You should also avoid close contact with arc welding, high-voltage transformers, and generators (things most of us don't encounter in daily life anyway). Contrary to early reports, iPods are safe; the electromagnetic field generated by an iPod is tiny and does not affect pacemakers. Cell phones are generally safe as well, but it is a good idea to hold the phone to the ear on the side opposite your pacemaker or defibrillator and to avoid keeping your phone in the pocket directly over the generator. Airport metal detectors have no effect on pacemakers or ICDs, although you will set them off if you walk through; carry your wallet-sized device identification card to help you manage this sort of situation. When somebody is screening you with a handheld wand, inform them of the generator location and ask them not to hold the wand over the area for more than thirty seconds.

Although the airport poses no risk to your pacemaker or ICD, the same cannot be said for the Gap or Abercrombie and Fitch. Theft detection scanners at the entrance of these and other stores can cause pacemaker or defibrillator malfunction. Walking between the surveillance pillars at a normal pace is fine, but lingering near these pillars can cause problems. If the new jeans that you must have are on a table near the theft detection apparatus, ask a salesperson to hunt through the pile to find your size and take them back to the safety of the dressing room.

When a person develops atrial fibrillation, the sinus node no longer functions as the heart's pacemaker. Instead, cells in the upper chambers generate 300 to 600 erratic impulses per minute (instead of the 60 to 100 beats normally initiated by the sinus node). These superfast stimuli cause the atria to quiver uncontrollably, diminishing the pumping function of the heart's upper chambers. Loss of forceful contraction of the atria slows blood flow, increasing the tendency of blood to clot in these upper chambers and reducing the heart's overall efficiency.

Clearly, a person cannot function at a heart rate of 300 to 600 beats per minute. Fortunately, the AV node usually performs its job as a way station, preventing most of these atrial impulses from reaching the ven-

SHOULD WE TURN OFF PACEMAKERS
AND DEFIBRILLATORS AT THE END OF LIFE?

How should we manage pacemakers and defibrillators in the person who is dying? Will these devices prolong the dying process and even cause harm by delivering inappropriate shocks? These questions have sparked debate among doctors, ethicists, and lawyers. Experts generally agree that it is okay to turn off a pacemaker or defibrillator if this is the patient's wish. This is also true for the person's medical power of attorney if the patient has made his or her desires known but is incapable of acting upon them.

However, it is not necessary to rush to deactivate these devices in all terminal patients. Pacemakers are unlikely to prolong life or suffering in the terminally ill patient, so they are usually not a concern. In contrast, defibrillators can prolong the dying process and cause discomfort by delivering harsh shocks. The patient has the right to discontinue this treatment, which is accomplished simply by waving a programming wand over the defibrillator. If the doctor is uncomfortable with deactivating the heart rhythm device, he or she must identify a doctor who will do so. In these situations, it is our medical obligation to follow the patient's wishes and to ensure that we provide comfort to the terminally ill.

tricles. Thanks to the AV node, most people with atrial fibrillation have a heart rate of 90 to 140 beats per minute before treatment; this may be uncomfortably fast, but the ventricles can keep up with this rate. Patients with atrial fibrillation may also notice that their heart rhythm is irregular, a result of the sporadic way the atrial impulses traverse the AV node.

Atrial fibrillation can be dangerous if not managed properly. People with atrial fibrillation tend to die earlier and are more prone to strokes, dementia, and congestive heart failure. They frequently suffer from loss of energy and reduced exercise capacity, which can diminish quality of life. With so many people experiencing atrial fibrillation and its associated complications, it is a huge contributor to health care costs. Annual expenditures to treat atrial fibrillation currently top $7 billion in the United States.

Can you prevent yourself from developing atrial fibrillation? Not entirely, as there is no single, clear-cut, modifiable risk factor that causes the arrhythmia. However, a variety of conditions are associated with atrial fibrillation, and you can control or treat many of them.

RISK FACTORS FOR ATRIAL FIBRILLATION

Modifiable risk factors

Hypertension

Diabetes

Obesity

Thyroid disease

Electrolyte imbalance

Tobacco abuse

Alcohol abuse (binge drinking, prolonged heavy drinking)

Medicines (asthma inhalers, some antidepressants)

Cardiac conditions

Heart valve disease

Heart attack

Congestive heart failure

Non-modifiable risk factors

Advanced age

Genes

If a person comes in with a first episode of atrial fibrillation, we draw blood to check for correctible, predisposing medical conditions that can cause the abnormal heart rhythm; these include an overactive thyroid and electrolyte imbalances. If these problems are present, correction is simple and will usually facilitate return to normal sinus rhythm. We also perform an echocardiogram to rule out heart valve disease, as atrial fibrillation is sometimes the first sign of an underlying problem with the mitral valve. If you have atrial fibrillation, make sure that your doctor carries out these studies. We have seen dozens of patients who have undergone years of treatment for atrial fibrillation without anyone ever recognizing that an underlying mitral valve abnormality or thyroid disease was the real culprit.

Knowing your family history is also important. If a first-degree relative— parent or sibling—develops atrial fibrillation, your risk is increased two- to threefold. The effect is particularly strong if the relative developed atrial fibrillation at a young age. People who have a family history of atrial fibrillation should take a couple of simple precautions. Request an EKG as part of your annual physical examination, and follow a lifestyle that minimizes the risk factors for atrial fibrillation. Finally, a recent study has suggested an association between atrial fibrillation and two common inflammatory diseases, rheumatoid arthritis and lupus, finding that patients with these diseases have a 60 percent higher risk for developing atrial fibrillation than the population at large. Although the findings are preliminary and a cause-and-effect relationship was not proven, having either of these two conditions should be cause for extra vigilance on your part.

DO ALCOHOL AND CAFFEINE CAUSE ATRIAL FIBRILLATION?

In 1978, a group of doctors noticed an increase in emergency room visits for atrial fibrillation among people who had been drinking heavily around Christmas and New Year's. Surmising a connection between binge drinking and atrial fibrillation, they coined the term "holiday heart syndrome." Subsequent observations suggested that binge drinking can precipitate atrial fibrillation in susceptible individuals and that chronic heavy drinkers are prone to arrhythmias. Moderate drinkers need not worry: having one to two drinks per day does not increase the risk of developing atrial fibrillation.

The relationship between coffee and atrial fibrillation has been studied more extensively than the alcohol connection. It is widely believed that caffeine causes atrial fibrillation. For the most part, this is a myth. While there are certainly a few people in whom caffeine triggers atrial fibrillation, in most of us it has no effect on heart rhythm, other than causing an occasional palpitation or a temporary increase in heart rate. Doctors frequently advise patients with atrial fibrillation to avoid caffeine, but we disagree with this wholesale recommendation. If you are one of the few people in whom caffeine causes atrial fibrillation, you should switch to decaf. But in most atrial fibrillation patients there is no relationship between coffee and heart rhythm; feel free to have your morning cup.

Diagnosis

Symptoms of atrial fibrillation include weariness or fatigue, shortness of breath, chest pain, decreased exercise capacity, and palpitations or a racing heartbeat. However, one-third of atrial fibrillation patients have no symptoms at all and are surprised and dismayed when a routine physical examination or EKG uncovers a heart rhythm abnormality. They should actually be glad that the atrial fibrillation has been identified before they suffered a serious complication such as a stroke.

Given that many people with atrial fibrillation have no symptoms, how can you tell if you are in atrial fibrillation? A definitive answer requires an EKG machine. But you can get a general idea just by taking your pulse.

Take the first two fingers of your right or left hand and place them in the center of your neck. Press in gently and slowly slide the fingers toward the side of your neck. They will enter a groove next to your Adam's apple. At that point, you should be able to feel the pulsation of your carotid artery. Each pulsation represents a heartbeat.

Feeling your pulse gives you information about your heart rhythm and your heart rate. First let's perform a rough assessment of your heart rhythm. Close your eyes as you feel your pulse. Do the pulsations occur at regular intervals? If so, you are probably not in atrial fibrillation. On the other hand, if the heartbeats come at irregular and unpredictable intervals, you may be in atrial fibrillation.

Next let's check your heart rate. Count the number of heartbeats in thirty seconds, and multiply by two. The product is your heart rate. A normal resting heart rate is 60 to 100 beats per minute. A resting heart rate greater than 100 may be caused by atrial fibrillation.

Make an appointment to see your doctor if your pulse is irregular or if your heart rate falls out of the normal 60-to-100-beats-per-minute range.

Treatment: Heart Rate and Rhythm

With 3 million Americans suffering from atrial fibrillation, you might think that we have treatment for this arrhythmia completely figured out. We don't. There is a great deal of controversy and, unfortunately, many patients receive incorrect treatment.

Treatment of atrial fibrillation is based upon three general principles:

1. *Control heart rate (all patients)*

2. *Correct heart rhythm (some patients)*

3. *Prevent strokes (all patients)*

The first priority in the person with atrial fibrillation is to ensure a normal heart rate. Too rapid a heart rate causes uncomfortable symptoms and, over time, can lead to permanent heart damage. The goal is to get the resting heart rate down to about eighty beats per minute or less. This is generally easily achieved with medicines, which usually include beta-blockers, calcium channel blockers, or occasionally digoxin.

Once the heart rate is controlled, the doctor and patient must tackle the big underlying question: what to do about the heart rhythm. The options are either to try to restore sinus rhythm or to leave you in atrial fibrillation with a well-controlled heart rate. For years, doctors and patients subscribed to the commonsense notion that restoring normal sinus rhythm should be the goal. After all, compared to people with atrial fibrillation, those in normal sinus rhythm live longer and do better. So our mission should be to get every patient with atrial fibrillation back into sinus rhythm, right?

Not so fast. Large randomized controlled trials have analyzed treatments for atrial fibrillation in thousands of patients and have uncovered no clear benefit to attempts to restore normal sinus rhythm in older people with limited or no symptoms—the majority of those with atrial fibrillation. This counterintuitive finding has been reproduced in several studies: most people with asymptomatic atrial fibrillation tend to do equally well whether we try to convert them to normal sinus rhythm or simply leave them in atrial fibrillation but control the heart rate.

This conclusion initially produced confusion, consternation, and controversy. But we now understand the reasons behind this surprising discovery. At issue is the group of medicines that we use to try to achieve sinus rhythm, which are called anti-arrhythmic drugs. They don't work very well and they have major side effects. In some cases, the medicine is worse than the disease.

After one year of treatment with anti-arrhythmic agents, only about half of patients have stayed in normal sinus rhythm. Eventually 20 to 30 percent of patients stop the medicine because of side effects, which range from nausea and vomiting to thyroid or liver problems and even blue skin. (That's right—long-term use of the potent anti-arrhythmic drug amiodarone can cause a person's skin to turn blue. This is uncommon, but it is striking—and often permanent.)

When anti-arrhythmic medicines restore sinus rhythm without causing side effects, people do tend to feel better. On the other hand, a strategy of controlling heart rate and leaving the person in atrial fibrillation is associated with fewer medication-induced side effects and hospital admissions. So which approach is better?

The answer depends upon the patient. In older people and those who are not bothered by the atrial fibrillation, controlling heart rate alone is often the preferred strategy. On the other hand, in a young person (younger than sixty) or someone who is very symptomatic, it is reasonable to try to restore sinus rhythm. You want your cardiologist to tailor the therapy to you, your symptoms, and your lifestyle.

Attempts to restore sinus rhythm may require electrical cardioversion. Using the same paddles that we apply in emergency situations, we deliver a small shock to the sedated patient, which "resets" the heart to normal sinus rhythm, much like rebooting your computer. However, it is not a cure, as 75 percent of patients return to atrial fibrillation within a year. Therefore, anti-arrhythmic medicines are generally prescribed after an electrical cardioversion to try to maintain sinus rhythm. If a medicine works initially and fails over time, we sometimes try a different medicine. But if two or three medicines fail or cause side effects, it is time to consider either leaving the person in atrial fibrillation and controlling heart rate, or pursuing an interventional strategy to restore sinus rhythm.

Ablation of Atrial Fibrillation

In recent years an innovative intervention, catheter ablation, has been increasingly used to restore sinus rhythm. In this procedure, an electrophysiologist threads a long, thin catheter through a vein in the leg and into the left atrium of the heart. This is done with X-ray guidance and does not require surgery. The doctor then delivers energy through the catheter to burn or freeze selected areas within the heart, to create scar tissue that strategically blocks abnormal impulses and their conduction. Successful treatment of atrial fibrillation is achieved in 60 to 85 percent of patients but depends greatly on the physician's skill and the patient's characteristics.

The ablation procedure is challenging for the doctor. It is like trying to hit a fastball thrown by a major-league pitcher; it can be done, but it requires an expert batter, not a Little Leaguer. You want an electrophysiologist with extensive experience with the procedure and a high success rate. In addition, you need to ensure that you are a good candidate for the procedure. The patients who do best are those who are relatively young and who have intermittent (paroxysmal) atrial fibrillation and no enlargement of the heart.

Before catheter ablation, you need to have realistic expectations. Don't be alarmed if the procedure does not immediately restore sinus rhythm. Atrial fibrillation recurrence in the first three months after catheter ablation is very common, though it frequently resolves with time and medicines. But if you are still having atrial fibrillation four months or more after the procedure, it is worth considering a repeat catheter ablation. About 30 percent of patients require a second catheter ablation, sometimes called a "touch-up." Your doctor should discuss these issues with you *before* the first ablation.

If catheter ablation works in 60 to 85 percent of atrial fibrillation patients, you might ask why we don't use it as first-line therapy. The answer is that it carries a risk of complications, just like any medical procedure. Overall, about 2 to 5 percent of patients suffer a complication as a result of catheter ablation. Death is rare, but other problems, including a buildup of fluid around the heart, damage to the blood vessels in the leg, scarring of the veins that enter the heart from the lungs, and injury to the nerves that control breathing (the phrenic nerves), occur occasionally and can be troublesome. This is the reason that we currently recommend catheter ablation only in selected patients who have symptoms from atrial fibrillation and for whom medical therapy fails to work.

LONE ATRIAL FIBRILLATION: A BETTER PROGNOSIS

In general, atrial fibrillation is associated with decreased longevity and increased risk of complications, most notably stroke. However, one group of atrial fibrillation patients does not have this unfavorable prognosis. Young patients (under sixty) who are otherwise healthy and have no other heart disease are said to have "lone atrial fibrillation," meaning that the arrhythmia is not associated with other conditions such as hypertension. In these people, atrial fibrillation carries only a minimally increased risk of stroke and no increased risk of death. When highly symptomatic, these patients are ideal candidates for catheter ablation.

Stroke Prevention

While controversy exists about whether we need to restore sinus rhythm in patients with atrial fibrillation, doctors agree that every patient with atrial fibrillation should have a plan to prevent stroke—the most feared complication of atrial fibrillation. Atrial fibrillation causes 15 to 20 percent of all strokes, accounting for 75,000 strokes per year in the United States. Strokes caused by atrial fibrillation tend to be larger than those caused by other conditions. One-third of the strokes caused by atrial fibrillation are fatal.

Why do people with atrial fibrillation suffer strokes? The strokes are caused by blood clots that form in the heart. These blood clots develop as a result of two factors: the slow movement of blood in the fibrillating atrium, giving the blood time to clot, and a general increased tendency for blood to clot in patients with atrial fibrillation. Blood tends to clot in an area of the heart called the left atrial appendage, which is like a little cul-de-sac, about as large as your thumb, attached to the heart. If a blood clot forms in the left atrial appendage and a piece of it breaks off, the clot enters the circulation and travels to the brain, where it wedges in one of the brain's arteries, cuts off blood flow, and causes a stroke.

Most strokes associated with atrial fibrillation are preventable. The key to prevention is taking medicines that reduce blood clotting. Warfarin (Coumadin) and aspirin are the two most commonly used medicines for this purpose. Warfarin prevents blood clotting by reducing the liver's production of several of the proteins that cause blood to clot, while aspirin works by inhibiting the action of platelets in the blood.

Warfarin is far more effective than aspirin. In atrial fibrillation patients, warfarin reduces the risk of stroke by about 60 percent, compared to only a 20 percent reduction with aspirin. In addition, warfarin is the only medicine proven to reduce the risk of dying among people with atrial fibrillation. But this efficacy comes with some downsides. Warfarin is associated with an increased risk of bleeding, ranging from about 1 to 10 percent per year, depending upon the patient. When bleeding occurs in the brain, it causes a stroke, the very outcome we try to prevent with warfarin. (A stroke caused by bleeding in the brain is called a hemorrhagic stroke; a stroke caused by a clot blocking an artery in the brain is called an ischemic stroke.)

Once again, individualizing therapy is the key. We need to balance the risk of ischemic stroke and the risk of bleeding. We focus first on the stroke side of the equation, as we choose between warfarin, aspirin, and no therapy. Without any preventive treatment, the average stroke risk is about 3 to 5 percent per year among patients with atrial fibrillation. However, this risk varies from person to person depending upon other characteristics. Patients at the highest risk, particularly those who have had a previous ischemic stroke, should take warfarin. On the other hand, those at the lowest risk should usually take aspirin. A simple scoring system can help you determine the right treatment for you.

Scoring System for Stroke Risk in Atrial Fibrillation

CONDITION	POINTS
Age 75 or older	1
High blood pressure (hypertension)	1
Diabetes	1
Congestive heart failure	1
History of ischemic stroke or transient ischemic attack (TIA, or mini-stroke)	2

Using the table, add up the points that correspond to your medical situation. If your score is 0—you have none of these conditions—you should probably take an aspirin a day (81 to 325 mg) for stroke prevention. If your score is 1, warfarin or aspirin is acceptable, although warfarin is preferred. If your score is 2 or greater, warfarin is generally the better choice.

Most people with atrial fibrillation have one or more of the conditions in the table, so warfarin is usually the obvious choice for stroke prevention. But what about the risk of bleeding? A history of bleeding from the gastrointestinal tract, other bleeding problems, or a high risk of trauma (particularly from falls in unsteady seniors) makes 25 percent of people unsuitable for warfarin. Such patients are treated with aspirin or aspirin plus clopidogrel, which are less effective than warfarin but have less risk of bleeding.

After weighing the risks of ischemic stroke and bleeding, we face additional challenges with warfarin treatment. Although we are generally clear on who should receive warfarin for stroke prevention, the medicine is underused. One-third of atrial fibrillation patients who should be taking warfarin do not take it. Sometimes a person simply refuses; in other cases the doctor fails to prescribe the medicine. For those who do take warfarin as recommended, it can be very difficult to maintain the required level of inhibition of blood clotting. In fact, at any given moment, only about half of patients on warfarin are getting the optimal effect. The problem is that warfarin is a difficult medicine for patients to take. It requires lifestyle changes and commitments that extend beyond filling a prescription and taking a pill.

CHALLENGES WITH WARFARIN THERAPY

Monthly (or more often) blood test is necessary to optimize dosing

Diet (especially leafy green vegetables) can interfere with warfarin action

Interacts with many other medicines

Dose is different for different people

Dose can vary for a given person over time

Takes several days to reach desired level of action

AN ALTERNATIVE TO WARFARIN

Warfarin was approved for use in 1954 and for more than fifty years was the only good option for stroke prevention in atrial fibrillation. But now, alternatives are emerging. As a result of a landmark FDA decision on October 18, 2010, we finally have a substitute. A study of 18,000 people demonstrated that the new drug dabigatran (Pradaxa) was equally effective as warfarin at preventing strokes in atrial fibrillation. Blocking blood clotting by a different mechanism than warfarin, dabigatran is a twice-a-day medicine that does not require any monitoring using blood tests. Unlike warfarin, the same dose is appropriate for nearly everyone (in the absence of kidney disease, where a lower dose is prescribed). If you currently take warfarin and have no problems with this medicine or complaints about the necessary blood tests, we recommend that you stick with that drug. However, if your warfarin has been difficult to regulate or the inconvenience associated with the medicine is great, ask your doctor about switching to dabigatran. One caveat, though: dabigatran is more expensive. The annual cost of dabigatran is $2,884, versus only $1,761 per year for one year of warfarin and the related blood tests.

The bottom line here is pretty simple. If you have atrial fibrillation, risk factors for stroke, and no strong medical reason not to take an anticoagulant such as warfarin, take this medicine! Warfarin is vastly underprescribed, particularly in the elderly. Older people stand to gain the largest benefit from warfarin or dabigatran and face the greatest risk if these medicines are not prescribed. Advanced age is not a reason not to take warfarin, unless the person has an unsteady gait and is prone to falls.

No matter what your age, if you have atrial fibrillation, discuss stroke prevention with your doctor, so that you can avoid the problems encountered by our patient Catherine Henry and keep dancing through life.

RX: KEEPING IN RHYTHM

Do not ignore palpitations or fainting spells if:

 They are accompanied by chest pain or shortness of breath

 They occur together

If you feel worse after receiving a pacemaker, ask your doctor about "pacemaker syndrome"

If you have severe heart damage or heart failure, ask your doctor if a pacemaker or defibrillator is right for you

If you have a pacemaker or defibrillator, avoid:

 MRI scans

 Lingering near theft detection devices at stores

If your pacemaker or defibrillator is recalled:

 Get the facts: manufacturer, model, device, serial number

 Realize that not all recalled devices must be replaced

 Develop a course of action with your doctor

Teach yourself, your friends, and your family how to help a person who collapses suddenly:

 Avoid delays, which can be deadly

 Perform chest compressions

 Learn how to use an automatic external defibrillator

If you have atrial fibrillation, discuss these three points with your doctor:

 Control of heart rate

 Prevention of stroke

 Return to sinus rhythm

CHAPTER 15

LIVING WITH HEART FAILURE

THE BIG PICTURE

"You have heart failure."

It sounds like a death sentence. Each year, more than 500,000 Americans are stunned to hear these words from their doctors. These new patients join the ranks of the nation's 5 million people living with heart failure. Our plan is to help both recently diagnosed heart failure patients and those who were previously diagnosed by explaining heart failure and detailing the many effective treatment options available.

The most important concept to understand about heart failure (also called congestive heart failure) is that receiving this diagnosis does not imply that the end is near. Simply put, congestive heart failure means that the heart is unable to fully meet the circulatory demands of the body. We will not stand before you like a doctor on *Grey's Anatomy* and offer a solemn pronouncement: "You have six months to live." (We must have missed the day in medical school when the professors explained how to precisely determine a person's life span.) But we do know this: with proper treatment, most heart failure patients can maintain a good quality of life and live for years.

HEART FAILURE AFTER A HEART ATTACK: CARL BRUCE GETS OUT OF THE WOODS

Carl Bruce and his wife came to us searching for a way to treat his heart failure and reclaim his life. A top-performing fifty-four-year-old real estate executive, Carl had suffered a seemingly uncomplicated heart attack three years earlier. The episode began one evening, shortly after a dinner meeting, when Carl noticed subtle chest tightness and mild shortness of breath. Attributing these symptoms to indigestion, he took an antacid and went to bed early.

After a restless night, Carl awoke in the morning feeling extremely tired and very short of breath. He called his family doctor, who directed him to the emergency department. Carl asked if he could wait until after work, as he was nearing the end of important negotiations to purchase a shopping center, but his doctor told him to go to the hospital immediately. Anticipating a brief interruption to his day, Carl donned a suit and grabbed his briefcase so that he would be prepared for his afternoon slate of meetings.

Within minutes of his arrival at the hospital, Carl had an EKG and a diagnosis. His EKG showed clear evidence of a recent heart attack, which had probably occurred during his bout of "indigestion" the night before. The doctors determined that Carl's heart attack was already over, with more than twelve hours having elapsed since an artery on his heart became blocked, so there was no reason to rush to the cardiac catheterization laboratory and place a stent to open the blocked artery. The doctors would instead focus on monitoring Carl and crafting a plan for his future cardiac care.

Carl did not make it to work that day. Exchanging his suit for a hospital gown with that special open-at-the-back feature, Carl settled in for a four-day hospital stay. A night in the coronary care unit confirmed a stable heart rhythm, so Carl spent the remaining three days on a regular hospital floor. Prior to discharge, his cardiologist performed a heart catheterization to determine the extent and severity of Carl's coronary artery blockages. The coronary angiogram showed a complete blockage of the left anterior descending coronary artery, the largest and most important artery on the heart. Carl's other two major coronary arteries had only minor narrowings. An echocardiogram showed the damage to Carl's heart. The front wall of the left ventricle no longer contracted vigorously with each heartbeat, and Carl's ejection fraction (a measure of heart function) was 45 percent, slightly below the normal value of 50 to 60 percent. The damage was not too extensive, and the doctors forecast an excellent prognosis. In a few weeks Carl could return to work and resume all of his previous activities.

Although the doctors were optimistic, Carl did not like the idea of living with heart damage. He wanted to know why his doctors could not perform a procedure to repair his heart. After all, he knew that cardiologists and surgeons had all kinds of interventions to treat heart problems. His doctors explained that they had no magic medicine to fix the damage caused by a heart attack. Going forward, there were two cardiac goals: to prevent Carl from having any more heart attacks and to avoid the development of heart failure.

Carl's heart team did well with heart attack prevention but missed critical opportunities to avoid heart failure. Spurred to action by his heart attack, Carl quit smoking, adopted a Mediterranean diet, and adhered to his prescriptions for daily doses of simvastatin (a statin drug) and aspirin. Six months later, his lipid panel showed excellent cholesterol levels and his EKG revealed no new problems. The cardiologist once again told Carl that his prognosis was excellent, recommended adding an exercise program, and told him to return for annual visits.

Carl thought that he was home free. For the next two years, he did well. He had no chest pain or shortness of breath, and the memories of his heart attack faded. He was physically active, although he never started an exercise program because of the demands of his job. His next two annual visits to the cardiologist were uneventful, each one ending with the advice to "keep doing what you are doing." But Carl would soon learn that these recommendations were insufficient.

About three years after his heart attack, Carl developed new symptoms. He was tired all of the time and he became short of breath when climbing stairs or walking uphill. With no chest pain, he figured that he was just getting older. But when a single flight of stairs began to feel like Mt. Everest, Carl finally called his cardiologist. The doctor listened to his story and performed an echocardiogram, Carl's first since the heart attack. The echo revealed an enlarged left ventricle and an ejection fraction of only 25 percent, meaning that his heart function was less than half of normal. The cardiologist next ordered a repeat cardiac catheterization to determine whether Carl's worsening symptoms and reduced heart function were due to new coronary blockages. The catheterization showed no changes in Carl's arteries.

Then the cardiologist dropped the bomb; Carl had congestive heart failure (CHF), meaning that his heart was unable to pump enough blood to meet his body's needs. To Carl and his wife, this was as stunning and scary a diagnosis as they could imagine. The cardiologist prescribed new medicines, including a diuretic to reduce the shortness of breath and a small dose of an angiotensin receptor blocker (ARB) to help with heart function. With these drugs, his shortness of breath improved, but Carl was still easily fatigued and he felt doomed. He became depressed. Finally he made an appointment to come to the Cleveland Clinic to see if anything more could be done.

We easily confirmed Carl's diagnosis of mild CHF. He appeared well, although he and his wife were very anxious. His blood pressure was 140/85 and his heart rate was eighty-six beats per minute. We wanted to see lower values for both. Carl's medical treatment was inadequate. He needed a medication overhaul, or, as we say, "a tune-up." We stopped his diuretic and ARB and put him on a better heart failure regimen that included an ACE inhibitor.

Within a month, Carl's blood pressure was down to 120/75 and his pulse had dropped to seventy-eight beats per minute. Carl felt better. His fatigue was gone and he could climb two flights of stairs without shortness of breath, although he still became a bit winded when walking briskly up the long hill near his house. We moved to the next step in his heart failure plan by starting him on a beta-blocker. The combination of a beta-blocker and an ACE inhibitor—the two critical medicines for heart failure patients—is essential to improving the prognosis of patients with heart failure. Most important, Carl reported that he felt good.

Over the next eight months, Carl stayed on his medications. We repeated his echocardiogram after a year and found that his ejection fraction had increased to 40 percent—certainly not normal, but much better than the 25 percent value he had when we first saw him. We helped him construct an aerobic exercise program to further increase his endurance; soon he was walking briskly for thirty to forty minutes five days a week and playing tennis on weekends. His depression disappeared. Four years after his heart attack, Carl reclaimed his life thanks to good heart failure treatments.

Carl Bruce's story illustrates many of the key issues in the management of congestive heart failure. It is critically important to remember that CHF is often preventable. Like Carl, many heart attack patients initially recover with reasonably normal heart function and only a mild decrease in the ejection fraction. But even so, many heart attack survivors need an ACE inhibitor, and all of them need a beta-blocker. Without appropriate medicines, over the ensuing months and years the heart undergoes structural changes (dilation) and its function often declines. Congestive heart failure can gradually develop in patients who thought that they were fine after surviving a heart attack.

Unfortunately, Carl Bruce did not receive the proper prophylactic treatment, and as a consequence developed CHF three years after his heart attack. Even after he presented with congestive heart failure, he received inadequate medical treatment that only partially relieved his symptoms. Fortunately, it was not too late for him. Today, more than two years after his initial diagnosis of congestive heart failure, Carl remains nearly symptom-free and has a positive outlook on life. While Carl thought that his improvement was nothing short of a miracle, we knew that it was a simple and predictable result of the right treatment. If you or a family member has congestive heart failure, we will help you improve your symptoms and prognosis so that you, like Carl, can live life to its fullest.

CONGESTIVE HEART FAILURE: WHAT IT IS AND WHAT CAUSES IT

As we have emphasized, congestive heart failure does not mean that your heart is about to stop beating and that death is imminent. It just means that the heart can't pump the full amount of blood the body needs.

The prognosis and treatment of CHF depend to some extent on the disease that originally caused the heart damage. Many disorders lead to heart failure; these include coronary heart disease, heart valve problems, high blood pressure, and cardiomyopathies (diseases of the heart muscle).

Coronary Heart Disease with a Heart Attack

Coronary heart disease is the most common cause of heart failure. Today's heart failure epidemic is actually attributable in large part to the great improvements in our treatment of heart attacks. Decades ago, up to 25 percent of heart attack victims died within a few days. Today, more than 90 percent survive, creating a growing population of people living with damaged hearts. Many of these individuals eventually develop heart failure.

The typical CHF patient has suffered one or more heart attacks that have severely damaged the heart muscle. Because heart muscle cells

HEART FUNCTION BY THE NUMBERS:
UNDERSTANDING YOUR EJECTION FRACTION

If you have congestive heart failure or almost any other important cardiac issue, you have probably had an echocardiogram. One of the key results of the echocardiogram is a measurement of your left ventricle's ejection fraction. The ejection fraction reflects the function of your left ventricle, your heart's main primary pumping chamber, and is the percentage of the blood in your left ventricle that is ejected with each heartbeat. A normal ejection fraction is 50 percent or greater; your heart does not squeeze out every drop of blood each time that it beats.

Although the ejection fraction is an important measurement of heart function, it does not tell the entire story when it comes to a person's cardiac status or prognosis. Patients often express great concern about a low ejection fraction, but we remind them not to focus excessively on this single measure of heart function. Every experienced heart doctor has encountered patients with an ejection fraction of 10 percent who function well, performing nearly all activities of daily living without difficulty. In addition, people are often confused by discrepancies in ejection fraction measured by different imaging studies; while we usually rely on echocardiography, doctors can also estimate this number from MRI scans, nuclear medicine studies, and cardiac catheterizations. Don't let minor variations in measurements from different types of tests worry you.

Each time you have an echocardiogram, note your ejection fraction. If it is falling, particularly in the setting of worsening symptoms, take the initiative and ask if there are ways to improve it. But if you are on the right medicines and your symptoms are stable and well controlled, don't let a falling ejection fraction send you into a psychological tailspin. How you feel and function is more important than the number.

---

cannot regenerate, damage is permanent. Loss of muscle mass due to multiple heart attacks is cumulative. Thus, a second or third heart attack further damages heart muscle, eventually compromising the heart's ability to contract vigorously, resulting in heart failure.

For most patients with CHF, the common pattern includes a series of heart attacks that produce sufficient cumulative damage to chronically impair heart function. But as in the case of Carl Bruce, even a single heart attack can sometimes cause enough muscle damage to result in CHF. Any heart attack should automatically trigger a plan devised by you and your doctor to prevent both future heart attacks and the development of CHF. Smoking cessation, control of cholesterol and high blood pressure, a good diet, and daily exercise are critically important. In addition, the right medical regimen, usually including an ACE inhibitor and a beta-blocker, is very important as part of post-heart-attack care; such a program might have prevented Carl's heart failure.

Coronary Heart Disease Without a Heart Attack

In some patients, coronary heart disease causes heart failure without permanently damaging heart muscle. Here's how this problem can occur. Patients may gradually develop coronary artery blockages that reduce blood flow to the heart muscle but never actually cause a heart attack. If a blockage in an artery becomes very severe, there may be inadequate blood flow to meet the needs of the heart muscle. The heart responds to this shortfall by reducing the force of contraction in the area with inadequate blood supply. This adaptive mechanism allows the heart muscle to continue to survive, albeit at a lower level of performance. If enough heart muscle is contracting poorly because of chronically inadequate blood flow, the patient develops CHF. The medical term for this living but dormant heart muscle is "hibernating myocardium."

It is important to recognize patients with this situation, because their heart failure is potentially reversible. Detection of hibernating but viable heart muscle is critically important when assessing heart failure patients with coronary heart disease. We often see patients who have been told that their heart failure is irreversible and their prognosis poor. However, in certain patients, correcting coronary blockages with stenting or bypass surgery can actually reverse CHF. When we bring a normal blood supply to the hibernating muscle, it contracts better and the CHF improves or even disappears.

If you have CHF and coronary heart disease, your doctor should look for muscle that is starved for blood. We have several imaging techniques to detect this sort of viable but dormant heart muscle, including PET scans and MRI scans. Identification of hibernating myocardium is particularly important if the degree of CHF seems excessive for the extent of heart muscle known to be damaged by previous heart attacks.

Heart Valve Disease

Heart valve disease is an important but often overlooked cause of CHF. In the first half of the twentieth century, heart valve damage due to rheumatic fever was a common cause of heart failure and was often fatal. Rheumatic fever is caused by a streptococcus infection, often related to something as innocuous as a strep throat. Two pivotal innovations in medicine lessened the cardiac toll of rheumatic fever: the development of penicillin in the 1940s and the advent of surgery to repair and replace heart valves in the 1950s. Penicillin, if given early after a strep infection and continued for at least ten days, effectively prevents development of rheumatic fever and heart valve damage. Don't ignore a persistent sore throat in your children.

When rheumatic fever does cause heart valve damage, we either repair the valve or replace it with an artificial valve. (See Chapter 13 for more on valve replacement surgery.) Today, rheumatic heart disease is on the decline, but other heart valve problems have taken its place, including spontaneous degeneration and bacterial infections of heart valves.

To prevent heart failure from heart valve disease, we need to fix the valve *before* the patient develops irreversible heart damage. While many patients and doctors withhold surgery until severe symptoms develop, this can be a costly strategy. We often see asymptomatic patients with irreversible heart damage. They have missed the best window for safe and effective surgery. In heart valve patients, routine echocardiograms—usually performed annually—often detect changes in heart function before symptoms occur. These cardiac changes represent the first signs of heart damage and should trigger surgical repair to prevent development of more serious damage. If you have known heart valve issues, don't skip your annual echocardiogram just because you feel fine.

We recognize that many patients want to put off having heart valve surgery for as long as possible. The good news here is that our techniques for fixing heart valves are becoming less and less invasive. We can now replace an aortic valve through a catheter in the leg, instead of having to do traditional open-chest surgery. We can perform mitral valve procedures through tiny incisions. These therapies are becoming increasingly common. Don't avoid your doctor; putting off heart valve surgery can open the door to heart damage and heart failure.

HEART FAILURE WITH "NORMAL" HEART FUNCTION

Most heart failure patients have heart damage that impairs the heart's ability to pump. We call this *systolic* heart failure because systole is the part of the cardiac cycle, or heartbeat, that includes ejection of blood. Other patients, particularly elderly patients with high blood pressure, suffer from *diastolic* heart failure, a condition in which the heart actually pumps well but has trouble relaxing enough to fill with blood before its next contraction. These heart failure patients often have entirely normal systolic left ventricular function and a normal ejection fraction.

The idea that that a person could have normal pumping function and heart failure at the same time initially made little sense to doctors, until we figured out that fully normal heart function requires that the heart both contract forcefully to eject blood and relax to fill with blood before each contraction. In patients with diastolic heart failure, stiff, abnormally thickened heart muscle does not relax completely, and blood backs up in the lungs, resulting in congestion and shortness of breath. If you have these symptoms, high blood pressure, and normal pumping function, the astute doctor will look beyond your ejection fraction and prescribe appropriate treatment to control your blood pressure and help you and your heart to relax and feel better.

High Blood Pressure

Hypertension remains an important cause of heart failure. Surprisingly, many patients with CHF due to hypertension have only a modest increase in blood pressure, although they have usually had elevated blood pressure for many years. When the heart is forced to pump against an elevated blood pressure, the muscle of the left ventricle gradually thickens. This process is similar to the increased muscle bulk produced by weight training. The thick left ventricle becomes stiff and difficult to fill with blood, which causes pressure in the heart to rise and leads to congestion in the lungs. This causes diastolic heart failure. Eventually, after years of pumping against an elevated pressure, the thickened left ventricle dilates and begins to fail, resulting in reduced pumping function and systolic heart failure.

We can prevent people with hypertension from developing heart failure if the elevated blood pressure is recognized and treated early. If the hypertensive patient does develop heart failure, appropriate treatments can still provide major benefits. CHF tends to stabilize if blood pressure is lowered to normal early in the disease process, and the heart muscle may even return to normal thickness.

Cardiomyopathies

Both coronary heart disease and hypertension are diseases that indirectly damage heart muscle, ultimately causing heart failure. In other patients, the heart fails because of disorders that directly affect the heart muscle. The term *cardiomyopathy* refers to a spectrum of diseases that attack the heart muscle and impair its structure and function. There are several types of this disorder, including dilated cardiomyopathy, in which all of the chambers are enlarged, and hypertrophic cardiomyopathy, in which the heart muscle is abnormally thickened. Some of these have a genetic basis, while in other cases the cause is unknown.

Viral cardiomyopathy is a particularly insidious condition in which a viral infection directly damages heart muscle, producing either temporary or permanent heart failure. Sometimes after a seemingly innocuous upper respiratory tract infection, viral damage to the heart muscle causes rapid development of CHF. Another, increasingly common cause of cardiomyopathy is cancer chemotherapy, which can directly damage heart muscle. Each of these heart muscle disorders has a different prognosis and may require somewhat different treatments. If you develop heart failure caused by a cardiomyopathy, you should see a heart failure specialist to ensure that you receive a medical regimen tailored to your specific cardiac condition.

TREATMENTS FOR CHF

Although CHF is a serious disorder, the prognosis for patients with heart failure has never been better. We have a wide and growing array of options that enable us to impact both quality and longevity of life in most patients.

HEART FAILURE TREATMENTS

Lifestyle

Low-salt diet

Aerobic exercise

Smoking cessation

General risk factor reduction

Medications

ACE inhibitor

Beta-blocker

ARB

Diuretic

Aldosterone antagonist

Electrical therapies

Special pacemaker

Implantable defibrillator

Surgical therapies

Ventricular assist device

Heart transplant

Medicines for Heart Failure

ACE Inhibitors and ARBs

Appropriate medical therapy represents the cornerstone of treatment for CHF. Once we started Carl Bruce on the right medicines, he improved dramatically. How did these medicines increase his heart function and reduce his symptoms?

The main pumping chamber of the heart, the left ventricle, ejects blood into the aorta, which then carries blood to all of the body's tissues. When it contracts, the left ventricle must overcome the blood pressure in the aorta, a force known as "afterload." By lowering blood pressure, we can reduce the force against which the heart must work, making the heart's job easier. This is the idea behind ACE inhibitors, which reduce blood pressure by causing blood vessels to relax and dilate. This drop in blood pressure re-

EXERCISE TO TREAT HEART FAILURE

Unfortunately, the myth that exercise is dangerous for the heart patient is a common misconception. Nearly all heart patients can benefit from exercise, and this holds true for patients with heart failure and heart damage.

Patients with congestive heart failure usually have reduced exercise capacity, and this obviously makes it harder to exercise. Our advice is to do whatever you must to find the motivation to exercise. Play the theme from *Rocky*. Watch *Chariots of Fire*. Tune in to *The Biggest Loser*. Or consider this: aerobic exercise significantly improves quality of life in heart failure patients.

The keys to safety and success are to start aerobic exercise slowly and to increase gradually. Walking is the ideal form of aerobic exercise for the heart failure patient. Resistance training confers little benefit, and heavy weight lifting may even be harmful in this subset of cardiac patients.

The benefits of aerobic exercise are actually not related to a direct effect on the heart. Aerobic exercise works by increasing muscle efficiency, improving the ability of the body's muscles to extract oxygen from the blood. For CHF patients with impaired heart function, this improved muscle efficiency increases exercise capacity, even though the ejection fraction remains low. With exercise training, you can do more with less.

duces the left ventricle's workload and increases its ability to eject blood. As a result, the ejection fraction goes up and an enlarged heart may even shrink toward normal size. ACE inhibitors, discussed in detail in Chapter 11, represent first-line therapy for CHF patients; if a patient cannot tolerate these medicines, we switch to the closely related angiotensin receptor blockers (ARBs), which act by a similar mechanism.

Why do ACE inhibitors and ARBs work so well in treating CHF? We turn to human evolution to answer this question. Over the course of thousands of years, our bodies developed systems designed to protect us from harm. Our ancient ancestors rarely suffered from coronary heart disease or atherosclerosis because of their lifestyles, which included fresh, low-calorie foods and high levels of physical activity. But their world was dangerous, and their greatest health danger was trauma. The tiger in the jungle was a much greater threat than a heart attack. So humans evolved reflexes and mechanisms to protect against blood loss from trauma, mechanisms that today often backfire and contribute to the development of CHF.

In the heart failure patient, the damaged heart does not pump the normal amount of blood. The body senses this reduced blood flow and "thinks" that the person is bleeding. A series of automatic reflexes causes the brain and kidneys to release hormones that constrict blood vessels, attempting to restore blood pressure. The most powerful chemical released by this reflex is angiotensin, the very substance blocked by ACE inhibitors and ARBs. While these adaptations help the trauma victim to survive, in the patient with CHF this cascade of events hurts instead of helps.

Although cardiac output is diminished, the CHF patient is not bleeding. The automatic and inappropriate constriction of blood vessels forces the heart to pump against a higher pressure, essentially making the heart work harder. This further reduces ejection fraction, leading to release of more angiotensin and a downward spiral that increases stress on the heart. ACE inhibitors break this vicious cycle.

When it comes to heart failure, ACE inhibitors have a dual role: *preventing* development of CHF in heart attack victims and *treating* heart failure in those with established CHF. If an ACE inhibitor is given prophylactically after a large heart attack, the heart's workload is reduced and the left ventricle is spared the gradual deterioration that results in CHF. Carl Bruce's doctors missed this opportunity. When we saw him, he already had heart failure. But ACE inhibitors still helped, easing his heart's work and improving its function. As his ejection fraction increased, his symptoms abated, and his left ventricle gradually returned toward normal size.

Using ACE inhibitors in the heart failure patient requires expertise and care. ACE inhibitors reduce blood pressure, which may present a dilemma because some CHF patients already have a relatively low blood pressure. As a consequence, after an ACE inhibitor is started, you may feel dizzy, particularly when standing suddenly (this is known as postural hypotension). Don't give up on the medicine if this happens. In patients with a low blood pressure, we may need to start ACE inhibitors at a low dosage and slowly increase the dose over weeks to months. Patience and persistence can make a big difference. When starting an ACE inhibitor, take care to stand up slowly and get out of bed in stages, first sitting for a minute or two and then standing up. In most patients, the body adjusts over time and dizziness subsides.

ACE inhibitors offer huge benefits in long-term treatment of CHF.

High-quality randomized clinical trials demonstrate that these drugs extend life and reduce the need for hospitalization. Additional studies confirm that ACE inhibitors improve symptoms and quality of life in CHF patients. However, many patients who might benefit from ACE inhibitors don't receive these drugs. One problem is that ACE inhibitors can acutely impair kidney function. Kidney insufficiency is common in CHF patients, often as a result of reduced blood flow to the kidneys, and many physicians are reluctant to use ACE inhibitors in patients with even a mild degree of preexisting kidney dysfunction. But this approach is shortsighted. Because ACE inhibitors improve heart function, many patients with mild to moderate kidney impairment will eventually show *improved* kidney function if treated long-term with these drugs. In most patients with mild to moderate kidney dysfunction, a trial of ACE inhibitors is warranted (with monitoring of the kidneys). If kidney function deteriorates, it will almost always return to normal if the ACE inhibitor is stopped.

About 5 to 10 percent of patients develop an annoying cough after starting an ACE inhibitor. If this symptom is mild, the substantial benefits of the drugs may be worth tolerating the side effect. However, in some patients the cough is intolerable. Fortunately, we have a pretty good alternative that does not cause coughing: angiotensin receptor blockers. Many doctors consider ARBs to be slightly less effective than ACE inhibitors in patients with congestive heart failure, and the data showing benefits of ARBs are less robust compared with studies of ACE inhibitors. Therefore, ACE inhibitors, if tolerated, are always preferred. Another reason we prefer ACE inhibitors is cost; most ARBs are still available only as brand-name drugs and are relatively expensive, although many will become generic in the next few years.

Recognizing that both ACE inhibitors and ARBs help patients with heart failure, physicians naturally wondered if we could double the benefit by giving patients both types of drugs. Randomized clinical trials examining this strategy produced mixed results, with some showing additional benefits and others identifying potentially dangerous side effects from the combination, including increased blood levels of potassium and greater impairment of kidney function in susceptible patients. We combine ACE inhibitors and ARBs only for selected patients with severe heart failure. We do not add the ARB until we have reached the maximum dose of the ACE inhibitor, and we closely monitor potassium levels and kidney function. ACE inhibitors and ARBs should be combined only under the direction of a specialist in congestive heart failure.

Beta-blockers

Beta-blockers are extraordinarily valuable in treating patients with congestive heart failure. Like ACE inhibitors, beta-blockers' effectiveness can be traced to our evolutionary development of lifesaving reflexes. As noted earlier, when the heart fails, the body interprets the reduced cardiac output as blood loss. The brain responds by triggering a critical reflex that increases blood levels of adrenaline (epinephrine), the hormone responsible for the fight-or-flight reaction, including the racing heart that we all experience when frightened or stressed. Unfortunately, in the heart failure patient, surging adrenaline levels actually damage the heart and cause muscle cells to die. This worsens heart failure.

Well-conducted studies have shown that using beta-blockers in heart failure patients blocks the effects of adrenaline and prevents further heart damage, allowing the heart to heal and eventually increasing the ability of the heart muscle to contract. This helps to extend life, significantly reduce hospitalizations, and improve exercise capacity and quality of life. Now beta-blockers have become the standard of care for most CHF patients.

Although heart failure patients derive enormous benefits from administration of beta-blockers, starting these drugs can be tricky. As we noted in Chapter 11, beta-blockers can acutely worsen CHF symptoms. The key to successful administration of these drugs in CHF is to start with a very low dose and increase it slowly while closely monitoring the patient for worsening symptoms. If you initially get worse when you begin beta-blocker therapy, don't become discouraged. Most patients will tolerate gradually increasing dosages. Abandoning beta-blockers too quickly is the wrong move.

Don't be alarmed if your doctor does not start a beta-blocker immediately after your initial diagnosis of heart failure. Beta-blockers are a long-term treatment for CHF. When patients are hospitalized for CHF, we focus on treating the most severe symptoms first, then add low-dose beta-blockers as part of the long-term management plan.

DRUGS TO AVOID IN CONGESTIVE HEART FAILURE

In addition to telling you which drugs heart failure patients should take, we must also highlight those that should be avoided. Some common medicines can trigger or worsen heart failure symptoms in susceptible patients. Among these, the non-steroidal anti-inflammatory drugs (NSAIDs) are notorious. These medicines include prescription and over-the-counter pain relievers such as ibuprofen (Motrin and Advil), naproxen (Aleve), celecoxib (Celebrex), and dozens of others. These drugs decrease the kidneys' ability to excrete salt and water, resulting in fluid accumulation that can trigger heart failure symptoms. Acetaminophen (Tylenol) does not have this property and therefore does not worsen heart failure.

Calcium channel blockers, a class of drugs used to treat high blood pressure, can also worsen CHF. Two of the calcium channel blockers, diltiazem (Cardizem and other brands) and verapamil (Calan and other brands), are particularly problematic. These agents decrease the contractile force of the left ventricle, which can worsen heart failure.

The medical management of heart failure is complex and precarious. Before starting a new medicine, whether prescribed by a doctor or plucked off the drugstore shelf to ease a sore back, check with your cardiologist to make sure that you are not endangering your heart.

Diuretics (Water Pills)

When the heart fails, it pumps less blood to all of the organs, including the kidneys; this impairs the kidneys' ability to perform one of their key jobs, the removal of salt and water from the body. Further compounding the problem, the kidneys in heart failure patients actually release hormones that cause retention of salt and water. The resulting increase in circulating fluid causes congestion in the lungs. When this happens, the patient experiences shortness of breath, particularly during exercising or when lying flat in bed at night. If enough fluid accumulates, the ankles and feet swell, a condition termed edema.

To help remove this excess fluid that accumulates in their lungs and ankles, many CHF patients require diuretics—medicines that stimulate the kidneys to excrete salt and water. With appropriate diuresis, a fluid-overloaded CHF patient may lose ten or more pounds of fluid in just a few days. With this fluid loss comes reduced shortness of breath and ankle swelling, often prompting patients to say, "I feel like a new person."

The most commonly used diuretic in CHF patients is furosemide (Lasix), a powerful drug that can be given orally or by injection. Within minutes of its administration, urine output increases dramatically. In fact, patients taking furosemide quickly learn that it is prudent to have access to a bathroom for the first hour or two after taking this drug. As with ACE inhibitors and beta-blockers, careful dose adjustment is important. If you take too little diuretic, your lungs become congested and your ankles swell; if you take too much, you'll become dehydrated. Overdiuresis can also impair kidney function (usually temporarily) and deplete your body of sodium, potassium, and other electrolytes such as magnesium.

Aldosterone Antagonists

Aldosterone antagonists work by influencing the same hormone system blocked by ACE inhibitors and ARBs. High-quality randomized controlled trials demonstrate that two of the most common of these drugs, spironolactone and its chemical cousin eplerenone, reduce the risks of death, hospitalization, and worsening symptoms when added to an ACE inhibitor in patients with severe congestive heart failure.

Despite these benefits, aldosterone antagonists are second-line agents. Their benefits are not as great as those of ACE inhibitors or beta-blockers, and their side effects can be troubling. They tend to increase potassium

DIET AND HEART FAILURE: LIMIT YOUR SALT

If you have heart failure and you can remember only one dietary tip to keep you out of the hospital, this is it: limit your salt. We all know that over the course of many years a high salt diet can cause high blood pressure. In the heart failure patient, the problem is more immediate. Over the course of just a few hours, a high salt meal can lead to shortness of breath, an ambulance ride to the emergency room, and several days in the hospital.

Inability to adequately excrete salt and water is a key feature of congestive heart failure. Dietary salt increases fluid retention, with resulting congestion of the lungs and shortness of breath. In patients with severe CHF, a single binge—like eating a bag of potato chips or a soft pretzel coated with salt—can result in hospital admission.

Avoiding salt requires vigilance and planning. Salt is ubiquitous in the American diet and is often hidden in canned products and prepared or restaurant foods. Patients with CHF should aim to limit salt intake to 1,500 mg per day. This is not so easy to do when you consider that a single can of chicken noodle soup may contain more than 1,000 mg of sodium!

Read labels carefully. Avoid foods prepared by others. Watch your daily sodium intake. Choose low-salt offerings: the low-salt chicken soup is right next to the standard soup. Follow these rules and you may keep yourself out of the hospital.

levels, which complicates management of the CHF patient. In addition, spironolactone, but not eplerenone, can cause gynecomastia (breast enlargement and tenderness) in men. Nevertheless, if CHF symptoms are not relieved by conventional medical treatments, we will sometimes add an aldosterone antagonist.

Medications in Heart Failure: The Take-Home Message

Nearly all CHF patients should receive both an ACE inhibitor and a beta-blocker. Data show that, taken together, these two classes of drugs reduce mortality, improve symptoms, increase ejection fraction, and help keep patients out of the hospital. But today in the United States many heart failure patients do not take an ACE inhibitor (or an ARB) and a beta-blocker. We are not providing heart failure patients with our best medical care.

Know Your Heart Failure Medicines

MEDICINE	COMMON EXAMPLES	COMMON BRAND NAMES
ACE inhibitor	Enalapril	Vasotec
	Lisinopril	Prinivil, Zestril
	Captopril	Capoten
Beta-blocker	Carvedilol	Coreg
	Metoprolol	Toprol XL
ARB	Candesartan	Atacand
	Valsartan	Diovan
	Losartan	Cozaar
Diuretic	Furosemide	Lasix
	Bumetanide	Bumex
	Torsemide	Demadex
Aldosterone antagonist	Spironolactone	Aldactone
	Eplerenone	Inspira

If you are a heart failure patient, check your medicines and discuss them with your doctor. Get involved with your care. The key to success in treating CHF is a partnership between you and your cardiologist to determine the optimal drugs and dosages to maximize your benefit. Expect frequent office visits: CHF is a chronic condition that requires flexible treatment strategies and periodic tweaking to get the best result.

Electrical Therapies for CHF

Although most of our focus is on the heart's pumping ability, sometimes abnormalities of the heart's conduction system (or electrical system) also contribute to the development and risks of CHF. Doctors' growing understanding of the role of the conduction system in CHF has opened up a whole world of new therapies.

Specialized Pacemakers: Cardiac Resynchronization Therapy

In normal patients, both of the heart's pumping chambers (the ventricles) contract simultaneously in a coordinated and rhythmic fashion. In patients with heart failure, enlargement of the heart and damage from heart attacks often block or slow the heart's electrical system, disrupting this synchronous contraction. The result is less efficient cardiac function in a person who already has a weakened heart muscle.

Recognizing that an uncoordinated electrical system contributes to heart failure, cardiologists set out to develop special pacemakers that could fix the heart rhythm. Crafting one of modern cardiology's greatest success stories, they produced biventricular pacemakers that simultaneously deliver electrical impulses to the right and left ventricles and coordinate their pumping. The implantation of these devices is known as cardiac resynchronization therapy. High-quality clinical trials showed that cardiac resynchronization therapy provides important benefits to many CHF patients, including improved heart function, reduced time in the hospital, fewer symptoms, and longer life.

Currently, about two-thirds of heart failure patients treated with these specialized pacemakers show measurable benefits. One of our current research goals is to better identify those patients who will benefit from cardiac resynchronization therapy. Meanwhile, if you have CHF, are currently treated using maximum medical therapy, but still have major symptoms, you may be a candidate for one of these special pacemakers.

Implantable Defibrillators

Despite our broad range of modern medical therapies for CHF, the mortality rate remains high. About half of the deaths in heart failure patients are caused by a sudden cardiac arrest, and the majority of these are due to a heart rhythm disturbance that originates in the left ventricle.

As noted earlier, damaged heart muscle does not conduct electrical impulses normally; this predisposes heart failure patients to a chaotic rhythm known as ventricular fibrillation. In patients with ventricular fibrillation, the heart does not contract well enough to pump any blood, and unconsciousness occurs within seconds. Immediate CPR saves a few patients by allowing time for emergency medical personnel to arrive and deliver an electrical shock. But if defibrillation is not performed within four to eight minutes, ventricular fibrillation is always fatal.

Recognizing the threat posed by ventricular fibrillation, pioneering cardiologists developed an extraordinary device, the implantable cardioverter defibrillator (ICD). As we discuss in Chapter 14, the ICD is a specialized type of pacemaker that continuously monitors the heart's electrical system. ICDs can correct several types of heart rhythm disturbances and, if necessary, deliver a powerful jolt of electricity to shock the heart out of life-threatening ventricular fibrillation. The electrical shock is unpleasant for patients, but preferable to the alternative—death. These devices store a record of the event, enabling the electrophysiologist to review what happened and adjust medical treatment to prevent future occurrences. To date, ICDs have saved many thousands of lives.

WHO NEEDS AN IMPLANTABLE CARDIOVERTER DEFIBRILLATOR (ICD)?

Survivors of sudden cardiac death

Patients with documented dangerous heart rhythms—ventricular tachycardia, ventricular fibrillation

People with severe heart damage caused by heart attack

Anyone with severe heart damage from causes other than heart attack

Controversy exists concerning which patients should receive an ICD. Perhaps as a consequence of this confusion, only about 40 percent of the people who should get an ICD actually receive one. If you have had a heart attack, find out how well your heart functions; you need this piece of information to determine with your doctor whether or not an ICD is right for you. Remember that we measure the pumping ability of the left ventricle by the ejection fraction. A normal ejection fraction is 50 to 60 percent. If your echocardiogram reveals an ejection fraction that is 35 percent or less, you may be a candidate for an ICD. Although the evidence is a bit weaker, patients with heart failure due to causes other than coronary heart disease (including cardiomyopathies) and an ejection fraction less than 35 percent should also receive a defibrillator. If you have heart failure or you have had a heart attack, ask your doctor if an ICD is right for you.

As with pacemakers, ICDs must be placed by electrophysiologists, the heart rhythm experts. These doctors ensure that the ICD is programmed correctly. Incorrect programming can lead to inappropriate shocks, and these are very troubling for the patient. In fact, 10 to 25 percent of patients experience an inappropriate shock within a year or two of receiving an

ICD. These shocks feel like being on the receiving end of a mule's hind legs; this is an acceptable trade-off if it saves your life, but not if it is the result of incorrect programming. Always alert your electrophysiologist if you receive a shock from your ICD.

The Best of Both Worlds

As you've learned, special pacemakers to resynchronize heart rhythm help people with CHF feel better and live longer, and ICDs prevent them from dying suddenly. Now, heart failure patients can get the best of both worlds. Following the example of multifunctional cell phones, we now have specialized devices that combine ICD function with special resynchronization pacing.

Transplantation and Mechanical Cardiac Assistance

Despite our impressive armamentarium of modern drugs and technologies, some CHF patients fail to improve, eventually reaching the point at which their quality of life is unacceptable. For carefully selected patients, heart transplantation or the placement of a mechanical device to assist the failing heart may represent the best option.

Heart Transplantation

First performed in 1967 by South African heart surgeon Christiaan Barnard, heart transplantation has improved dramatically over the last five decades. For a heart transplant team, the procedure and care are now routine. In the best centers, about 90 percent of transplant recipients survive at least one year, more than 80 percent live at least three years after transplant, and 75 percent live five or more years. When the operation goes well and patients meticulously follow a precise medical regimen, quality of life after heart transplantation can be superb. Some heart transplant recipients have actually run a full marathon!

The transplant recipient requires frequent and careful medical follow-up to prevent complications. The immunosuppressive drugs used to prevent rejection of the new heart make transplant recipients more vulnerable to certain cancers and to infections, both of which can be life-threatening.

ACUTE HEART FAILURE: "I CAN'T BREATHE!"

You need more air. Struggling to breathe as deeply as possible, panic creeps in, and the air hunger intensifies. You are starved for air and nothing you do makes it better. And it is getting worse with every passing minute.

Any CHF patient who has experienced an acute heart failure exacerbation understands this frightening but common experience. Worsening heart failure of this sort is the number one reason for hospitalization of Medicare patients in the United States.

The factors leading to such episodes are sometimes elusive, but several themes are common. CHF exacerbations may occur after dietary indiscretions involving salt, missed doses of medications, or failure to promptly refill prescriptions. Each of these causes leads to a predictable series of events.

Mild to moderate fluid overload triggers shortness of breath. Difficulty breathing is scary and causes a surge in adrenaline and other hormones, elevating blood pressure. Increased blood pressure means that the heart has to work harder, and this further worsens the congestive heart failure. More fluid accumulates in the lungs, increasing the shortness of breath and even causing pulmonary edema (severe lung congestion). The downward spiral lands the patient in the emergency room.

Prevention and early intervention can save you from this terrifying sequence. Fill your prescriptions. Take your medicines as directed. Avoid salt. Intervene early if fluid begins to accumulate. If you have a history of heart failure and you notice weight gain (more than two pounds in two days), ankle swelling, or increasing shortness of breath, call your doctor early so that you do not have to call 911 later.

A particularly challenging complication after heart transplantation is development of accelerated coronary heart disease in the new heart. This results from damage to the lining of the coronary arteries from chronic low-level rejection, which promotes plaque buildup. Since the nerves to the heart are severed after transplantation, patients who develop coronary heart disease or suffer a heart attack in the transplanted heart never have any chest pain.

Despite major advances in cardiac transplantation and excellent results, this operation is still relatively uncommon. Only about 3,500 heart transplants are performed in the world each year, with 2,300 in the United States. The major problem is availability of donor hearts. The typical donor is an unfortunate young person involved in a motor vehicle accident, who survives the initial trauma but has an irreversible brain injury. Criteria for brain death are very rigorous, and only a small proportion of trauma victims meet these standards. Of these, only a few acceptable hearts are actually donated because it is difficult for families to donate a relative's organs while still grieving for their loss. Given the scarcity of donor hearts, we have developed an elaborate system to ensure fair allocation of the few available organs to the neediest recipients. Hospitalized heart failure patients requiring powerful drugs or artificial pumps to stay alive receive the highest priority. Less sick patients often wait for many months or years, and some die while waiting for transplantation.

Left Ventricular Assist Devices

To address the problem of the limited availability of donor hearts, several companies, in collaboration with physicians and surgeons, have developed implantable pumps to support blood circulation in patients with advanced heart failure. The most common category of pump is the left ventricular assist device (LVAD), which does exactly what its name suggests: supplements the pumping action of the damaged left ventricle, taking over the majority of its workload. LVADs are suitable only for patients with primary failure of the left ventricle; they don't work for right-sided heart failure. For patients with failure of both the right and left ventricles, a total artificial heart is available in a few centers but is used infrequently because of the complexity of the device and high complication rates.

Although rejection is not a consideration with LVADs, other complications are significant, including the potential for strokes due to formation of blood clots within the pump, which can break loose and travel to the brain. And because there are connections between the pump and an external power source, bacteria may enter the body and cause serious infections.

Engineering advances have gradually improved LVADs over the last decade, enhancing pump reliability and lowering complication rates. Early LVADs required a refrigerator-sized external console to support the device, severely limiting patient mobility and keeping many patients trapped in the hospital until a donor heart became available for heart transplant. Recent improvements now allow patients to function more independently by carrying a battery belt that powers the LVAD. The next generation of devices will transmit power through intact skin, eliminating some of the infection risk. Many of our latest devices pump blood continuously, rather than in a pulsating fashion; as a consequence, these LVAD patients do not have a pulse!

LVADs were initially approved for a situation known as "bridge to transplant," meaning that the device is used to keep the patient alive until a matching donor organ becomes available. However, as these devices improved and became more reliable, heart failure specialists extended their use. Currently, the most common pattern of usage is known as "destination therapy," which means that the LVAD is intended as a long-term treatment with no expectation of later heart transplantation. Patients selected for destination therapy usually do not meet the stringent criteria for transplantation but have the potential for a better quality of life with a permanent LVAD. As these devices improve, many authorities expect destination therapy to increase dramatically in coming years.

A final, growing category of LVAD usage is termed "bridge to recovery." These patients have severe heart failure, but their physicians believe that the cause of CHF may be temporary. The LVAD is used to buy time, maintaining life while the heart heals. Once the heart has recovered, surgeons remove the LVAD and the patient survives with his or her own heart.

Today, we are placing more LVADs than ever before. A recent study of LVAD patients made headlines with its finding that, against medical advice, many patients continue to drive after receiving their heart pumps. Some patients even report changing their LVAD batteries while behind the wheel. We recognize that driving and maintaining a measure of independence are quality-of-life issues, but safety comes first. At least for now, we advise those with LVADs to sit in the passenger seat.

LIVING WITH HEART FAILURE: DICK CHENEY

Although he spent a long, tough eight years as the forty-sixth vice president of the United States, Dick Cheney freely admits that the biggest battle of his life has been the one that he has waged against heart disease and heart failure. Starting with his first heart attack on Father's Day weekend in 1978, Cheney has suffered a total of five heart attacks; for unclear reasons, each heart attack occurred during an election year. The cumulative damage to his heart caused a severe drop in his ejection fraction and left him a heart failure patient.

Although some may disagree with Cheney's politics, no one can dispute the excellent cardiac care that he has received. Cheney has run the gamut of therapies to manage his heart failure. He has received medicines, an internal defibrillator, and even a left ventricular assist device. He and his doctors are contemplating a heart transplant as the next step.

Cheney's story illustrates the success of our vast armamentarium for helping the heart failure patient. In addition, he demonstrates that the heart failure patient can pursue his dreams with vigor. Speaking to a group of cardiologists, Cheney summed up his treatment this way: "Many of the opportunities I've had would never have come to me at all were it not for steady advances in the practice of cardiology.... I guess what I'm saying is that, for those who wish Dick Cheney had called it quits a long time ago, they can blame it all on you [cardiologists]."

RX: CONGESTIVE HEART FAILURE

Heart failure is not a death sentence

Prevent heart failure—if you or a family member has a heart attack, ask your cardiologist about:

The extent of heart damage

Your ejection fraction

Whether or not you will receive an ACE inhibitor and a beta-blocker

Treat diagnosed heart failure:

Follow a heart-healthy lifestyle

Aerobic exercise

Low-salt diet

Stop smoking

Check your medicines to ensure that they include an ACE inhibitor and a beta-blocker

Ask your cardiologist if you are a candidate for a defibrillator

If your heart failure does not improve with standard medicines:

Get a second opinion to ensure that you are on the right medicines at the right doses

Explore the option of specialized biventricular pacing

If you remain severely limited, inquire about left ventricular assist devices and heart transplantation

CHAPTER 16

VITAMINS AND SUPPLEMENTS: TRICK OR TREATMENT?

THE BIG PICTURE

If this were a category on *Jeopardy*, the clues would include:

- More than 100 million Americans take them
- We spend $27 billion per year purchasing them
- People consider them safe because they are "natural"
- They are largely unregulated (FDA approval *not* required)
- Touted benefits include treatment or prevention of heart disease, cancer, and almost every other ailment known to humankind

The answer: "What are vitamins and supplements?"

⦓⦓⦓⦓⦓

Medicinal supplements, ranging from herbal concoctions to bat guano, have been around for centuries. Once these supplements were the only medicines available, but today vitamins and supplements compete with prescribed medicines as people search for ways to treat and prevent disease.

Supplements and vitamins generate so much public interest that the NIH has awarded $250 million in grants to study them. Traditional medical doctors are not necessarily opposed to the use of supplements; some of these agents may actually benefit patients. But if they are going to be used as medicines, vitamins and supplements must be evaluated using the same rigorous standards that we apply for drugs such as Lipitor and Plavix. This means that we need to understand their biological actions and prove their value to patients. Along the way, we must also determine their side effects. Just because many of these compounds are natural does not mean that their safety is guaranteed; poison ivy and arsenic are natural, too.

Over the last two decades, large numbers of heart patients have turned to supplements to replace or augment standard medications. In addition, some doctors prescribe them to their patients, often with an incomplete understanding of the latest scientific data on these supplements. In many cases, the patients' and doctors' enthusiasm for vitamins and supplements is based upon observational data rather than upon carefully designed clinical trials that demonstrate concrete benefits. For example, studies demonstrate that people with heart disease often have low levels of vitamin D; people inferred from this that vitamin D supplementation might reduce heart disease. Current clinical evidence—the result of large, well-designed scientific studies—suggests that it probably does not.

As with vitamin D, the use of supplements often seems logical. For example, we know that people with heart disease frequently have elevated levels of a chemical called homocysteine in their blood. Since B vitamins decrease homocysteine levels, one might reasonably suppose that B vitamins improve heart health. But they do not. In other instances, such as the widespread use of antioxidants, supplements aimed at heart health are embraced for theoretical benefits, rather than real clinical proof that they help people. And in some cases, their use can actually cause significant harm.

We become particularly worried when our well-intentioned patients add a few supplements to their shopping carts when they visit the local pharmacy to pick up their monthly prescriptions. As our patient Susan Fremer learned, the practice of combining supplements with prescription medicines can be as dangerous as mixing drinking and driving.

"I THOUGHT THEY WERE HARMLESS"

Before heart surgery to replace a defective aortic valve, Susan Fremer filled out the usual questionnaire asking her to list all the medications she was currently taking. Answering the question did not take much time: she simply wrote, "None." When the anesthesiologist completed his pre-surgery history and physical, he made sure to repeat the question. Again Susan answered, "I don't take any medicines. Aside from this heart problem, I'm perfectly healthy."

The following Monday we took Susan to the OR for her heart surgery. Replacing an aortic valve is a fairly straightforward procedure, and the operation went well. After restarting her heart, we looked at an echocardiogram to confirm that her new valve—a cow valve—was functioning well. It was. The operation was almost over.

We encountered just one problem: we couldn't stop the bleeding. There was blood everywhere—it spurted from suture lines on her heart and dripped from the skin edges. The operative field was a sea of red. Our suction device had to work overtime to prevent the blood from welling up out of the incision and cascading to the floor. We decided to wait a few more minutes for the blood to begin to clot. But sixty minutes later, Susan was still bleeding from every surface.

Now we pulled out our big guns, several powerful agents that help blood to clot—platelets, plasma, and a variety of clotting factors. We used the everything-but-the-kitchen-sink approach, giving Susan every conceivable medicine or product that enhances clotting. Three hours later, she was still bleeding, and with her chest open in the cold operating room, Susan's body temperature was falling (which further impairs blood clotting). We had to get her out of the OR—fast. We could not close her chest, because the accumulating blood would compress her heart. So we placed a sterile plastic cover over the incision in her sternum and took her up to the ICU.

Over the next six hours, Susan bled steadily. The two drainage tubes that we had left in her chest—each about half as thick as a garden hose—steadily filled with blood. We gave her a total of twenty units of red blood cells to replace those that she lost, and continued to supply clotting factors. Baffled, we called in a hematologist to help us understand the problem.

The first thing that he did was to ask Susan's daughter if Susan took any medicines. Confirming what her mother had told us, she answered no. Persisting, the hematologist asked, "Does she take any medicines or supplements at all?" At which point Susan's daughter reached into her purse and pulled out a Ziploc bag. Handing it to him, she said, "Mom doesn't take any medications. But she does take these."

The bag contained *thirteen* different supplements and vitamins. Included among them were the culprits that caused the bleeding: garlic, vitamin E, ginkgo biloba, and fish oil capsules. Each of these substances interferes with blood clotting. Their combination, all taken in high doses, had created a life-threatening problem.

With the hematologist's help, we hit on the right combination of treatments and were able to stop the bleeding over the next few hours. The following day, Tuesday, we returned Susan to the operating room and closed her incision. We woke her up on Wednesday. Her first words were, "I'm here. I guess that means that the surgery went well." Saving the details for a future discussion, we assured her that she was doing fine.

Three days later, we filled Susan in on the details. She was surprised, to put it mildly. She had not thought of her supplements as real medicines and had had no idea that they could cause complications. In fact, she'd been sure that they protected her heart and strengthened her body. Susan asked us what she should do with her Ziploc full of supplements. Here are our answers.

WHO REGULATES VITAMINS AND SUPPLEMENTS?

One of the most important misunderstandings concerning vitamins and supplements regards their government regulation—or, more precisely, the relative *lack* of government control. Because they come in pill form, are sold in the same shape of container as prescription medicines, and are arrayed on the pharmacy shelves, it is easy to assume that supplements go through the same regulatory process as prescription medicines, gaining FDA approval only after rigorous testing. Even many physicians believe this to be the case. But it is not.

Today, more than 30,000 dietary supplements are sold in the United States. They are not FDA-approved to treat diseases, and their safety is not FDA-assured. They are regulated according to the Dietary Supplement Health and Education Act (DSHEA) of 1994. As long as a company does not make a specific health claim (e.g., the product prevents or treats a disease or medical condition), it may bring a supplement to market without FDA approval. This law creates a loophole for companies that manufacture supplements. For example, the makers of Enzyte can get away with marketing Enzyte for "male enhancement." But they are not permitted to claim that their product treats erectile dysfunction or enlarges your penis, although they hint at these benefits. By positioning the pill as a supplement rather than as a medicine, Enzyte's manufacturers avoided the scrutiny that comes with the FDA approval process. As a result, they are able to sell a drug that has potentially serious side effects, one of which is a worrisome change in the heart's conduction system.

Why are patients and physicians so easily misled concerning the limited benefits and potential risks of many supplements? The DSHEA places responsibility for ensuring the truthfulness of advertisements for dietary supplements with the Federal Trade Commission (FTC), not the FDA. Of course, the FTC knows nothing about drugs, so supplement manufacturers often take advantage of this situation and impute benefits to their products that have never been confirmed by formal clinical studies. And many of the bill's principal sponsors in Congress were from states where many of the companies selling supplements are headquartered.

The FDA does retain some regulatory authority over vitamins and supplements. If the FDA can prove that a dietary supplement is dangerous, they can force its removal from the market, but proving that danger is exceedingly difficult. A potentially greater problem than dangerous supplement side effects occurs when patients are lulled into believing that they can replace prescription medicines with ineffective supplements. In many cases, doing so leaves their medical condition untreated.

Supplements do not undergo rigorous safety testing by regulatory authorities prior to marketing. Unlike the case of prescription drugs, no federal agency is responsible for determining if dietary supplements actually contain the ingredients listed on their labels. In fact, many supplements contain different amounts of active ingredients than promised. A large proportion of supplements, perhaps as much as 40 percent, contains contaminants, including lead, bacteria, and pesticides.

Nearly two decades after DSHEA, the marketed array of worthless or harmful dietary supplements is growing by the day. A quick Google search of "dietary supplements for heart health" yielded 1.1 million hits. You can visit the vitamin section of your local pharmacy and see hundreds of these supplements, many labeled with the claim that they "promote heart health." In the pharmaceutical world, these products are commonly called "nutraceuticals" because they are often derived from foods. As described in the *Washington Monthly* by author Stephanie Mencimer:

Since DSHEA became law, substances as varied as paint stripper, bat shit, toad venom, and lamb placenta have all been imported from overseas, bottled up—often by people with no scientific or health backgrounds—and marketed as dietary supplements to unsuspecting American consumers. Many supplements have been tainted with salmonella, arsenic, lead, pesticides, unapproved foreign prescription drugs, as well as garden-variety carcinogens. And despite their New-Age health aura, a significant portion of these "natural supplements" are stimulants, depressants, and other mood-enhancers that some medical experts believe would be classified as drugs if they were synthetic. A surprising number of these products are addictive.

Fortunately, both scientists and the FDA are becoming increasingly focused on supplements and vitamins, working together to ensure the public's safety. The FDA has recently assumed a more active role in the regulation of supplements, taking action against companies that make unsubstantiated health claims or have inadequate safeguards against contamination in their manufacturing processes. Meanwhile, scientists have performed detailed scientific studies of the cardiac (and other health) effects of many supplements and vitamins, aimed at answering critical questions about their safety and effectiveness.

You should think of supplements as drugs and consider their benefits and risks accordingly. Don't get your medical advice from a health food store. Never take any supplements without discussing them with your doctor.

FISH OIL AND OMEGA-3 FATTY ACIDS

Between 2008 and 2011, fish oil use jumped by more than 50 percent, meaning that today tens of millions of Americans take fish oil. Their reason? Heart health.

The story tying fish oil to heart health began more than fifty years ago. In 1944, scientists recognized that a diet high in whale, seal, and fish seemed to protect Greenland Inuit people from developing coronary heart disease. Later studies showed that their seafood-heavy diets contributed to the Inuit's excellent cholesterol and lipid profiles. Upon further examination, scientists found that greater fish consumption was associated with a lowered risk of heart disease, whether you lived in Norway, Holland, Japan, the United States, or any other country. Fish appeared to protect the heart. Subsequent research suggested that the active ingredients in fish were the special omega-3 fatty acids eicosapentaenoic acid (EPA) and docosahexae-noic acid (DHA).

Scientists have confirmed that these omega-3s are biologically active, meaning that they cause measurable changes in the body, including blood vessel relaxation, reduced blood clotting, reduced inflammation, and possibly stabilization of heart rhythm. With this list, it is logical to conclude that omega-3s should be good for the heart. But, as we will show you, the evidence of cardiac benefit is not conclusive.

Omega-3s in People with Heart Disease

A single large, randomized controlled trial supports the concept that daily administration of 1 gram of an EPA/DHA combination may benefit patients with coronary heart disease who have suffered a heart attack. When started early after a heart attack, omega-3s were reported to reduce the risks of death and dangerous heart rhythms. Other trials suggest that omega-3s may also reduce future cardiac events in those with coronary heart disease but without a previous heart attack. A small number of trials suggests that omega-3s may help patients with heart failure to avoid hospital admission and live longer.

Although these data concerning fish oil and the heart appear promising, they are not yet conclusive. Some scientists take issue with the design and conduct of the studies that suggest a benefit from fish oil supplements in heart patients. Proponents don't talk about it much, but we also have studies in heart patients that have failed to confirm benefits of the omega-3s. While it is true that many of these negative studies had potential flaws that could explain their negative results (doses that were too low, starting the medicines too late after heart attacks), they do open the door to reasonable doubt. In addition, fish oil studies suffer from publication bias, where studies with favorable results are more likely to be published than those with negative results.

Given that we have some question concerning their effectiveness, the safety of fish oil supplements is particularly important. Fortunately, fish oil is considered reasonably safe, but there remain important issues. Some brands are contaminated with mercury, and others do not contain the amount of active ingredients promised by their labels. If a patient decides to take over-the-counter fish oil supplements, we suggest Carlson Super Omega3; independent testing has confirmed that this brand is mercury-free and contains the stated dosage of fish oil.

Like any medicine, fish oil supplements have potential side effects. Fish oil has a mild anticoagulant (blood-thinning) effect and should not be given routinely to patients who are taking blood thinners or who have a propensity for bleeding. Administration of omega-3s can cause indigestion and "fishy" burps, which can be prevented by taking the supplements at bedtime or with meals and by using enteric-coated products. (Some people also recommend keeping fish oil capsules in the freezer, but manufacturers discourage this practice.)

Taking all of the evidence together, we cannot recommend omega-3 supplements for all patients with coronary heart disease. Although the American Heart Association recommends that patients with coronary heart disease take supplements to get a combined total of 1 gram of EPA/DHA per day, we are concerned about potential side effects (bleeding and mercury contamination) and the relative weakness of the evidence supporting a real benefit. While it is possible that fish oil helps heart patients, medicines with a stronger and proven track record, including statins, aspirin, and beta-blockers, are far more important.

Omega-3s in People Without Heart Disease

What about use of omega-3s to prevent the *development* of coronary heart disease in the first place? Recently we asked the ten members of our operating room team if they took omega-3 supplements. Only one of them has coronary heart disease, but he and six others used the supplements (a rate that was just about average, as studies suggest that up to 75 percent of Americans take them). The six without heart problems said that they took the omega-3s to prevent them from having to trade places with the heart patient on the operating room table. Were they correct? Can omega-3 supplements prevent the development of coronary heart disease?

To date, no large randomized controlled clinical trial has shown a cardiovascular benefit to omega-3s in people without known heart disease, although in epidemiological studies, people who consume the most fish tend to be the least likely to develop heart disease. Adding weight to this finding, scientists observe that high levels of omega-3s in the blood correlate

FISH OR FISH OIL SUPPLEMENTS: HOW SHOULD I GET MY OMEGA-3S?

While some people maintain that consuming large amounts of fish is the more natural way of getting omega-3s—and also provides you with other nutrients—opponents argue that increased fish consumption brings with it greater exposure to mercury and pesticides. In fact, the risk of ingesting toxic levels of mercury and pesticides by eating fish is very low and can be minimized by avoiding shark, swordfish, king mackerel, and tilefish, which have the greatest mercury concentrations. Although it may seem attractive to take fish oil via a supplement, increasing fish consumption may make more sense for many people.

If you do take a supplement, which brand makes the most sense? The prescription-only FDA-approved version of fish oil, Lovaza, has a high concentration of omega-3s, but it is very expensive compared with over-the-counter versions. It is acceptable to use a non-prescription omega-3 supplement, but you should understand that Lovaza supplies 4 grams of EPA/DHA per day. Getting that much from an over-the-counter fish oil supplement might require 10 capsules per day (which adds 100 extra calories). If the goal is 1 gram per day, check the label to determine how many capsules you need to get this amount of EPA/DHA. And don't worry about fish allergies; fish oil capsules will not cause a reaction in those allergic to fish.

with a reduced risk of suffering a heart attack. These observations create a circumstantial case supporting the use of omega-3s to prevent the development of heart disease. But we need the gold standard data from randomized, controlled clinical trials in order to definitively confirm (or refute) this hypothesis. Such clinical trials will be completed in the next few years. Right now, the scientific proof is not strong enough for us to recommend routine omega-3 supplements in people without known heart disease. But we do encourage replacing dishes high in saturated fat (hamburgers, hot dogs, pizza) with fish (especially salmon, albacore tuna, lake trout, and other fatty fish) at least twice a week. At the very least, this dietary choice replaces something unfavorable with a host of nutrients with theoretical benefits, including omega-3s.

Omega-3s, Cholesterol, and Triglycerides

Members of our operating room team who took omega-3 supplements gave two related reasons for doing so: preventing heart disease and improving cholesterol levels. But in fact, in most studies omega-3s have been associated with small increases in LDL cholesterol with no change in HDL cholesterol. Don't count on omega-3s to improve your cholesterol levels.

On the other hand, omega-3s have a real effect on triglyceride levels. In patients with very high triglyceride levels (500 mg/dL or greater), taking 4 grams per day of omega-3s produces a 25 to 50 percent drop in triglycerides. However, in these patients, fish oil also significantly increases LDL cholesterol levels, which is undesirable. Therefore, it is best to combine omega-3s with a statin in the patient with coronary heart disease and elevated triglyceride and cholesterol levels.

Omega-3s: The Bottom Line

Large clinical trials enrolling a total of more than 30,000 patients confirm that omega-3s are probably safe in most people. We have consistent, but weak, evidence for potential benefits for patients with coronary heart disease or congestive heart failure. Therefore, these supplements may have some role in our management of cardiac patients. More answers will be forthcoming over the next few years as researchers examine the impact of omega-3s, particularly in patients without known heart disease. In a 1987 editorial discussing the health implications of fish oil, Dr. J. A. Rogan wrote, "Fish oil is a whale of a story that not surprisingly gets bigger with every telling." His comment holds true today.

SUPPLEMENTS TO LOWER YOUR CHOLESTEROL?

Many of our patients are reluctant to take statin drugs to help them reduce their cholesterol. Much of their concern is based upon folklore, but we feel that it is also fueled by the dietary supplement industry promoting a variety of remedies to lower cholesterol. Unfortunately, none of these supplements is as effective as a program that includes a healthy diet, exercise, and, for many people, a statin.

Who Needs Omega-3 Supplements?	
CONDITION	**OMEGA-3 DOSE**
Known coronary heart disease	Possible benefit seen in studies using 1 gram daily dosage
No coronary heart disease	Evidence for supplements inconclusive; eat oily fish twice per week
Congestive heart failure	Possible benefit seen in studies using 1 gram daily dosage
Severely elevated triglycerides	4 grams per day via prescription fish oil

One of the most popular anti-cholesterol supplements is red yeast rice, which actually contains a statin indistinguishable from lovastatin, the first statin marketed in the United States. However, the amount of statin contained in these products is uncontrolled and unpredictable. In addition, one-third of red yeast rice preparations contain contaminants that can be toxic to the kidneys. Recognizing the potential danger of taking a random, uncontrolled dosage of a statin, the FDA has repeatedly attempted to ban the sale of red yeast rice products. There is no conceivable benefit to taking this natural but unpredictable statin-containing supplement; the stakes are too high to trust your LDL cholesterol level to these compounds. Consuming red yeast rice for high cholesterol is a little like playing Russian roulette: you might get a blank or you might get a bullet.

A variety of other supplements are widely promoted to support healthy cholesterol. Plant stanols and sterols (also known as phytosterols) block intestinal absorption of cholesterol and can therefore lower LDL cholesterol slightly (5 to 8 percent). By itself, this is not a large enough change to make a significant difference in most patients with very high cholesterol levels. Nevertheless, today many foods, particularly certain margarines, are fortified with phytosterols promising to lower your cholesterol. The FDA has offered a weak endorsement for phytosterols, but we are still awaiting data examining the effects of plant stanols and sterols on the risks of hard outcomes like heart attack and stroke.

There is some evidence for a favorable effect of certain forms of soluble fiber—particularly psyllium seed, the main ingredient in the laxative Metamucil—on cholesterol levels. These products do slightly lower LDL cholesterol and triglycerides, but there are no high-quality randomized controlled trials demonstrating improvement in outcomes for heart patients. But if you do need a laxative, Metamucil and other generic brands of psyllium seed are safe.

An almost endless variety of other supplements make claims to promote healthy cholesterol levels. Policosanol, an alcohol derived from sugarcane, has been widely promoted as lowering LDL cholesterol; however, a high-quality randomized controlled trial showed no effect whatsoever. Similarly, garlic is widely touted as a cholesterol-lowering supplement but has no demonstrated benefits. Guggulipids (extracted from the bark of the mukul myrrh tree, which grows in India) are also promoted to improve cholesterol, but in a randomized controlled study this product actually *increased* LDL cholesterol levels. Lecithin is sometimes promoted for heart health, but studies show that it has no real benefit.

VITAMIN D AND CALCIUM

Everybody knows that calcium and vitamin D influence bone health, but in recent years scientists have linked these two compounds to an ever-increasing list of other health conditions, ranging from breast cancer to diabetes to heart disease. The more studies and headlines published about this topic, the greater the confusion. In 2010, a *New York Times* story predicted that vitamin D would be the "supplement of the decade." Will the science bear this out? Let's look at what we know so far.

How Much Vitamin D and Calcium Do You Need?

This seems like a simple question, but scientists and doctors argue forcefully about the answer. The Institute of Medicine recently reviewed all of the current data on health outcomes related to vitamin D and calcium and published recommended dietary allowances based on their findings. Although most of our vitamin D comes from sun exposure, the committee assumed minimal time in the sun when they came up with their dietary recommendations.

Recommended Dietary Allowances for Calcium and Vitamin D		
LIFE STAGE	CALCIUM (MG/DAY)	VITAMIN D (IU/DAY)
1–3 years	700	600
4–8 years	1,000	600
9–13 years	1,300	600
14–18 years	1,300	600
19–50 years	1,000	600
51–70 years, male	1,000	600
51–70 years, female	1,200	600
71 years or older	1,200	800
Pregnant or lactating female	1,000	600

Overall, the panel of experts concluded that the majority of Americans receive adequate amounts of calcium and vitamin D, with the exception of nine- to eighteen-year-old girls, who often do not get enough calcium. Most adults without osteoporosis do not need supplements. They also considered the risk of complications, which begins to mount when vitamin D intake surpasses 4,000 IU per day and when calcium intake exceeds 2,000 mg per day. In particular, too much calcium can lead to kidney stones.

These pronouncements by the Institute of Medicine set off a firestorm of controversy, with other experts contending that our calcium and vitamin D intakes fall far short of desirable levels and recommending routine supplements in all adults. For many people, particularly women who fear osteoporosis, the issue is extremely important. The final word is not yet in, but based upon the data available today, it appears that millions of us may be taking supplements that we just don't need.

Calcium, Vitamin D, and Osteoporosis

There is no question that calcium and vitamin D are essential to bone health. Calcium is critical for bone architecture and strength, and vitamin D helps the intestine absorb calcium. Osteoporosis is a disorder in which bone density decreases and bone architecture changes, putting the patient at risk for fractures, especially of the hip and vertebrae. Osteoporosis is

Sources of Vitamin D	
VITAMIN D SOURCE	**VITAMIN D CONTENT (IU)**
Salmon (fresh, wild, 3.5 oz)	600–1,000
Salmon (farmed, 3.5 oz)	100–250
Tuna (canned, 3.6 oz)	230
Egg yolk	20
Fortified milk (8 fl oz)	100
Fortified orange juice (8 fl oz)	100
Fortified yogurt (8 oz)	100
Fortified breakfast cereal (1 serving)	100
Multivitamin (standard)	400
Sunlight: 10 minutes of exposure to arms and legs	3,000

common. If you are currently fifty years old, the chance that you will some-day suffer an osteoporosis-related fracture is 50 percent if you are female and 13 percent if you are male. Overall, osteoporosis affects one-third of women who are sixty to seventy years old and two-thirds of women who are eighty or older. Declining estrogen production after menopause and a lower peak bone mass to start with make osteoporosis more prevalent in women.

Can taking extra calcium and vitamin D prevent you from developing osteoporosis? If you are like most adults, you probably already get enough of these nutrients from dietary sources and sun exposure, and increasing your daily intake of them has not been shown to help. On the other hand, if you already have osteoporosis—diagnosed by your doctor with a bone density test or by a previous fracture—you need calcium and vitamin D supplements, along with special medicines to prevent further bone loss.

Do Vitamin D Supplements Prevent Other Diseases?

Years ago, doctors found that vitamin D deficiency caused rickets, a bone disease, and that taking vitamin D supplements prevented the problem. This was a nice, tidy package, and many doctors thought that we had the vitamin D equation completely solved. Enamored with this special sun-light-related vitamin, scientists investigated further, finding receptors for it in cells throughout the body, indicating that its purpose might extend beyond bone health. In fact, vitamin D deficiency has been linked to a wide variety of serious illnesses, including various types of cancer, heart disease, diabetes, high blood pressure, and autoimmune diseases such as multiple sclerosis. These findings from observational studies raised an important question: could extra vitamin D ward off a whole host of medical problems?

The debate over this question is white-hot and ongoing. Spurred by scientific articles and corresponding media stories linking vitamin D deficiency to health problems, Americans spent $430 million on this supplement in 2009, representing an 82 percent increase from the previous year. Many doctors still claim that millions of Americans are vitamin D deficient and, consequently, exposing themselves to serious health risks. But looking at the science, we find more questions than answers. In fact, experts cannot even agree on what blood level of vitamin D represents a deficiency. At this time, we agree with the Institute of Medicine's conclusion: we do not have enough evidence to support taking vitamin D supplements to prevent or treat diseases other than osteoporosis.

Do Calcium and Vitamin D Supplements Cause Heart Disease?

Talk about another hot-button question. The scientific papers on this topic are all over the map. Because plaques that block arteries and cause heart attacks and strokes usually contain calcium, it might seem logical to assume that taking extra calcium could favor plaque formation. Recent, widely publicized studies (some of them randomized controlled trials) do suggest that calcium and vitamin D supplements cause slight increases in the risks of heart attack and stroke. On the other hand, we have observational studies identifying associations between vitamin D deficiency and development of coronary heart disease, death from heart failure, and fatal strokes. Large studies designed to clarify these issues are under way, but final results won't be available for at least five years.

Meanwhile, when we consider the available data as a whole, rather than focusing only on this week's revelation, we find a cardiovascular trend that is worth considering: wholesale administration of calcium (with or without vitamin D) to large groups of people might cause a modest increase in the numbers of heart attacks and strokes. We emphasize "modest" here. Taking calcium and vitamin D does not pose the same danger as smoking cigarettes or gaining fifty pounds. What this means is—no surprise—we need to think of these supplements as medicines, using them where the likely benefit outweighs the possible risk. When we combine the available data with this basic principle, we arrive at good, evidence-based conclusions:

♥ *Most healthy adults do not need calcium or vitamin D supplements.*

♥ *There is no evidence that natural sources of calcium or vitamin D influence cardiovascular risk, so watch your diet and habits to ensure that you meet intake goals the old-fashioned and best way: through diet and sunlight.*
  - Eat low-fat dairy products and fortified foods.
  - Get ten minutes of sun exposure on your arms and legs (not face) two or three times a week in the summer.

♥ *If you don't get adequate calcium or vitamin D from natural sources, ask your doctor about a supplement.*

♥ *Avoid mega-doses of these supplements, as they may cause complications including kidney stones.*

♥ *If you have osteoporosis, keep these points in mind:*
  - The benefit of taking supplements (with your other osteoporosis medicines) outweighs the possible risks.
  - Remember that smoking, excessive consumption of alcohol, and lack of exercise reduce bone density and make osteoporosis worse.
  - Exercise, in particular resistance training, can prevent bone loss and increase bone density.

THE B VITAMINS GET A GRADE OF F

Like nearly every other vitamin under the sun, B vitamins had their fifteen minutes of fame when it comes to heart health. Actually, their period of fame lasted for years, based on some reasonable scientific thinking but only weak circumstantial evidence. Scientists have long recognized that high blood levels of the amino acid homocysteine are associated with increased risks for

MULTIVITAMINS: ONE A DAY?

Half of all Americans take a multivitamin every day. Promising to promote health, prevent disease, boost immunity, and increase energy levels, these preparations generally contain an impressive list of ten to twenty-five isolated vitamins and other nutrients, often fortified with "bonuses" such as antioxidants. The annual price tag for these purported benefits: $5 billion. They don't make you sick and they don't (always) taste bad. But do multivitamins make you healthier?

As recently as 2002, authorities thought so. Since then, scientists have completed a number of large studies searching for a health benefit of multivitamins. They do satisfy the first rule of medicine, "Do no harm." Unfortunately, they don't do much good, either. A recent study of more than 180,000 people found that multivitamin use had no effect on the risks of dying from cancer or cardiovascular disease. The Women's Health Initiative came to similar conclusions in its study of more than 160,000 postmenopausal women.

Based upon these and other studies, the National Institutes of Health recommend the use of multivitamins only for adults with illnesses that cause vitamin deficiencies, including certain digestive diseases that limit food intake or vitamin absorption. Pregnant women also benefit from special supplements. As for kids, a sea change is under way. Many pediatricians now advise leaving the fruit-flavored gummy or character-shaped vitamins on the store shelves, recommending that kids take multivitamins only if they participate in strenuous and demanding sports, have very poor diets, or suffer from an eating disorder. Otherwise, a diet that includes dairy, fruits and vegetables, protein, and whole grains provides all of the vitamins and nutrients that kids need. Of these, fresh fruits and vegetables contain the most vitamins.

Popping multivitamins may seem virtuous and healthy, but they do not prevent disease or make up for a poor diet. For most of us, a good and varied diet provides all of the vitamins and nutrients that we need. If you take multivitamins, the excess vitamins are simply excreted in the urine. As a result, one famous nutritionist once quipped, "Americans have the most expensive urine in the world."

heart disease and strokes. It turns out that the combination of folic acid (vitamin B_9) and vitamin B_{12} reduces homocysteine levels. Therefore, it seemed logical to conclude that these vitamins would protect the heart, and many doctors prescribed them expressly for this purpose.

Fortunately, a group of English researchers decided to perform a rigorous examination of this hypothesis, comparing the folic acid/vitamin B_{12} combination to a placebo for 10,000 heart attack survivors over a seven-year period. They confirmed that the B vitamins reduced blood homocysteine levels by 28 percent but that this reduction had no effect on the risks of heart attack, stroke, or death. At about the same time, another trial enrolling more than 8,000 stroke patients reached similar conclusions. One bright spot of this study: folic acid and other B vitamin supplements had no impact on the risk of cancer, laying to rest previous concerns. We recommend including an adequate supply of these vitamins in your diet, and adding supplements in certain situations (e.g., pregnancy or nutritional deficiencies), but we do not endorse their use specifically for heart health.

ANTIOXIDANTS AND OTHER SUPPLEMENTS

The widespread use of antioxidants such as vitamin E is one of the most troubling examples of misuse of dietary supplements. The theory underlying using vitamin E to prevent or treat heart disease seems sensible. We know that oxidation of LDL is a key step in the development of plaques in the walls of arteries. Logically, preventing oxidation would be expected to prevent the buildup of artery-blocking cholesterol deposits. Based on some promising experiments using animal subjects, the hope (and hype) was that vitamin E could inhibit cholesterol oxidation and thereby help prevent or treat atherosclerosis in humans.

This concept was so widely promoted that for many years most of our patients took large doses of vitamin E to prevent or treat coronary heart disease. For a while it seemed that everybody was on antioxidants. Then some disturbing findings began to emerge. In patients taking statins, niacin, or both, adding vitamin E reduced their levels of "good" cholesterol (HDL) and actually seemed to *promote* plaque growth. Eventually, scientists performed large-scale randomized clinical trials to ascertain whether or not vitamin E benefits patients with heart disease. Not even a hint of a benefit was found. The critical lesson to be learned from the vitamin E story? Don't be surprised if today's trendy supplement becomes tomorrow's culprit.

Coenzyme Q_{10} (coQ_{10}) is one of the hottest supplements receiving public attention. Necessary for energy production in our cells, coQ_{10} is also a weak antioxidant. We get about half of our coQ_{10} from dietary fat, and the other half is produced by our bodies. In theory, a deficiency of coQ_{10} could lead to depleted energy stores in heart muscle, reduced heart function, and cellular damage, which has led some to suggest that coQ_{10} supplements can protect the heart. But there are very few data to support the hypothesis. There are also studies suggesting that coQ_{10} lowers blood pressure, but if this effect exists at all, it is minor.

Large studies show that statins lower coQ_{10} concentrations. Some scientists wonder if this might make statins dangerous, but these same studies show that this property causes no harmful effects on the heart. But there *is* a potential use for coQ_{10} related to statins. Limited research shows that 60–200 mg of coQ_{10} supplements per day may reduce the muscle aches that some patients experience as a result of statins. Our take: coQ_{10} supplements are probably safe, but the benefits remain unproven. If you have muscle pain while taking a statin, it is reasonable to try taking 100 mg of coQ_{10} daily.

A large variety of other supplements are promoted with too-good-to-be-true claims of benefits for the heart. The evidence for most of these claims is very weak. A quick Internet search reveals websites touting green tea extract, ginkgo biloba, cinnamon, yarrow, holy basil, grape seed extract, hawthorne berry, and artichoke leaf extract. The array of purported health benefits is astounding. But when we search the medical literature for data to support the claims, we find nothing. If it appears too good to be true, it probably is. You have no way of knowing whether the supplements contain the promised ingredients, or whether the products will benefit you. And don't forget the risks—these supplements may interact with your other medications and make you sick.

CHELATION

Our former neighbor Steve Robinson is lucky to be alive. When he developed an odd sensation of pressure in his chest while walking his St. Bernard, he came over to ask if we thought it could be his heart. Steve was fifty-seven years old and a little overweight. He had mild diabetes. And now he had chest pressure with exertion. Steve was definitely a candidate for coronary heart disease.

The next day, Steve came in to the hospital for testing. A cardiac catheterization showed that he had a 90 percent narrowing of the left main coronary artery; we call this particular blockage "the widow-maker" because it usually results in a fatal heart attack. We recommended bypass surgery to save Steve's life, but a friend at work talked him into a three-month course of chelation therapy instead, to "cleanse" Steve's blood and make the blockages go away.

Six weeks later, Steve came to the emergency room with crushing chest pain and an evolving heart attack. We performed emergency surgery, and Steve survived. He was one of the lucky ones. Chelation therapy cost him $6,000, but it did not cost him his life.

Chelation therapy is an FDA-approved procedure for treating lead and mercury poisoning. The idea is to administer an intravenous infusion of a chemical that binds to the toxic metal, enabling its removal in the urine. Because a commonly used chelating agent (EDTA) also binds to calcium, which is a major component of arterial plaques, some scientists hypothesized that chelation might remove the calcium from plaques and cause them to melt away. But the small number of studies assessing chelation therapy in heart patients showed no benefit. Worse, chelation therapy poses real medical risks, including kidney damage, bone marrow depression, low blood pressure, allergic reactions, and even death. Chelation therapy is *not* FDA-approved for treating the heart. If you have coronary heart disease, save your money and your life by getting real treatment.

RUNNING INTERFERENCE: SUPPLEMENTS AND HERBAL REMEDIES THAT INTERACT WITH TRADITIONAL HEART MEDICINES

Millions of Americans take standard medicines for their hearts, but hundreds of millions—three-quarters of the population—take supplements. While occasionally there may be good, non-cardiac-related reasons to use certain supplements, it is critically important to remember that supplements are medicines. Just like prescription medicines, supplements influence bodily processes. And like prescription medicines, they can interact with other drugs, causing potentially serious harmful effects.

Before deciding to take any supplement, talk to your doctor. Make sure that you are not setting yourself up for a dangerous drug interaction. And if you already take any supplements, now is the time to let your doctor know. Remember what Susan Fremer learned the hard way: just because something is "natural" does not guarantee that it's safe.

Of the ten most widely used supplements, eight of them interact with the blood thinner warfarin (Coumadin). Warfarin has a narrow therapeutic window, which means that you can quickly run into trouble by taking either a little too much (increased risk of bleeding) or a little too little (inadequate thinning of the blood). And trouble with warfarin can lead to serious problems, including a stroke or a life-threatening blood clot. If you take warfarin or other anticoagulants, be especially careful about starting any supplements or new medicines.

Supplements That Interact with Warfarin (Coumadin)*		
SUPPLEMENT	INCREASES BLEEDING RISK	INCREASES CLOTTING RISK
Alfalfa	✓	
Angelica (dong quai)	✓	
Bilberry	✓	
Fenugreek	✓	
Garlic	✓	
Ginger	✓	
Ginkgo biloba	✓	
Glucosamine/chondroitin	✓	
Saw palmetto	✓	
Coenzyme Q_{10}		✓
Ginseng		✓
Melatonin		✓
Soy		✓
St. John's wort		✓

* This list contains many of the most popular supplements, but other agents may interfere with warfarin's action. Check with your doctor before starting any supplement.

RX: VITAMINS AND SUPPLEMENTS

Vitamins and supplements are medicines:

 They cause biological changes

 They can interact with other medicines

"All natural" does not guarantee safety

Do not take a supplement without telling your doctor, especially if you take a blood thinner such as warfarin (Coumadin)

Fish oil supplements may be good for you:

 Their best-supported use is in heart patients with both elevated triglyceride and elevated LDL cholesterol levels

 Omege-3 supplements may be of benefit in other patients with coronary heart disease, but further research is needed to confirm this

 Current data do not support fish oil supplements for the prevention of heart disease

 Including oily fish in your diet, particularly as a replacement for red meats, is associated with a reduced risk of developing coronary heart disease

Do not count on supplements to lower your cholesterol:

 A healthy diet, exercise, and, when necessary, a statin are safer and more effective

PERSONAL PLANS

CHAPTER 17

THE MYSTERIES OF VENUS: UNDERSTANDING THE HEARTS OF WOMEN

THE BIG PICTURE

Ask a woman what disease she fears most, and most likely she will answer "breast cancer." But while breast cancer is a highly visible risk, *heart disease is actually the leading cause of death among women of all ages.* This startling revelation has spurred two decades of careful study of the causes, symptoms, treatments, and outcomes of heart disease in women.

The media have overemphasized disparities between the sexes, creating the perception of vast differences between women and men when it comes to coronary heart disease. But the truth is there are actually more similarities than differences between the sexes. Most important, women need to understand that the primary symptom of coronary heart disease, chest pain, and the principal strategies for prevention and treatment—healthy lifestyle, medicine, angioplasty, and surgery—apply equally to women and men.

But the scope of heart disease is broad, and questions and controversies abound when it comes to heart disease in women. Do women *always* experience the same sort of chest pain as men during a heart attack? Are women undertreated when it comes to heart disease? After a heart attack, why do women tend to fare worse than men? Does hormone replacement therapy protect or hurt the hearts of postmenopausal women? What are the special cardiac risks associated with pregnancy and menopause?

Understanding the answers to these questions will arm women and their partners with the knowledge they need to prevent heart disease and to ensure that they receive appropriate treatment if heart problems develop.

THE KNOWLEDGE GAP

Scientists' focus on heart disease in women is relatively new. During the first eighty years of the twentieth century, male doctors studied and treated heart disease in men. This sounds a bit self-serving on the part of male physicians, but this approach was based upon the widely held belief that estrogen provided women with lasting protection from heart disease. Today, we recognize the error in this thinking.

Women are not immune to coronary heart disease. The numbers tell the story. Today, 6.5 million American women suffer from heart disease. In fact, in every year since 1984, more American women than men have died from coronary heart disease. And women have benefited less than men from the medical community's advances in preventing and treating heart disease. A 2010 study revealed that the proportion of men between thirty-five and fifty-four suffering a heart attack has decreased in recent years, while the percentage of women experiencing a heart attack has actually increased. Clearly, we still have work to do.

Why is progress slower in the treatment of women? A knowledge gap is partly to blame, as well as failure to disseminate the knowledge that doctors and scientists do have. It is all too common for women and their doctors to ignore the threat posed by heart disease. The biggest mistake they make is to place too much faith in the power of estrogen. It is true that estrogen affords premenopausal women a certain amount of protection from coronary heart disease. This is one reason that, compared to young men, young women are less likely to get heart disease. But by age sixty-five women catch up, achieving an unwanted equality as they develop heart disease at a rate equal to that of men.

Let us restate the key message: heart disease is the leading killer of women of *all* ages. One in three women will die from cardiovascular disease. This is six times the number who will die from breast cancer.

Yet many women do not recognize the threat that they face. A 2009 study of more than 2,000 women revealed that only slightly more than half of women correctly identified heart disease as the leading cause of death among women. This is up from just 30 percent in 1994, but represents a slight decline from 2006. Awareness was particularly low among minority women.

This survey also demonstrated that recognition of heart attack warning signs has not improved since 1997. Only about half of women correctly identified chest pain and pain in the neck, shoulder, and arm as potential symptoms of a heart attack. Even more remarkably, when asked what they would do if they thought they were having a heart attack, only half reported that they would call 911.

The study also revealed tremendous confusion about strategies to prevent heart disease. Most women believe that antioxidants and multivitamins can prevent heart disease (they do not) while 29 percent cited aromatherapy and 19 percent hormone therapy as preventive strategies. Aromatherapy is worthless in the management of heart disease. And while hormone therapy is complicated—more on this later—it should not be relied upon to prevent heart disease.

Why is there so much misinformation? The majority of women surveyed obtained their information from television and magazines, and 42 percent said that their confusion stemmed from media reports. Fewer than half of them had discussed heart disease with their doctors.

We can bridge the knowledge gap and fix this problem. We will put you on the path to heart healthiness by clearing the confusion, busting the myths, and providing the critical information that Sandy and Marvin Seidman wish they had known before heart disease intruded into their lives.

SANDY AND MARVIN

Sandy Seidman's heart problems began when she was seventy-two years old. We had first met Sandy twelve years earlier, when her husband, Marvin, suffered a heart attack at age sixty. At the time, he was helped by clot-busting drugs, which opened up a blocked artery on his heart. Sandy nursed him through the subsequent bypass surgery intended to prevent him from having another heart attack.

Over the next decade, we aggressively managed Marvin's risk factors for heart disease. Under our direction, he stopped smoking and started an exercise program. Diet and a statin reduced his LDL and total cholesterol levels. A simple diuretic corrected his high blood pressure. Hovering like a mother hen (Marvin called this "nagging"), Sandy ensured that Marvin followed his diet, filled his prescriptions, and exercised daily.

In addition to being a good patient, Marvin was punctual. So we were surprised one Wednesday when he and Sandy did not show up for their scheduled appointment. Marvin rescheduled for the following week. When we entered the examining room, the change was clear. Sandy was pale, her breathing was shallow, and she looked fragile—a real contrast to the robust, outspoken person we had come to know.

Sandy explained that she had been feeling very tired and a little short of breath for about a month. The day before Marvin's scheduled appointment, she developed stabbing chest pain that would come and go. Initially she ignored it, thinking it was most likely just a pulled muscle from playing with her grandchildren. By evening Sandy felt more tired, and Marvin noticed that she was pale.

He drove her to the emergency room, where she waited for two hours before she was seen for a presumed "flu-like illness." The young emergency room doctor was surprised by her high heart rate and low blood pressure. An abnormal EKG and blood test confirmed his suspicion: Sandy had suffered a heart attack. She was admitted to the hospital and spent three days undergoing tests, which revealed that her cholesterol was high (230 mg/dL) and she had diabetes. Once the testing was completed and Sandy felt a little better, she was given a handful of prescriptions and discharged. Although she took her medicines faithfully, Sandy complained that she still felt tired and weak.

After finishing her story, Sandy asked if we could take care of her as we had Marvin. Could we help her find her energy, avoid a second heart attack, and reclaim her life? Of course we agreed. We had spent more than a decade educating Marvin and Sandy about Marvin's heart but had simply assumed that Sandy's primary doctor was providing the counseling about heart health that every woman needs. As it turned out, Sandy and Marvin had shared their risk factors for heart disease. Before Marvin's heart attack, they had both been sedentary smokers who enjoyed diets high in calories and saturated fats. But unlike Marvin's, Sandy's risk was ignored.

Believing that heart disease was a male problem, Sandy dismissed key warning signs of her impending heart attack (unusual fatigue and shortness of breath) and the stabbing chest pain that signaled the heart attack itself.

Like many women, Sandy put off going to the hospital and encountered delays in the emergency room. She was discharged with little information about what to do next. In addition, like most women who suffer a heart attack, Sandy was not referred to a cardiac rehab program.

Determined to take care of Sandy as we had taken care of Marvin, we adjusted her medicines to give her the best treatments for diabetes and high cholesterol. We prescribed a program of cardiac rehab. Most important, we educated her.

Back to her old energetic self, Sandy now understands her heart, and can be proactive as she takes care of both herself and Marvin. Sandy and Marvin shared everything, including the experience of a heart attack. But today they also share a heart-healthy lifestyle that will ensure their future heart health.

SIGNS AND SYMPTOMS YOU CANNOT IGNORE

Chest Pain

As the Seidmans now both understand, chest pain is the single most common symptom of coronary heart disease in both women and men. Do not ignore it. Until proven otherwise, you must assume that chest pain means heart disease.

Chest pain arising from the heart comes in two varieties: angina, which is caused by temporary inadequate blood flow to the heart muscle, and which does not result in permanent damage; and heart attack, in which limited blood flow causes the death of heart cells and permanent muscle damage.

While a heart attack is usually the first sign of heart disease in men, the first symptom in women is more commonly angina without a heart attack. Each year, 4 million women are hospitalized for chest pain. Although an episode of chest pain does not *always* represent a heart attack, it often serves as an early warning sign. Paying attention to chest pain can help you avoid a heart attack down the road.

Angina is usually described as discomfort, heaviness, and squeezing or fullness in the chest that generally occurs with exercise or stress and is relieved by rest or nitroglycerin. The pain may travel to the arm, shoulders, jaw, neck, back, or upper part of the abdomen. Because this description is based largely on the experience of middle-aged white men with heart disease, some question whether it applies to women. *It is a myth that typical chest pain never occurs in women. In fact, chest pain is the most common cardiac symptom in both men and women.*

While most women with coronary heart disease experience typical chest pain, women are somewhat more likely than men to report "atypical" chest pain. Atypical chest pain may be burning or sharp; it is often of shorter duration and lesser severity than typical chest pain. In some cases, atypical chest pain can be reproduced simply by pressing on the chest, but don't be fooled into thinking that this means the pain is coming from the muscles or bones, rather than from the heart.

So how can you tell if your chest pain—typical or atypical—is from the heart? You can't. Be suspicious of all chest pain. If you have chest pain, get help.

CLASSIC HEART SYMPTOMS IN WOMEN AND MEN

Canadian researchers devised a clever experiment to determine whether men and women experience similar symptoms when an artery on the heart becomes blocked. They examined 305 heart patients (121 women, 204 men) who were undergoing cardiac catheterization and angioplasty, in which a small balloon is inflated in an artery of the heart, temporarily blocking blood flow—similar to the way a blood clot blocks blood flow during a heart attack.

During the part of the procedure in which an artery was blocked, researchers asked patients what they were feeling. The most common answer was—you guessed it—chest pain! Yet women were more likely than men to report additional symptoms, including throat, jaw, and neck discomfort. Don't let these other symptoms fool you into thinking that your chest pain is not heart-related.

Heart Attack

What symptoms should alert women to the possibility that they are experiencing a heart attack? Again, chest pain of any sort is number one on the list. But the sexes do not always experience heart attacks identically. Women are more likely than men to have additional symptoms, including shortness of breath, back pain, neck pain, jaw pain, nausea and vomiting, dizziness, and fatigue. Of these, shortness of breath is the most common additional symptom. Don't let additional symptoms confuse you—assume that all chest pain is heart-related, and get immediate help.

Heart Attack: Symptoms in Women

SYMPTOM	PERCENTAGE OF WOMEN WITH SYMPTOM
Chest pain or discomfort	70
Shortness of breath	58
Weakness	55
Fatigue	43
Cold sweat	39
Dizziness	39
Nausea	36
Back pain	21

Is it possible to have a heart attack without chest pain? The answer is yes. About 25 percent of heart attack victims do not experience chest pain, and this is more common in women than in men.

If you don't have chest pain, how do you know if you are having a heart attack? Shortness of breath is an important clue. Other heart attack symptoms that can occur without chest pain include indigestion, nausea and vomiting, sweating, fatigue, and dizziness. If these symptoms begin with no apparent reason (e.g., you feel like you have indigestion but you have not eaten recently, or you are experiencing shortness of breath that feels out of the ordinary for you) and don't resolve within a few minutes, call 911.

Women and their doctors often initially ignore chest pain and shortness of breath. Women wait longer than men before seeking treatment for a heart attack, and when they finally seek help, they are more likely to go to a doctor's office instead of heading straight to the emergency room. Once they finally reach the emergency room, they face greater delays in diagnosis than do men. Meanwhile, as the minutes tick by, muscle cells are dying and heart function is deteriorating. Rapid treatment is the key to rescuing the heart from the damaging effects of a heart attack.

Not all heart attacks occur suddenly. Many women experience very early warnings of heart problems. Signs of an impending heart attack—what physicians call prodromal symptoms—occur more commonly in women than in men. In fact, more than 80 percent of women report having experienced warning symptoms one month or more before a heart attack compared with 50 percent of men.

Heart Attack: Early Warning in Women	
SYMPTOM	PERCENTAGE OF WOMEN WITH SYMPTOM *BEFORE* A HEART ATTACK
Unusual fatigue	72
Sleep disturbance	48
Shortness of breath	42
Indigestion	39
Anxiety	36
Chest discomfort	30

Some women might scan this list and say to themselves, "I have those symptoms all the time." The key here is *change*. Do not ignore new onset of fatigue, writing it off to a busy schedule—especially if your schedule is always busy but the tiredness is new. Press your doctor to explore your symptoms. You may avert a heart attack.

TESTING, TREATMENTS, AND OUTCOMES: WORSE RESULTS IN WOMEN?

Women with chronic angina get less relief from medical therapy than do men. Women who experience heart attacks are more likely to die than are men who suffer heart attacks. Why do women with coronary heart disease fare worse than men?

Some blame it on a combination of undertreatment and misdiagnosis of women with heart disease. Although this is not the entire story, there is some support for this argument. Studies from the 1980s and 1990s showed that women with heart disease received fewer medical tests, less frequent administration of appropriate medicines, and fewer referrals for angioplasty and bypass surgery.

Are women better-off today? While there has been definite improvement in the care of women with heart disease, some gaps in treatment remain. We will help you take charge of your care, focusing on the two most common scenarios, women suffering from angina and those who actually have a heart attack.

BREAKING THE LAW: WOMEN IN CLINICAL TRIALS

Most studies of heart disease focus on men. In the 156 randomized clinical trials that form the basis for the American Heart Association's 2007 Guidelines for the Prevention of Cardiovascular Disease in Women, only 30 percent of patients enrolled were female. In addition, only one-third of the trials reported results for men and women separately.

The NIH Revitalization Act of 1993 states that NIH must include women and minorities in major clinical trials in sufficient numbers to determine whether treatment effects differ in these groups. But today women represent only 27 percent of subjects enrolled in NIH-sponsored studies of cardiovascular disease. If we want to understand the gender-specific features of cardiovascular disease and its treatment, we will need to do better than that. Some scientists claim that women are underrepresented because they are reluctant to participate in studies and more likely to withdraw from them. Prove these statements wrong—if your doctor offers you a spot in a clinical trial, take the time to consider it.

ANGINA: CHEST PAIN WITHOUT A HEART ATTACK

First let's consider women who have not had heart attacks, but who have chest pain caused by coronary heart disease. This chest pain usually occurs with exertion or exercise, but as we have discussed, it may have atypical features. Chest pain in women is often a sign of impending trouble. Women with coronary heart disease who suffer from chronic chest pain are more than twice as likely to suffer death or heart attack as their male counterparts.

A recent European study of nearly 4,000 patients with chronic chest pain found that women were substantially less likely to be referred for an exercise stress test or a cardiac catheterization. Even after coronary heart disease was identified, women were less likely to receive appropriate medical therapy, which should include taking a daily aspirin and a statin, and in some cases angioplasty or bypass surgery.

Is this underuse of medical testing and therapies in women inappropriate or is it medically justified? The answer is probably somewhere in the middle. Many hospitals and doctors fail to appropriately utilize medical resources when treating women with heart disease. But there are also important differences between the arteries of men and women, whether diseased or healthy, and these can (and should) influence strategies for testing and therapy.

Because of biological differences, some common tests and therapies do not perform as well in women and therefore should be used more selectively. One of our most common diagnostic tools, the standard exercise cardiac stress test, is less reliable in women, generating more false positive results; this reduces the likelihood that doctors will order this test in women. When women undergo another common procedure, cardiac catheterization, the identification of arteries requiring stenting or bypass is less common than in men, and the risks of bleeding and damage to an artery of the leg or heart are higher. The less favorable risk-to-benefit ratio in women may influence a physician's decision about whether to perform a cardiac catheterization. These findings mandate that doctors should not always treat men and women exactly the same way. There *are* differences between the sexes—after all, women don't get prostate exams and men don't undergo regular mammograms.

One of our biggest challenges when it comes to heart tests in women is that we don't completely understand the biology of women's chest pain. Some women with chest pain who have a positive stress test—indicating inadequate blood flow to the heart—do not have significant blockage of an artery on the heart. Confirming our ignorance about what causes this scenario, the medical community calls this "syndrome X." No, we're not kidding: we really use this term.

We are not sure what causes syndrome X, but we do know that women who have it are often deeply troubled by it and limited by their pain. And despite their normal-appearing coronary arteries, women with syndrome X have a high likelihood of experiencing future heart attacks—30 percent of them develop blockages in the coronary arteries within a decade. Unfortunately, the most common "treatment" of syndrome X is a bit of reassurance and a prescription for a tranquilizer.

This is where you must be proactive. If your primary care doctor writes your chest pain off as "nerves," make sure that you see a cardiologist. If your cardiologist suggests an exercise stress test, ask if another test—such as a nuclear or echo stress test—might be a better choice. If you have a positive nuclear stress test, your doctor should consider cardiac catheterization. Whether or not you have blockages, if your chest pain is from your heart, you will probably benefit from standard therapy, including a healthy lifestyle and medicines such as statins, beta-blockers, and nitroglycerin. Exercise is particularly effective at reducing chest pain in women with syndrome X. The most important thing to remember is that if your doctor tells you "It's not your heart," respond with the question "Are you sure?"

CHEST PAIN: TAKE CHARGE WITH A FEW EASY STEPS

See a cardiologist

Ask "Could it be my heart?"

Ask about a nuclear or echo stress test instead of a standard exercise stress test

Consider a cardiac catheterization if the nuclear or echo stress test is positive

Ensure you get the correct medicines (statins, beta-blockers, nitrates) if chest pain is cardiac-related

Exercise and follow a heart-healthy lifestyle no matter what the tests show

If you are told it's not your heart, ask "Could it be my heart?" again, just to make sure

HEART ATTACK

Although syndrome X remains mysterious, we have fewer blind spots when it comes to diagnosing and treating a heart attack. Clear guidelines from the American Heart Association and the American College of Cardiology spell out the treatments for heart attack victims. Yet it seems as if women have worse outcomes than men after a heart attack. Every major cardiology conference generates media headlines such as "Post-Heart-Attack Fatalities Higher in Women than Men."

These headlines don't tell the whole story. After a heart attack, 10 percent of women and 5 percent of men die in the hospital. Within one year of a heart attack, 38 percent of women and 25 percent of men have died. The raw numbers speak for themselves. But we need more careful analysis to tell us why women fare worse, which women do worse, and what we can do about it.

The most important factor responsible for the sex difference in heart attack survival rates is the higher risk profile of the average female heart attack patient. On average, female heart attack patients are five to ten years older than male heart attack victims and tend to have more serious health problems, including diabetes, high blood pressure, and heart failure. If we account for the advanced age and additional health problems in women who have heart attacks—factors we call "co-morbidities"—we see that gender is not the primary problem. In other words, women's worse outcomes are caused mainly by the co-morbidities they possess. Most researchers have come to believe that if a man and a woman with similar health profiles suffer identical heart attacks, their outcomes will be similar, too.

Younger women—less than fifty years old—deserve special attention. While heart attacks are not particularly common in this age group, they are devastating when they do occur. Compared to young men, young women who suffer a heart attack tend to be more critically ill at hospital admission and to have more risk factors, including diabetes, hypertension, and history of stroke. Once hospitalized, they have twice the risk of dying in the hospital than men of a similar age. Some scientists believe that younger women have unusually aggressive coronary heart disease, insofar as it is able to overcome the protective effect of circulating estrogen. Compounding these issues, young women are also more likely to experience delays in treatment, either because they do not go to the hospital or because doctors miss the diagnosis. But we are making progress. Over the last ten years, outcomes after heart attack have improved among young women.

Although gender-associated differences in risk profiles are well documented, some experts still claim that the primary explanation for women's poor outcomes is treatment inequality, namely, under-treatment of women with heart attacks. Unfortunately, there may be some truth to this argument. As we mentioned earlier, many studies confirm that women receive less aggressive treatment and are less likely to receive a timely EKG, see a cardiologist, and receive appropriate medications. They are also at least 20 percent less likely to receive invasive therapies, including cardiac catheterization and stenting.

When we perform angioplasty to treat a heart attack, we carefully track the "door-to-balloon time," the interval from hospital arrival to deployment of an angioplasty balloon in the blocked artery. The American Heart Association recommends a door-to-balloon time of 90 minutes or less. In one study, the average door-to-balloon time was 95 minutes for men versus 103 minutes for women. We need to speed the process for all heart attack patients, but particularly for women.

While inequalities in treating coronary heart disease still exist, we are doing better at making sure that we offer our most advanced therapies to women. This leads to the next question: do our best therapies work as well in women? Women have smaller arteries than men, so opening up a blocked artery (angioplasty and stenting) or sewing a new artery or vein downstream as a bypass to carry blood (coronary artery bypass grafting) is technically more difficult. Historically, women have had worse outcomes with both stenting and bypass surgery. In 1985, the risk of death after angioplasty was several fold greater for women than for men. Today, though, results are better. After accounting for other health problems, the overall risk of death is similarly low for both men and women undergoing angioplasty/stenting or bypass surgery. However, women have more bleeding complications with angioplasty and a longer and more difficult recovery after bypass surgery.

Where does this leave us? Women should be vigilant and proactive when they go to the hospital with chest pain and a possible heart attack. Ask the right questions, and ask them early. Most significant differences in outcomes between men and women occur within twenty-four hours.

On arrival at the emergency room with chest pain, make sure that you have an EKG and a blood test for your troponin level. If the results do indicate a possible heart attack, ask to see a cardiologist and whether a cardiac catheterization will be done. Not everybody with a heart attack needs an urgent cardiac catheterization, but it may be the right test for you. Ask.

Finally, when you are discharged from the hospital, make sure that plans for recovery and what you need to do to prevent future cardiac events are in place. Make certain that your medicines include a statin, aspirin, and a beta-blocker. If you do not get these prescriptions, ask why not (there may be a perfectly good medical reason). Ask for a doctor's referral to a cardiac rehab program. Finally, ensure that you have a follow-up appointment with a cardiologist. These steps for your heart health must be taken *before* leaving the hospital.

HEART ATTACK: TAKE CHARGE WITH SIX KEY QUESTIONS

"What does my EKG show?"

"Is my troponin blood test normal?"

"Do I need a cardiac catheterization?"

"When is the cardiologist coming by?"

"Am I on aspirin, a statin, and a beta-blocker?"

"Where should I go for my cardiac rehab?"

RISK FACTORS FOR HEART DISEASE IN WOMEN: ROUNDING UP THE USUAL SUSPECTS

The very best way to take charge of chest pain or a heart attack is to avoid these problems in the first place. We are heart doctors, so we love seeing you, talking to you, and helping you. But wouldn't you rather avoid the anxious visits to our offices? This is where it's important to understand the traditional risk factors for heart disease—smoking, unhealthful diet, physical inactivity, cholesterol and lipid abnormalities, high blood pressure, obesity, diabetes—and their subtle variations in women.

Conventional risk factors are the primary causes of coronary heart disease in both women and men. There is no mystery here. Among people with coronary heart disease, 85 percent of women and 81 percent of men have one or more of the standard risk factors. A study of more than 84,000 women confirmed that a heart-healthy lifestyle (no smoking, good diet, maintenance of normal weight, and exercise) can potentially prevent up to 80 percent of heart attacks.

We know that men have heart attacks at an earlier age than women (average age of fifty-six for men versus sixty-five for women). While many believe that the protective effect of estrogen explains the delay in women, differences in standard risk factors also play a major role. There is strong evidence that men develop heart disease earlier than women because men accumulate more risk factors at an earlier age. Minimizing the importance of estrogen, some experts argue that women manifest their heart disease at a later age simply because it takes them a few extra years to develop high blood pressure, lipid abnormalities, diabetes, obesity, and other damaging conditions.

Our take on this is that conventional risk factors, sex hormones (estrogen), and sex-based differences in anatomy and physiology all play important roles in women's heart health. But because standard risk factors for heart disease can be improved by simple lifestyle strategies, it is critical to understand the modifiable behaviors that contribute to heart disease in women.

Although heart problems usually occur later in life, risk begins to accumulate early. By age forty, more than half of women have at least one risk factor. While all of the risk factors are bad, some of them are especially dangerous for women. Smoking is a key preventable cause of coronary heart disease in both women and men. Smoking cigarettes doubles the risk of a heart attack. But the combination of smoking and taking birth control pills increases the risk of a heart attack twentyfold in women under thirty-five.

Both women and men get diabetes, but the cardiac danger from the disease is greater in women, who have a greater risk of dying from coronary heart disease. The best ways to avoid diabetes are simple—weight management and exercise. In fact, physical fitness appears to be more important than body weight itself in preventing heart disease in women.

Blood lipid levels also hold different implications in women. For women, decreased HDL cholesterol (less than 50 mg/dL) appears to be a stronger risk factor than elevated LDL cholesterol (greater than 130 mg/dL), which is the most important target in men. Nevertheless, the smartest strategy for a woman is to keep all lipid levels in a favorable range.

DO STATINS WORK EQUALLY WELL FOR MEN AND WOMEN?

On March 29, 2010, an article in *Time* addressing whether statins work just as well in women as in men set off a firestorm of controversy. The writer, Catherine Elton, described complications of statin therapy in two middle-aged women and concluded that the risk-to-benefit ratio does not support broad use of statins to prevent heart disease in women. Fear and uncertainty reigned among the 12 million American women taking statins. Many called their doctors. Some simply stopped taking the medicines.

The American Heart Association and cardiologists responded quickly, reminding us that our largest studies of statins support their use both in women with coronary heart disease and in many of those at risk for cardiovascular disease. A meta-analysis in the prestigious journal *Lancet* confirmed the beneficial impact of statins. And the more recent Jupiter Trial revealed that statin use in women at risk for heart disease reduced subsequent needs for coronary artery stenting and bypass surgery.

Elton was correct in her assertion that we have more evidence for a benefit of statins in men than in women. But we have plenty of data demonstrating important cardiovascular benefits in women. The bottom line is that statins *are* effective in the treatment and prevention of coronary heart disease in both women and men.

Because the relative impact of conventional risk factors differs for men and women, the American Heart Association has created a female-specific approach to heart disease screening. Unlike previous screening tools, this one is easy to apply and does not require your doctor's input. You can assess your own risk right now.

Assessing a Woman's Risk of Heart Attack and Heart Disease

RISK CATEGORY	CHARACTERISTIC
High risk	Known cardiovascular disease (heart attack, angioplasty, bypass surgery, coronary heart disease, stroke, peripheral arterial disease)
	Diabetes
	Chronic kidney disease/dialysis
At risk	Cigarette smoking
	Poor diet (more than 7 percent of calories from saturated fat)
	Physical inactivity (no exercise)
	Poor exercise capacity (cannot climb 2 flights of stairs without stopping)
	Obesity (waist size > 35 inches)
	Family history of early cardiovascular disease in a first-degree male relative under 55 or female relative under 65
	High blood pressure
	Lipid abnormalities (HDL < 50 mg/dL, triglycerides > 150 mg/dL, LDL cholesterol > 100 mg/dL)
Optimal risk	None of the above
	Healthy diet (<7 percent of calories from saturated fat)
	Exercise at least 30 minutes per day

Only 4 percent of women fall into the optimal risk category. Where do you fit?

THE SCIENCE BEHIND THE DIFFERENCES: ESTROGEN, BLOOD VESSELS, AND THE BIOLOGY OF WOMEN

We have identified key differences in the sexes' risk factors and treatments for heart disease, including the increased frequencies of syndrome X and atypical heart attack symptoms as well as a later age of onset. Many of these differences are rooted in the unique biology of women.

The most obvious cardiac difference between women and men is the fact that women have smaller hearts and coronary arteries. Small arteries in women are more than a simple reflection of smaller body size. When men and women of similar size are compared, the coronary arteries of women are still smaller. An artery that is smaller in diameter can be blocked by less plaque or clot, and is more challenging to repair with angioplasty or bypass surgery. This size difference accounts for some of the disparity in outcomes between women and men with coronary heart disease.

HEART TRANSPLANTS, TRANSSEXUALS, AND CORONARY ARTERIES

Why are women's arteries smaller? The answer relates in part to the actions of circulating sex hormones (estrogen, progesterone, testosterone) in men and women. This concept is supported by interesting observations involving heart transplants. When a heart from a woman is transplanted into the body of a man, exposure to male hormones causes the coronary arteries to enlarge. However, when a female-to-female heart transplant occurs, there is no change in arterial caliber. Studies of arteries' size in transsexuals further illustrate the influence of hormones. When transsexual men (males transitioning to female) take estrogen, arteries in the arm (and presumably the heart) shrink. In contrast, when a transsexual woman takes male hormones (androgens such as testosterone), the arteries enlarge. A person's sex and sex hormones clearly influence artery size. These factors also affect arteries' physiology in ways that can be particularly harmful to women.

All over the body, the smaller blood vessels of women have distinct vulnerabilities. Several diseases related to blood vessel function occur exclusively in women, including hypertensive disorders of pregnancy, diabetes associated with pregnancy, and polycystic ovarian syndrome. Each of these conditions is related to the development of cardiovascular disease in women. Other vascular problems, including migraine headaches and inflammatory diseases such as lupus and rheumatoid arthritis, are far more common in women than in men. Given the large number of problems involving blood vessels and inflammation, it is no surprise that women have gender-specific issues with the arteries of the heart.

Let's continue our scientific comparison of the sexes by examining the most common cardiac problem, atherosclerotic plaque. Most heart attacks in both women and men are caused by plaque-based blockage of an artery on the heart. Like men, women develop classic coronary artery lesions, consisting of cholesterol-filled plaques that grow inside arteries and impede blood flow. But in regard to their distribution and composition, these plaques often differ in women when compared to men.

Although women with coronary heart disease tend to have more risk factors than men, they have a lower plaque burden, meaning that they have a lower overall volume of plaque in their coronary arteries. Their disease also tends to involve fewer coronary arteries—one or two of the heart's arteries, rather than all three. While plaques in men are more likely to contain calcium, women's tend to be less dense and non-calcified, appearing "soft." These soft plaques may be more dangerous, increasing the risk of a heart attack.

We mentioned earlier that obstructing plaques are not the sole cause of coronary artery problems. Thirty percent of women who undergo cardiac catheterization, whether for chest pain or a heart attack, have apparently normal coronary arteries. Many of these women have syndrome X—inadequate blood flow to the heart without obstructing plaque in the arteries. For the most part, this problem is a women's disease.

Many scientists believe that heart symptoms and heart attacks with normal-appearing coronary arteries are caused by the abnormal function of very small, downstream arteries on the heart. This is termed "microvascular dysfunction," and it may result from spasm of the smaller arteries or failure of the arteries to expand when additional blood flow is needed. Inflammation may contribute to this problem. When these tiny arteries constrict, the heart muscle receives inadequate blood flow, which can cause chest pain and a heart attack.

Inflammation, small vessel spasm, and microvascular dysfunction are thought to be more important in women's heart disease than in men's. This means that we need to think beyond the classic obstructing plaque when treating heart disease in women. Of course, there is something else going on with women: the estrogen question. When it comes to heart health, there are two key questions concerning a woman's natural estrogen: (1) whether estrogen protects younger women from heart disease, and (2) whether estrogen decline at menopause contributes to heart disease in middle-aged and older women. The simple answer to both of these questions is yes. But the complete answer is more complicated. For one thing, not all of estrogen's effects are good for the heart.

Cardiovascular Effects of Estrogen: A Mixed Picture

POTENTIALLY BENEFICIAL	POTENTIALLY HARMFUL
Decreased LDL cholesterol	Increased triglycerides
Increased HDL cholesterol	Increased inflammation
Blood vessel dilation	
Protection against vascular injury	
Inhibition of atherosclerosis	
New blood vessel formation (angiogenesis)	

Estrogen has a variety of biological effects, some beneficial and some harmful. While decreased LDL cholesterol and increased HDL cholesterol are certainly positive effects of estrogen, the increased triglycerides and inflammation caused by estrogen count as negatives. Estrogen's effect on blood clotting is controversial, with some studies pointing toward increased clotting and other evidence suggesting clot prevention.

Overall, these biological mechanisms, coupled with the observation that premenopausal women rarely develop coronary heart disease, support the theory of a protective role for estrogen in young women. The finding that women with diseases associated with very low levels of estrogen have a sevenfold increase in the risk of developing coronary heart disease further supported this concept.

High circulating estrogen levels and a relatively low number of standard cardiac risk factors delay the appearance of coronary heart disease in most young women. But everything changes at menopause. Estrogen levels drop by 90 percent and the type of estrogen in the body changes, with most of the estrogen being produced by fat cells (estrone) rather than by the ovaries (estradiol). This major hormonal shift contributes to the increased risk of coronary artery disease that begins soon after menopause.

MENOPAUSE AND HEART DISEASE: CHECK YOUR RISK FACTORS

Menopause causes a variety of changes that can be bad for the heart. In the year surrounding the beginning of menopause, total and LDL cholesterol levels increase, and many women also experience a decrease in HDL cholesterol. In addition, clusters of risk factors, including obesity, diabetes, and hypertension, tend to appear around the time of menopause, putting women on a collision course with cardiovascular disease. The incidence of coronary heart disease climbs rapidly in the first few years after menopause. But this sequence of events is not inevitable. The average age at menopause is fifty-one, and the average life expectancy of women in developed countries is eighty-two years. Women live more than one-third of their lives in the postmenopausal state. The goal is to be healthy and functional during this third of life. The onset of menopause is a time to assess your risk factors for heart disease and to work with your doctor to develop a heart-healthy plan, including exercise, a low-salt Mediterranean-style diet, and annual checks of blood lipids and blood pressure. Don't accept excess risk of heart disease simply because you hit menopause. Be proactive and reduce your risk.

These observations concerning the cardiac benefit of natural estrogen set up the next big question for doctors. If estrogen decline at menopause contributes to development of coronary heart disease, why not simply treat postmenopausal women with supplemental estrogen? Wouldn't this protect their hearts, just like natural estrogen protects the hearts of younger women? Doctors did not wait for rigorous scientific studies to answer these questions. They rushed for their prescription pads on the basis of compelling circumstantial evidence. For decades doctors thought that taking hormones after menopause was helping the hearts of women. They were wrong.

HORMONE REPLACEMENT THERAPY: A BIG MISTAKE?

The story of hormone replacement therapy—administration of estrogen or estrogen plus progesterone—to postmenopausal women is long, convoluted, and still evolving. Based upon the data we have so far, we know that postmenopausal women should not take estrogen to try to prevent heart disease. But short-term hormone replacement therapy to relieve hot flashes and night sweats in recently menopausal women is reasonably safe.

No topic in women's health has generated as much controversy and confusion as the role of hormone replacement therapy. Early observational studies suggested that postmenopausal women on HRT cut their risk of developing cardiovascular disease by 30 to 50 percent. Some researchers questioned this observation, suggesting that it resulted from "healthy user syndrome"—that is, women who took hormones were prone to be more health conscious in general. If that were the case, the improved heart health in HRT users would be a consequence of their overall better health.

This debate prompted more rigorous studies. When women were randomly assigned to receive HRT or a placebo, HRT reduced LDL cholesterol by 15 percent and increased HDL cholesterol by 15 percent. With these positive effects on lipids, HRT was deemed "good for the heart" by most women and their doctors. As a consequence, by 2000, Premarin (an estrogen) was the second most commonly prescribed drug in the United States, with 46 million prescriptions filled in 2000 at a cost of more than $1 billion. Prempro, a combination of estrogen and progesterone, was not far behind, with 22 million prescriptions written in 2000.

Critically thinking doctors remained skeptical. Estrogen-based HRT improved certain risk factors for coronary heart disease, but most studies examined only these indirect benefits. The key question remained unanswered: did HRT actually influence the progression or development of coronary heart disease itself?

The Heart and Estrogen/Progestin Replacement Study (HERS) was the first big study to look at the impact of HRT on hard clinical outcomes—heart attack and death. In this trial, women with established coronary heart disease were randomly assigned to receive either HRT or placebo. As expected, women who received HRT had a decrease in LDL cholesterol and an increase in HDL cholesterol. But women receiving HRT were actually shown to have an *increased* risk of heart attack in the first year. They also had higher risks of gallbladder disease and serious blood clots in their veins. Another study demonstrated that HRT failed to slow the progression of atherosclerotic plaque in women with coronary heart disease. The take-home message was surprising: HRT offered no protection to women who already had coronary heart disease.

But what about women without heart problems? Would HRT prevent them from developing coronary heart disease?

The massive NIH-sponsored Women's Health Initiative addressed this question. In these studies, 27,000 women without heart disease, ages fifty to seventy-nine, were randomly assigned to receive HRT or a placebo. HRT consisted of estrogen alone in women who had had a hysterectomy, and estrogen plus progesterone in women who still had a uterus (the addition of progesterone prevents overgrowth of the lining of the uterus, which can lead to endometrial cancer). The results of the studies were startling: HRT was harmful in women with no history of heart disease. Although HRT improved LDL and HDL cholesterol levels, once again these improved levels did not translate into a cardiac benefit.

The estrogen-plus-progesterone part of the study was stopped three years early because of an overall negative health impact: women receiving HRT had increased risks of invasive breast cancer and serious cardiac events. As in previous studies, the increased risk of heart problems became evident in the first year. HRT did produce some health benefits, including increased bone density and fewer fractures, and a lower risk of colon cancer. But overall risk outweighed these benefits.

Risks of Hormone Replacement Therapy: Estrogen plus Progesterone	
HARMFUL EFFECT	**INCREASE IN RISK**
Breast cancer	26 percent
Heart attack or death from heart disease	29 percent
Stroke	41 percent
Blood clot in the lung	200 percent
Ovarian cancer	58 percent

Study authors estimated that if 10,000 people took HRT for one year, there would be 7 additional events from coronary heart disease, 8 additional strokes, 8 blood clots in the lung, and 8 cases of invasive breast cancer. Overall, 1 of every 100 women would have a serious complication within five years of beginning HRT.

Next came a study of estrogen therapy in women who had previously undergone hysterectomy. This study, too, was halted early, in this case because stroke was the primary problem. Women receiving HRT had a 39 percent increase in the risk of stroke, amounting to an additional 12 per 10,000 women per year.

Like the combination of estrogen and progesterone, estrogen alone increased the risk of blood clots in veins (33 percent) and decreased the risk of hip fractures (30 percent). There was no apparent beneficial effect on heart disease. Interestingly, though, there appeared to be a slight decrease in the risk of breast cancer (23 percent) among the women receiving estrogen. Doctors still debate whether this effect on breast cancer is a true benefit or a chance finding.

These two large-scale studies of HRT made headlines. By mid-2004, the answers seemed clear: HRT did not confer cardiac protection to post-menopausal women, and treatment was associated with a variety of adverse outcomes, including heart attack, stroke, blood clots to the lungs, and breast cancer. Additional studies demonstrated that HRT failed to correct other issues associated with menopause, including cognitive and sexual dysfunction, depression, and insomnia. HRT was finished. Or was it?

Subsequent analyses of these data, and corresponding media reports, have created tremendous confusion. Scientists have taken a variety of approaches as they have reexamined the volumes of data generated by the Women's Health Initiative. Each report has produced a slightly different answer. We have to take all of these studies together to arrive at our best advice on HRT.

Our conclusion is that HRT should not be used to protect the heart. But careful analysis reveals that HRT poses little to no risk when used for short periods (six months) by women who are within ten years of menopause. In these women, HRT is effective at relieving hot flashes and night sweats. In contrast, in older women and those more than ten years from menopause, HRT is riskier—it increases the likelihood of heart attack and death from heart disease.

These different effects of HRT according to time since menopause have been termed "the timing hypothesis." The idea is that HRT has neutral (or possibly even slightly beneficial) cardiac effects in younger women, who generally have little or no preexisting coronary heart disease. In these women, who went through menopause relatively recently, HRT's positive effects on cholesterol and blood vessel function are thought to dominate. In contrast, when administered to older women who already have coronary artery plaque, the negative effects of estrogen, including increased inflammation and increased tendency of blood to clot, lead to heart attacks.

Although the timing hypothesis is controversial, we believe that it makes sense. HRT is a medicine. Like any medicine, it is not right (or wrong) for everybody. Patient characteristics, including the time since menopause and the state of the coronary arteries, play a role in deciding whether to use HRT for relief of menopausal symptoms. HRT should not be prescribed in women over the age of sixty or in women with a history of heart attack, stroke, breast cancer, or blood clots to the lung.

Today, HRT can be used to relieve menopausal symptoms in women between fifty to fifty-nine who are within ten years of menopause. In these women, the risk associated with HRT is low, and the benefit in terms of quality of life may be substantial. Recognizing this, 64 percent of postmenopausal female doctors (and 74 percent of the wives of male ob/gyn physicians) use HRT. HRT should be started at the lowest possible dose, and patients should be weaned off it after six months, if possible.

ORAL CONTRACEPTIVES: DIFFERENT FROM HORMONE REPLACEMENT THERAPY

The controversy concerning hormone replacement therapy for postmenopausal women has created confusion about the relationship of oral contraceptives and cardiovascular disease. More than 10 million American women use oral contraceptives. Today's oral contraceptives contain very low doses of hormones—a quarter of the estrogen and a tenth of the progesterone present in original preparations of the pill. Do current oral contraceptives carry cardiovascular risks? The answer is yes, but the risks are very small.

Oral contraceptives cause a slight increase in the risk of blood clots in veins of the legs and in the lungs. The increased risk of stroke associated with modern oral contraceptives is modest. Oral contraceptives also cause a moderate increase in the risk of heart attack. But if a woman takes oral contraceptives and smokes, the risk of heart attack is increased as much as twentyfold.

PREGNANCY: DANGEROUS FOR THE HEART?

Let's consider the cardiac implications of pregnancy, another uniquely female event. Pregnancy affects every part of a woman's body, including the cardiovascular system. If not recognized and addressed, some of these effects may jeopardize future cardiac health.

High blood pressure is the most common unfavorable cardiovascular consequence of pregnancy. During pregnancy, 10 percent of women develop hypertension (blood pressure greater than 140/90). By itself, this condition is easily managed. A more serious condition, preeclampsia, is present when a woman develops the combination of hypertension and protein in the urine at twenty weeks of pregnancy or beyond. Preeclampsia affects 3 to 5 percent of pregnant women and can be fatal if untreated.

The good news is that both hypertension and preeclampsia disappear after the child is born. The bad news is that they may leave lasting effects. Hypertension during pregnancy (termed "gestational hypertension") is associated with a small increase in later cardiovascular disease. The long-term risk is far greater with preeclampsia. Of special concern are women with preeclampsia who deliver early; they have an eightfold increase in the risk of death from later cardiovascular disease.

You can take steps to prevent pregnancy from creating heart problems down the road. It all comes back to managing the usual suspects—those risk factors we keep discussing. Limiting weight gain to twenty-five to thirty-five pounds reduces the risk of developing hypertension. If a woman does develop hypertension or preeclampsia during pregnancy, she should schedule a full checkup six months after delivery to assess her weight, BMI, blood pressure, blood glucose, and blood lipids. When cardiovascular events occur in women with a history of preeclampsia, the average age is thirty-eight. The message here is to intervene early. Don't wait until menopause for your first assessment of risk factors—do it soon after delivery.

Although a woman with hypertensive disorders of pregnancy may not have symptoms, other, more threatening conditions leave clues when they develop. We all know that swelling of the ankles, shortness of breath, and fatigue are common in pregnancy. But if they arise or worsen suddenly in the last trimester of pregnancy or within five months after delivery, they may be symptoms of peripartum cardiomyopathy, a life-threatening problem that causes a dramatic reduction in heart function. Although it occurs in only one of 3,000 live births, peripartum cardiomyopathy is sixteen times more common in African American women, particularly those with high blood pressure.

The clue to diagnosis of peripartum cardiomyopathy is the *sudden* development or worsening of symptoms—swelling of the ankles, shortness of breath, fatigue—in an otherwise normal pregnancy. An echocardiogram can confirm the diagnosis. The key to recovery is to start medical therapy early. With appropriate treatment, 94 percent of women survive at least five years, and more than half recover full heart function. But the condition is prone to recur with subsequent pregnancies. Women whose heart function does not recover should not become pregnant again.

The most serious cardiovascular complication of pregnancy is aortic dissection, a tear in the aorta. Women with Marfan syndrome or a bicuspid aortic valve are at particular risk for this problem during pregnancy. If you have a heart murmur, Marfan syndrome, or a known aortic valve abnormality, you *must* see a cardiologist for an echocardiogram before becoming pregnant. If an enlarged aorta is detected, fixing it before becoming pregnant is the safest course.

When aortic dissection occurs, it causes sharp, tearing pain in the chest or back. If a pregnant woman develops severe, unrelenting chest or back pain that comes on suddenly, it must not be ignored. While this condition requires emergency open heart surgery, advances in surgical technique enable us to save both the mother and the baby in most cases.

BREAST-FEEDING: GOOD FOR THE BABY, GOOD FOR THE MOTHER

Not all aspects of pregnancy and child-rearing pose dangers to the heart. For the health of the child, the American Academy of Pediatrics recommends breast-feeding for the first twelve months of a baby's life. Breast-feeding decreases the risks of ear infection, asthma, diabetes, and sudden infant death syndrome. Breast-feeding is also good for the mother, with potential improvements in heart health topping the list of benefits. Expending an average of 480 calories per day, breast-feeding helps deplete the fat stores accumulated during pregnancy and restore an ideal weight. Observational studies suggest that breast-feeding lowers blood pressure and improves cholesterol levels, which could translate into a reduced risk of future heart disease. The message: breast-feeding is the right choice for both baby and mother.

A couple of final thoughts about pregnancy. For more than 90 percent of women, pregnancy has no long-term cardiovascular consequences. But development of hypertension or preeclampsia mandates lifelong attention to the mother's heart and cardiovascular risk factors. Typical cardiac symptoms such as chest pain, shortness of breath, and ankle swelling must not be ignored during pregnancy, as they may be clues to serious underlying problems. Enjoy your pregnancy, but be attentive to the needs of your own heart.

RX: THE HEARTS OF WOMEN

Know your risk:
Be aware: heart disease is the number one killer of women
Take the American Heart Association quiz to determine your own risk
Even if your numbers have been good, have them checked again at menopause

Reduce your risk:
Don't count on estrogen to protect your heart
Don't ignore your heart health just because you are young
Don't smoke
Don't let menopause get to your heart: one-third of your life is ahead of you

Be aggressive:
Take chest pain seriously
Don't ignore new fatigue or shortness of breath
If you develop heart disease:
• Ask the right questions
• Make a plan with your doctor
• Make sure that you get appropriate—and equal—treatment

CHAPTER 18

HEART DISEASE IN MEN: IT *IS* ~~ALL~~ PARTLY ABOUT SEX

THE BIG PICTURE

Ninety percent of coronary heart disease is preventable. We know the risk factors, warning signs, and strategies for prevention. As a result, the risk of dying from heart disease has dropped by 50 percent over the last twenty years. But before we congratulate ourselves, we need to examine a few sobering numbers.

Heart and vascular disease remains the number one challenge in medicine: it kills more people than any other health condition. One in three men will die from cardiovascular disease. In 2010, 400,000 men experienced their first heart attack, and 250,000 had their second (or third, or fourth). If you are a forty-year-old man who looks and feels healthy, *you still face a 50 percent chance of developing heart disease* sometime in your life. In fact, chances are you already have some plaque lurking undetected in your coronary arteries.

So how can you avoid joining the friends, relatives, and millions of other men on the road to heart disease? Our goal is to guide you to a different path. We will detail a simple strategy that will both secure your health and make you feel good. Along the way, we will highlight points of special interest, explaining the important links between the heart and issues such as erectile dysfunction and the safety of sex.

Our plan is to make this easy and to help you avoid surprises down the road. Surprises in men with coronary heart disease can be particularly devastating—half of the men who die from heart attacks have no warning signs or previous symptoms. Like famed newscaster Tim Russert, they are struck down suddenly. Understanding the genesis of heart disease and managing your risk factors may prevent you from suffering a similar fate.

TIM RUSSERT: A PREVENTABLE DEATH

After an illustrious career in TV news, Tim Russert himself became the nation's biggest story in June 2008 when at the age of fifty-eight he suffered a fatal heart attack at his desk.

The media and the viewing public were stunned. Russert was brilliant, always brimming with energy. He was a fixture at key media events, an incisive analyst of every presidential election in recent memory. A man in his position was presumably receiving the very best health care. How could this happen?

The problem was that on the inside, Russert was just like many of the rest of us. He was a middle-aged man with risk factors for coronary heart disease, including increased weight, elevated triglycerides, and very low HDL cholesterol levels. In fact, Russert's doctors knew that he had coronary heart disease. His cardiologist had prescribed medicines and exercise. Russert had even taken a stress test just two or three months before, and his condition appeared stable. But it wasn't.

In this modern age of high-tech cardiac imaging, highly effective drugs, and lifesaving angioplasty and stenting, like nearly 300,000 Americans every year, Russert succumbed to sudden cardiac death as a result of an old-fashioned heart attack. This is primarily a male problem: 80 to 90 percent of the people who suffer sudden cardiac death are men.

The chain of events that occurred in Russert's heart is, unfortunately, very common. For reasons that we will never know, a plaque in Russert's left anterior descending coronary artery suddenly ruptured, causing a blood clot to form at the site. The clot blocked the artery, limiting blood flow to the heart muscle. His heart's response to the sudden lack of blood flow was ventricular fibrillation, an abnormal heart rhythm in which the heart muscle stops its rhythmic contraction. Blood flow to the body ceased, and death occurred in minutes. This is the most common pattern producing sudden cardiac death in middle-aged and older men.

This tragedy did not have to happen. Prevention starts with you. The key is to understand the risk factors for heart disease and do your best to banish them from your life. You must know the signs of heart problems and avoid the all-too-common practice of trying to wish them away. We will provide the road map, marked with simple, preventive prescriptions to unseat heart disease from its position as the number one killer of men.

RISK FACTORS, SIGNS, AND SYMPTOMS THAT YOU MUST KNOW

On average, women live about six years longer than men. The reason for this disparity is that men develop cardiovascular disease at a younger age than do women, which causes them to die earlier.

Many doctors have built their careers trying to explain why heart disease occurs earlier in men than in women. They usually blame hormones, proposing that estrogen protects women and testosterone hurts men. This is an appealing concept, but it is also, for the most part, unproven. The primary reason a man or woman suffers from heart disease can be explained by risk factors. Media reports frequently state that half of heart attacks occur in men with no risk factors. Nonsense! We can't blame heart attacks on simple bad luck. They are preventable. And prevention begins with understanding traditional risk factors.

The table lists the key modifiable risk factors for heart disease. Take a

Coronary Heart Disease: Traditional Risk Factors	
RISK FACTOR	PERCENTAGE OF MEN WITH THIS RISK FACTOR
Smoking	23 percent
Failure to exercise five days per week	59 percent
Overweight or obese	72 percent
Diabetes	15 percent
High blood pressure (> 140/90)	34 percent
Total cholesterol > 200	45 percent

moment to determine which of these apply to you. Fewer than 10 percent of men are free of all of these risk factors; they are the healthiest men among us. Are you in that 10 percent?

The table contains conditions that *you* can influence by *your* lifestyle choices. True, genetics and a family history of heart disease contribute to risk, but those are things you cannot change. Nevertheless, you should be aware of your family history, particularly if close relatives have developed cardiovascular disease at a young age—under fifty-five. If you do have a family history of heart disease, making good lifestyle choices becomes even more important. The key is targeting those risk factors that you *can* improve.

Some people are skeptical that improving risk factors can have much of an impact on your chances of developing heart disease. But we have very strong evidence that managing risk factors bears fruit. Landmark studies from the United States, Canada, and Europe clearly demonstrate that the risk of dying from coronary heart disease has dropping steadily over the past twenty-five years. Some of this can be explained by improved treatment for people who already have heart disease, but careful analyses demonstrate that medical advances account for only about half of our progress. The other half is a direct consequence of people living healthier lifestyles.

The greatest improvements have come from reducing cholesterol levels, controlling blood pressure, increasing physical activity, and limiting smoking. These trends are the good news. But there is also bad news. Increased obesity and the associated increase in diabetes threaten decades of progress. Left unchecked, these two factors will likely reverse the decades-long trend of reduced mortality from coronary heart disease.

Our prescription for optimizing your risk factor profile is simple. We have five easy steps you can take to avoid becoming the next Tim Russert.

THE BIG FIVE: FIVE THINGS YOU CAN DO TO PREVENT HEART DISEASE

Don't smoke

Exercise daily

Healthy diet (Mediterranean)

Check your blood pressure

Get a lipid profile

Let's start with the obvious—smoking. Nearly one-quarter of adult men smoke. We find this statistic almost unbelievable. On a daily basis, we witness the ravages of heart disease in smokers and see the impact on their families. Smoking doubles your risk of dying from heart disease. If you smoke, we are not here to judge you. But we are here to tell you to do everything in your power to stop. If you quit smoking right now, your arteries will begin to return to normal quickly. Over the next five years, your risk of heart attack will plummet, approaching the same level as that of somebody who has never smoked. It's never too late to do your arteries a favor. Quit now!

In Chapter 7 we outline the cardiac benefits of exercise, both aerobic and resistance training. A consistent exercise program is one of the most important steps you can take to secure your heart health. And a $75 pair of running shoes is a lot less expensive than a $40,000 post-heart-attack hospital bill. At a minimum, walk briskly for thirty minutes every day. Even better, exercise to the point of sweating or breathing hard at least five days per week, and add resistance training twice a week. You will notice effects on your energy level, your mood, and your waistline. Your heart will experience benefits as well, a consequence of lower blood pressure, better cholesterol levels, and improved blood sugar levels.

Physical activity must be coupled with a heart-healthy diet. But which diet? Choices abound, but it is actually pretty straightforward. A heart-healthy diet should follow a few simple rules related to calories and composition. The calorie part is easy—don't consume too many calories. The composition component involves minimizing saturated fats and added sugars while emphasizing mono- and polyunsaturated fats, whole grains, fruits, and vegetables. Put the salt shaker down. The most reliable scientific evidence suggest that a Mediterranean-style diet is best for heart health. We spell out our diet recommendations in Chapter 5. The key point is to use common sense when it comes to food. Look at your portion size, especially when you are eating out. Do you really need that much food? Do you truly believe that a daily dose of french fries is a good idea? Is dessert necessary? You know when you have gone too far. If you finish a meal and need to loosen your belt a notch, you know that you could have done better.

The combination of exercise and a healthy diet will improve your fitness and reduce your fatness. A healthy waist size is less than 36 inches for most men. If your waist size is greater than 40 inches, you have abdominal obesity, which is strongly linked to heart disease.

But what if you are physically active and still overweight? We all know people who fit this description. Every weekend, we play tennis with Sam. Sam is fifty years old and fifty pounds overweight. But he is a great tennis player and he has excellent endurance. Even though he is big, he plays like he is physically fit. Should we give Sam a free pass on the weight issue because he is athletic?

A recent study published in the *Journal of the American Medical Association* tried to tease out the relative importance of fatness versus fitness in heart health. The two are closely linked, but they are not the same. In this study, the authors concluded that obesity was more strongly related to cardiovascular risk factors than was fitness. What this means is that being physically active does not cancel the negatives associated with being overweight. You need both—physical fitness and a healthy body weight.

It is your responsibility to take care of yourself, but you need a doctor to help you. Beginning at age forty, have an annual checkup. Don't skip a year just because you feel good—one in ten heart attacks occurs in men under the age of forty-five. If you have no heart symptoms, you don't need any complicated procedures, but a few simple tests will go a long way in helping you understand your personal risk factor profile.

Get your blood pressure checked. Hypertension is painless, so people may not know that their arteries are under relentless attack. Increased pressure damages every artery, including those in the heart, brain, and kidneys. You want your blood pressure to be 120 over 80 or less.

While you are at the doctor's office, make sure that you also get a lipid panel, which measures your cholesterol (total, LDL, and HDL cholesterol) and triglycerides. Compare these values to the recommended ranges we outline in Chapter 3. Like high blood pressure, high cholesterol does not cause symptoms—until you have a major problem, like a heart attack.

A healthy lifestyle, coupled with targeted information from your annual checkup, will help you manage your risk factors and prevent coronary heart disease. But what if you are among the millions of men who already have coronary heart disease? The five steps we outlined above will still help you slow or halt progression of the disease. Whether you have heart disease or not, you also need to know five key warning signs.

FIVE WARNING SIGNS OF HEART DISEASE

Chest pain, discomfort, or heaviness

Jaw, arm, or shoulder pain—particularly on the left side

Back pain

Shortness of breath

Feeling light-headed, faint, or weak

BALDNESS AND HEART DISEASE: YOUR HAIR AND YOUR HEART

No man likes to lose his hair. But is baldness more than a cosmetic issue? Large observational studies suggest that baldness affecting the crown of the head is associated with an increased risk of developing heart disease. In contrast, frontal baldness (the common receding hair line) has not been linked to heart disease. Some researchers have suggested that increased testosterone levels in bald men may be the link between the scalp and the heart. However, men with the *lowest* testosterone levels have the *greatest* risk of heart disease, so testosterone levels do not explain the correlation.

A careful review of the evidence reveals that the association between baldness and heart disease is not a causal relationship. We don't think that bald men should worry more, or less, about their hearts than men with a full head of hair. But the 57 percent of men who develop baldness by the age of fifty should follow the same heart-healthy lifestyle recommended for everybody.

Heart disease and heart attacks don't always announce themselves with the traditional Hollywood-style heart attack—crushing chest pain accompanied by a heavenward gaze. Many heart attacks are not nearly that dramatic. Pain caused by heart problems does not have to be in the chest—it can affect the jaw, arm, shoulder, or back. Some people with heart disease and heart attacks experience other symptoms, such as shortness of breath or generalized weakness.

If you are a man forty years of age or older, be suspicious if you develop any of these symptoms. You should be especially wary if you have both symptoms *and* risk factors for heart disease—such as smoking, diabetes, high blood pressure, or obesity. The onset of these symptoms can mean a heart attack may be imminent—or, even worse, that you are actually in the middle of one. If you develop any of these symptoms, seek medical attention today. Not tomorrow. Today

Delays are deadly. While businesspeople claim that "time is money," we doctors say that "time is heart muscle." When a person has a heart attack, heart muscle cells start dying within thirty minutes. It is imperative to get to the hospital immediately, where a doctor can open the blocked artery and restore blood flow to the heart muscle.

What do most people do when they develop new chest, arm, jaw, or back pain or shortness of breath? Usually they wait an average of two to three hours before going to the hospital. Over the last twenty years, there has been virtually no improvement in the speed with which heart attack victims get to the hospital. The elderly are particularly prone to delaying care. No matter what your age, but particularly if you are seventy years or older, make sure that you get to the hospital or call 911 if you develop suspicious symptoms. Chest pain and shortness of breath are *not* normal parts of aging.

ERECTILE DYSFUNCTION: THE HEART OF THE MATTER

The heart and the penis are closely linked. While some men may believe that the heart's most important function is to pump blood to the penis, the relationship is, we think, a little more complicated. And understanding the close relationship between your heart and your penis could save your life.

Erectile dysfunction (ED) is the most important link between sex and the heart. Ten million to 20 million American men suffer from ED. Later we will discuss the treatments for ED. But first we want to emphasize a critical issue: overt erectile dysfunction is frequently a sign of covert heart disease.

The appearance of ED may threaten your sex life, but it also portends a much greater threat to your entire life. Over a five-year period, a man with ED has about a 50 percent increase in his risk of having a heart attack or of requiring hospitalization for heart disease. This risk is even higher in men under fifty, suggesting that ED is a particularly worrisome sign of bad heart health in younger men. The more severe the ED, the higher the risk of developing heart disease.

ED is also a bad sign in men who already have coronary heart disease. Half of men with coronary heart disease either have or will develop ED—and those that do have a worse prognosis than their counterparts without ED. The bottom line: ED and coronary heart disease travel together.

The medical link between erections and heart health involves atherosclerosis and blood vessel endothelial dysfunction. Atherosclerosis is a systemic problem that affects arteries throughout the body, from those in the penis to those in the kidneys, brain, legs, and heart. One of the first steps in atherosclerosis, which occurs before the formation of obstructing plaque, is abnormal function of the endothelial cells that line the inside of arteries and help control blood flow by causing arteries to dilate or constrict. Just like the heart's pumping, the penis's erection depends on normal function of these cells and the arteries that they regulate.

Erection is a vascular event. For an erection to occur, arteries in the penis must dilate (enlarge), enabling extra blood flow into the penis. This can occur only if the endothelium functions properly. The most common reason that a man cannot develop or maintain an erection is that the arteries fail to dilate because of endothelial dysfunction. And if the arteries in the penis are damaged by this early stage of atherosclerosis, the odds are high that arteries in the heart have been affected as well.

Although the underlying mechanism—damage or dysfunction of arteries—is the same, it is common for ED to develop *before* symptoms of coronary heart disease. Why? The arteries in the penis are smaller (1 mm, versus 3 to 5 mm in the heart), so it takes less endothelial dysfunction and less plaque to impair blood flow. In addition, unlike the heart, the penis, when faced with decreased blood flow, does not have the capability to form new arteries. On average, ED precedes coronary heart disease by about three years. The message here is that ED often serves as a warning of impending heart disease. A man with ED should be considered a heart patient until proven otherwise.

If you develop ED, you need to think above the waistline. Discuss it ASAP with your doctor, who can help with both your ED and your heart. But the heart comes first. The first thing your doctor will do is to assess your risk factors for heart disease. It turns out that—no surprise—most of the risk factors for heart disease are the very same conditions associated with development of ED.

COMMON RISK FACTORS: ED AND HEART DISEASE

Increased age

Smoking

Obesity

Diabetes

High blood pressure

Physical inactivity

High cholesterol (LDL and total)

Depression

A lifestyle that minimizes these risk factors reduces the chances of developing both ED and coronary artery disease. Conversely, an unfavorable risk factor profile for the heart also means bad news for the penis. So if we have not convinced you to adopt a heart-healthy lifestyle, perhaps we can persuade you to follow an erection-healthy lifestyle; they are the same thing.

In assessing your ED and associated risk factors, your doctor will perform a standard physical examination. He or she will also order routine blood tests, including a lipid panel and a glucose test. Further testing is generally not necessary. Unlike some doctors, we do not recommend a stress test for all men with ED. A stress test should be obtained only if you have specific cardiac symptoms, such as chest, neck, back, or arm pain or shortness of breath.

The most important step to take for both your heart health and your sex life is to optimize your risk factors. But what if you already have ED? ED often improves with a heart- and erection-friendly lifestyle. In a landmark study of obese men with ED, scientists demonstrated the favorable impact of lifestyle on sexual function. Men were randomly assigned to a group that followed a detailed weight loss program of diet and exercise, or to a group that was given only general dietary and exercise information. Over a two-year period, men who followed a healthy lifestyle lost an average of thirty pounds and had across-the-board improvements in risk factors, including reduced inflammation and better cholesterol levels. And there were corresponding benefits in erectile function: in one-third of the subjects, ED disappeared altogether. The program required commitment—treated men exercised about three hours per week. But we would guess that subjects thought the effort was justified, given the good result.

We intentionally chose to address lifestyle before filling you in on the medicines often prescribed for ED. Taking a pill for ED does nothing to improve risk factors or help the heart. These drugs must be used in conjunction with lifestyle changes. There are three medicines currently available for treatment of ED—Viagra (sildenafil), Levitra (vardenafil), and Cialis (tadalafil). They are among the most popular drugs in the world, with annual sales topping $1.5 billion.

The story of Viagra's discovery is emblematic of the link between heart disease and ED. In the mid-1980s, researchers were looking for a drug that would reduce chest pain in heart patients by improving blood flow in the coronary arteries. In 1989, they observed that sildenafil citrate (later named Viagra) looked promising in laboratory experiments. In a large study in which heart patients received either Viagra or a placebo (a

CIGARETTES AND ERECTILE DYSFUNCTION

It is a familiar movie scene: after sex, satisfied and relaxed, a man leans back against his pillow and lights up a cigarette. That cigarette (and every cigarette) affects blood vessels in every part of the body, including in the penis. And we know what happens when blood vessels in the penis don't function properly. Smoking is strongly associated with development of ED. But, just like weight loss, quitting smoking often makes ED go away. Within twenty-four hours of smoking cessation, blood flow to the penis improves. Within one year of quitting, ED improves in at least 25 percent of people. Enjoy and prolong a healthy sex life—don't light up that cigarette.

sugar pill), Viagra did cause a slight increase in coronary blood flow, but did not result in improvement of heart symptoms. But you can guess the interesting side effect that men noticed. Although Viagra lost its place as a heart medicine, in 1998 it became the first drug approved by the FDA for treatment of ED.

Today, once a man's heart and risk factors are assessed, Viagra, Levitra, or Cialis is prescribed as first-line medical therapy for ED. These agents work by blocking a protein that normally breaks down cyclic GMP, an important vasodilator in the penile arteries. When the breakdown protein is blocked, the penile arteries can relax, blood flow is increased, and an erection can develop. These medicines don't fix the endothelial dysfunction and early atherosclerosis that prevent normal erections; they simply provide a way around the problem.

Viagra, Levitra, and Cialis are effective in 80 percent of men with ED. They are safe in men with and without coronary heart disease. Although initial reports suggested cardiac danger, large studies confirmed that these medicines do not increase the risk of heart attack. The most common side effects are headache, flushing, and a runny nose, all caused by dilation of arteries elsewhere in the body. The medicines do cause a small decrease in blood pressure, but this is usually not significant.

One important caveat: men who take nitrate pills (nitroglycerin) for chest pain *must not* take drugs for ED at the same time. Like medicines for ED, nitrates cause arteries and veins to dilate, and the combination of the two may cause a dangerous drop in blood pressure. Now you understand the warning that accompanies every television commercial for these drugs. Men on Viagra or Levitra should not take nitrates for at least twenty-four hours after the last dose, and men on Cialis must wait forty-eight hours before taking nitrates. If you are taken to the hospital for chest pain, always tell the doctors and nurses if you take an ED medicine. This will prevent them from giving you a potentially life-threatening nitrate.

For us doctors, ED stands for "early detection." Asking our patients if they have erectile dysfunction is a cheap and effective screening test for cardiovascular disease. We have very effective therapies available for men with ED. But before getting out our prescription pads, we must consider the heart. After considering their cardiovascular risk factors, most men with ED can take appropriate medicines and enjoy a normal sex life.

SEX AND THE HEART PATIENT

Erectile dysfunction gets the most press. But another common fear is that sex is dangerous for men with heart disease, particularly those who have suffered heart attacks. This is simply not true.

Sexual activity is associated with minimal cardiac risk. Less than 1 percent of all heart attacks are triggered by sex, compared to 5 percent that are brought on by heavy physical activity and 3 percent by anger. A 1996 study in the *Journal of the American Medical Association* calculated that in healthy individuals without a history of heart disease, the chance of sexual activity causing a heart attack is about two in a million. In a person with a history of prior heart attack, the risk of experiencing another heart attack as a consequence of sexual activity is still extremely low—about twenty in a million. This risk is even lower among heart patients who exercise regularly.

But heart patients and their spouses do worry, and doctors frequently fail to address their concerns. A 2010 study from the University of Chicago demonstrated that after suffering a heart attack, only about half of men and a third of women received discharge instructions regarding sexual activity. In the year following a heart attack, fewer than 40 percent of men and 20 percent of women talked frankly with their doctors about sex. But among those who did, that conversation had an impact—they were 30 to 40 percent more likely to resume sexual activity after the heart attack. After discharge, in addition to getting your stack of prescriptions and asking when you can start driving a car, ask your doctor about sex as well.

Because doctors often feel uncomfortable bringing up the subject, you, the patient (or spouse), might need to be the one to broach it.

So is sex safe after a heart attack? Almost always, the answer is yes. Most people can resume sex as soon as they feel well and can walk up two flights of stairs or do moderate exercise, usually in about two weeks. The same principles apply to those who have undergone angioplasty or bypass surgery. Resumption of sexual activity after both of these procedures is safe for most people.

Only a small number of heart patients need to see a cardiologist before resuming sexual activity. A panel convened at Princeton University compiled a series of conditions (which we have modified somewhat) that mandate a trip to the cardiologist before sex or before beginning a drug for ED. For the most part, these recommendations are obvious. If you are experiencing severe chest pain or shortness of breath, you are probably thinking more about a visit to the hospital than about a trip to the bedroom.

SEE A DOCTOR BEFORE SEXUAL ACTIVITY IF YOU HAVE ANY OF THESE CONDITIONS

Severe chest pain

Chest pain that comes on at rest

Severe congestive heart failure: shortness of breath at rest, ankles very swollen

Uncontrolled high blood pressure

Hypertrophic obstructive cardiomyopathy (diagnosed by echocardiogram)

Severe aortic stenosis (diagnosed by echocardiogram)

One of the reasons that heart patients are often wary of sex is the perception that sexual activity is associated with maximal or even supermaximal exertion. Alas, this is usually not the case. For a middle-aged man, the average workload associated with sexual activity is the equivalent of walking a mile in twenty minutes or climbing two flights of stairs in ten seconds. If you can do both of these activities without developing chest pain, you will likely be fine during sex as well.

Yet sexual activity does involve some exertion, and as a consequence it causes a cardiovascular response. During sex, there is a modest increase in heart rate that varies with position—with the man on top, the average maximum heart rate is 127 beats per minute, versus 110 beats per minute with the man on the bottom. (No kidding—scientists really did this experiment.) But these heart rate changes are not large enough for a doctor to intrude into your bedroom and advise a change in position. At the time of orgasm, blood pressure spikes briefly, generally reaching about 160/90. This is not even close to the maximum values attainable by middle-aged men during heavy exertion; shoveling snow places a far greater strain on the cardiovascular system.

Certain situations have been associated with greater physiologic changes during sex and, perhaps, a higher risk of heart attack: having sex after a heavy intake of food and alcohol, as well as engaging in sex in an unfamiliar setting or with an unfamiliar partner. A 1981 report described the experience of a middle-aged man who was wearing a heart rate monitor as part of his cardiac rehabilitation program. At noon, he had sex with his girlfriend, and his heart rate went from 96 beats per minute to 150 beats per minute. That night, during sex with his wife, his heart rate increased from 72 beats per minute to only 92 beats per minute.

A German study supports the idea that sexual activity outside of a person's normal routine can elevate cardiovascular stress and risk. Researchers identified thirty-seven men and two women who died during sex, presumably of heart attacks, and found that 82 percent of the men who died did so while engaging in extramarital sex. While this observational study does not rise to the level of scientific proof, it does suggest that situations that increase excitement, heart rate, and blood pressure may also increase risk for the heart patient. It also provides a scientific rationale for marital fidelity.

After a careful analysis of the data, we can say that sex is safe for nearly all heart patients, whether a man has angina or has had a heart attack, angioplasty, or bypass surgery. Heart disease should not be allowed to kill a man's sex life. But for a variety of reasons, it is probably safest to stay true to your usual partner.

DOES TESTOSTERONE HELP OR HURT THE HEART?

Continuing our discussion of the relationships between organs above and below the belt, we now turn our attention to testosterone, the male sex hormone that is necessary for a boy to develop during puberty and for a man to maintain adult male features and normal sexual function. In addition, natural testosterone exerts a wide variety of effects on the cardiovascular system. Cells in the heart and in arteries throughout the body have specific testosterone receptors on their surfaces, which supports the idea that testosterone is "meant" to affect our arteries.

So is testosterone good or bad for cardiovascular health? Given that millions of men take testosterone supplements to build muscle mass or enhance sexual performance, this is a very important question.

The idea that naturally produced testosterone causes heart disease in men has been around for a long time, but extensive research shows that high testosterone levels are *not* responsible for the increased risk of heart disease in men compared to women. Still, we don't yet have all of the answers about how testosterone affects the heart. At this point, our understanding of the relationship between testosterone and heart health is similar to the knowledge we had in the late 1990s concerning estrogen and women's hearts.

TESTOSTERONE'S CARDIOVASCULAR EFFECTS

Dilation of arteries in heart and elsewhere, increasing blood flow

Enhanced arterial repair

Decreased inflammation

Improved insulin sensitivity and glucose control

Decreased body fat, and increased lean mass

Small decreases in LDL cholesterol and total cholesterol

Variable effect on HDL cholesterol

Variable effect on blood clotting

Overall, these effects appear to add up to a favorable impact of testosterone on the heart and its arteries. Relaxation of the heart's arteries with a resulting increase in blood flow is generally a good thing. Improved insulin sensitivity leads to lower blood glucose levels and, possibly, to a lower risk of developing diabetes. The effects on cholesterol remain a bit murky, but we can state with confidence that testosterone does not have major negative effects on cholesterol levels.

As a man ages, his risk of heart disease increases, while at the same time his serum testosterone level (the amount of testosterone in his body, as determined by a test of blood serum) falls. This observation supports the notion that testosterone does not cause heart disease. Starting at about age thirty, serum testosterone levels decline by about 1 percent per year. General consequences of lower testosterone levels include reduced muscle strength and mass, increased fat, weight gain, and, in some men, erectile dysfunction, mood changes, and decreased quality of life.

As testosterone levels fall, bad things also happen to the cardiovascular system. Men who experience the greatest declines in testosterone levels tend to have particularly unfavorable cardiovascular risk factor profiles, including more diabetes and obesity, higher levels of total and LDL cholesterol, higher levels of inflammation markers, lower levels of HDL cholesterol, and more endothelial dysfunction. It is logical to conclude that a low blood testosterone level in a middle-aged or older man is bad news for heart health.

Indeed, large medical studies suggest a link between low testosterone and heart disease. Men with low testosterone tend to develop systemic signs of atherosclerosis, including plaque in the aorta and a thickening of the wall of the carotid artery in the neck. Low testosterone levels seem to put men at increased risk of heart attack and death. Over a ten-year period, men with the lowest testosterone values have a 25 percent greater risk of dying from heart disease. In addition, nearly one-quarter of men with coronary heart disease have abnormally low testosterone levels, and the more extensive the coronary heart disease, the lower the testosterone. Among men with coronary heart disease, those with the lowest testosterone levels face an increased risk of premature death.

The big question is whether a low testosterone level actually *causes* coronary heart disease, or whether it is simply a marker of generally poor health that includes heart disease. Unfortunately, we don't have the final answer. Nevertheless, based upon strong circumstantial evidence, some cardiologists suggest that testosterone levels, like cholesterol values, should be assessed routinely as a risk factor for heart disease. We are not quite ready to go that far.

If men with low testosterone levels have more risk factors, more heart disease, and earlier deaths, the next key question is whether doctors should connect the dots and prescribe these patients supplemental testosterone to protect their hearts. Animal experiments suggest that this might be a good idea. Administering testosterone to male rabbits has been shown to protect their arteries and prevents them from developing atherosclerotic plaques.

We have some data describing the impact of administered testosterone on the hearts of human males. When testosterone is given to men with coronary heart disease, arteries on the heart dilate and blood flow increases. There is a corresponding increase in the amount of physical activity a man can perform before he develops signs of inadequate blood flow and chest pain. In men with severe heart damage (heart failure), testosterone supplementation seems to increase their activity levels and independence. These benefits are greatest in men who have low testosterone levels to start.

So should all older men receive testosterone supplements to prevent or treat heart disease? Our answer is no. We don't have long-term studies with enough patients to determine the real impact of testosterone on hard clinical endpoints such as heart attack and death. While researchers have completed studies of the cardiac effect of hormone replacement therapy in women, there are no plans to conduct such research in men—a rare example of men being underserved in the battle against heart disease.

Although we do not have strong data to support a cardiovascular benefit, today millions of men regularly use prescription testosterone products or take supplements such as DHEA, a steroid that mimics some of the effects of testosterone. Over the last two decades, sales of these hormones have increased more than twentyfold. Some men take the supplements because they have been touted as "superhormones" that prevent aging and

DO STATINS LOWER TESTOSTERONE AND LIBIDO?

Few things are as important to men as sexual prowess and libido. So when the April 2010 edition of the *Journal of Sexual Medicine* published a report suggesting that statin medications reduce testosterone levels and decrease libido, international headlines followed. This unsubstantiated report from an obscure journal caused a great deal of anxiety among the 16 percent of U.S. men who take a lifesaving statin medication. Let's set the record straight.

The finding that men on statins have low testosterone is not a cause-and-effect relationship. The body manufactures testosterone from cholesterol, and it is true that statins reduce cholesterol levels. But statins do not lower the concentration of circulating, biologically active testosterone. People who receive statins have cardiovascular disease. We know that men with cardiovascular disease tend to have reduced testosterone levels, although we do not know the cause. Low testosterone levels in men on statins likely precede the administration of the drugs.

As for libido, most evidence shows that statin therapy actually enhances sexual function. A study from the Mayo Clinic suggested that men who took statins were less likely to develop erectile dysfunction. And a study from the University of Pennsylvania demonstrated that statins improved the response to Viagra in men with ED who initially did not respond to therapy with that drug. If your doctor prescribes a statin, don't worry about your sex life. Follow the prescription; it could save your life.

restore virility. Others believe testosterone and related steroids will protect their hearts. We don't recommend these practices.

Today the only common real indication for testosterone supplementation in adult men is to treat andropause, a condition in which older men have both low testosterone levels and symptoms attributable to testosterone deficiency—including fatigue, loss of energy, decreased libido, mood changes, hot flashes, and erectile dysfunction. Except for the last one, these symptoms sounds a lot like menopause in women. Doctors generally agree that it is reasonable to offer testosterone supplements to men who have both low testosterone and some or all of these symptoms. The goal here is to get testosterone levels back to normal. Testosterone supplements, most frequently administered as a gel or patch, relieve the symptoms in many of these men. Most notably, men with ED and low testosterone levels who fail to respond to standard medicines often attain sexual function when they take a testosterone supplement.

However, a recent randomized controlled trial raised important concerns about the use of testosterone supplements in older men. In the Testosterone in Older Men with Mobility Limitations Trial, 209 men sixty-five years of age or older with chronic illnesses and limited mobility were randomly assigned to receive daily testosterone supplements or a placebo for a six-month period. Doctors believed that these sick, frail men had the most to gain from testosterone therapy. As expected, men treated with testosterone improved their muscle strength, endurance, and mobility. But they also experienced a higher risk of cardiovascular complications, leading study organizers to halt the trial early. While investigators cautioned that these results of relatively high dose testosterone supplementation in older men might not apply to younger men receiving lower doses of the hormone, the study raised important questions about the safety of testosterone supplements.

Our take on this evidence is that testosterone replacement is relatively safe in selected men with andropause. However, until we have more data, it should be avoided in men who have heart disease or risk factors for heart disease (diabetes, high blood pressure, abnormal lipid values). Testosterone should not be used to try to prevent heart disease or to reverse or slow aging. It is not a "superhormone." Oral testosterone supplements can cause liver damage and should not be taken.

If a doctor does place a man on testosterone supplements, it is crucial to monitor the heart and vascular system. Blood counts and a lipid panel should be done before therapy, at one, three, six, and twelve months after treatment, and annually thereafter. Contrary to early reports, testosterone supplementation does not appear to increase the risk of developing prostate cancer. However, it is prudent to check the PSA level before beginning testosterone therapy and according to the schedule above once therapy is started. But again, unless you have an abnormally low blood testosterone level and symptoms, testosterone supplements are not for you.

UNLIKELY BEDFELLOWS: THE PROSTATE AND THE HEART

Until recently, cardiologists did not think much about the prostate, and urologists did not worry about the heart. But today the potential cardiac side effects of treatments for prostate cancer have engendered a great deal

ANABOLIC STEROIDS: IS EXTRA TESTOSTERONE BAD FOR THE HEART?

The chemical structure of testosterone was discovered in 1932, enabling scientists to create a new class of drugs with similar structure and function—androgenic anabolic steroids. These testosterone-like steroids were first used in 1939 to treat a variety of medical conditions, including impotence, depression, and starvation. Because these drugs increase strength and muscle mass, their subsequent abuse was almost guaranteed. The first abuses occurred during World War II, when they were administered to Nazi soldiers to increase their physical performance and aggression. Next came the beginning of the long relationship between sports and steroids. By 1970, use of anabolic steroids was a well-established practice among competitive weight lifters, cyclists, and track-and-field athletes. Soon these drugs infiltrated high schools and middle schools. Today the annual market for androgenic anabolic steroids exceeds $1 billion.

These substances are dangerous, with side effects that include liver damage, liver cancer, stroke, infertility, lipid abnormalities, and, of course, cardiac effects—heart attack, abnormal heart rhythms, damage to heart muscle fibers (cardiomyopathy) and sudden cardiac death. In fact, when the media report the sudden death of a young athlete, abuse of anabolic steroids is always near the top of the list of potential causes. Although we do not have enough data to quantify these risks, they are real. Beyond fair play, avoiding damage to the heart and other organs is another compelling reason not to take anabolic steroids.

of discussion across specialties—and confusion and fear among men with prostate cancer. In this section, we will explain why a man with prostate cancer must be especially conscious of his heart health.

This conversation is important to a very large number of men. Screening for PSA (prostate-specific antigen) has created an explosion in the number of diagnoses of prostate cancer—250,000 new diagnoses per year in the United States alone. One in five men will be diagnosed with prostate cancer at some point in his life.

For the majority of men with prostate cancer, their disease has not spread to other parts of the body at the time of diagnosis. This is good news, since men in this situation have nearly a 100 percent chance of living at least five years. The picture is not as optimistic for men who have more advanced cancer as a result of either distant spread (metastases) or extensive local growth. It is in the treatment of these men that heart health enters the picture.

Once again, we turn our attention to testosterone. Testosterone is the link between prostate cancer treatments and the heart. Prostate cancers grow more quickly in the presence of testosterone. In men with advanced or metastatic prostate cancer, medicines that reduce blood levels of testosterone can help limit cancer growth and even cause regression. This treatment, called androgen deprivation therapy, usually relies on a class of medicines called GnRH agonists, which include leuprolide, goserelin, and triptorelin. In men with advanced prostate cancer, they improve prognosis. However, these testosterone-lowering agents are unproven, and probably overprescribed, in men with local cancers, as well as in men who simply have an elevated PSA after initial treatment of prostate cancer.

Today, more than 600,000 men receive androgen deprivation therapy to lower blood testosterone levels. In the last section, we told you that men with naturally low testosterone levels have increased risks of heart disease and diabetes. So what do you think happens when we use medicines to lower testosterone levels in middle-aged and elderly men?

Once androgen deprivation therapy became standard for men with prostate cancer, doctors noticed an alarming but predictable trend. Men in whom testosterone levels were intentionally reduced seemed to develop more heart disease and diabetes. Large studies suggested that men undergoing androgen deprivation therapy had a 20 to 30 percent increase in the risk of heart attack, stroke, and sudden cardiac death over a period of one to four years, as well as increases in total cholesterol, LDL cholesterol, and triglycerides. They also saw decreased insulin sensitivity and unfavorable changes in body fat. Many of these changes were evident within three months of starting therapy.

In short, there are many dangerous cardiovascular similarities between men with naturally low testosterone levels and those treated with agents that intentionally lower testosterone levels. While the cardiovascular impact of androgen deprivation therapy remains a matter of some debate, we think that the available evidence suggests a link between this therapy and diabetes and heart disease. The FDA agrees, requiring that the GnRH agonists used to treat prostate cancer carry a warning about increased risks of diabetes and cardiovascular disease.

So what is a man with prostate cancer to do? Treating your cancer is the first priority, but you need to make sure that your prescribed therapy is the right choice. If you are diagnosed with prostate cancer and your urologist or oncologist recommends androgen deprivation therapy, ask if this treatment is of proven benefit for your type and stage of cancer—you want this therapy only if it is going to help you beat the cancer. Ask how it will influence your heart. Before starting therapy, you and your doctor should assess your cardiac risk factors and optimize them. Blood pressure, lipid levels, blood glucose, and weight should be recorded before beginning therapy, at three months, and annually thereafter. In most cases, though, there is no need for more advanced cardiac testing, such as a stress test or cardiac CT scan.

If you are placed on androgen deprivation therapy, be proactive about your overall health. You don't want to win the battle against cancer only to lose a war with heart disease or diabetes. The therapy is likely to make you lose muscle mass and gain fat; combat these trends with a healthy diet and exercise. Stop smoking. Make sure that your doctor checks your blood sugar and lipid levels at regular intervals. Once again, you need the knowledge and the will to take charge of your cardiac risk factors.

RX: THE HEARTS OF MEN

Risk factor reduction: the big five:
  Don't smoke
  Exercise daily
  Eat a heart-healthy Mediterranean diet
  Check your blood pressure
  Get a lipid profile

Erectile dysfunction:
  Remember that erection is a vascular event
  Think about your heart—ED also stands for "early detection" of heart disease

Testosterone:
  Testosterone is an important hormone but not a "superhormone"
  Do not take testosterone supplements to try to protect the heart or reverse aging

Prostate cancer:
  Ask if the treatment will affect your heart
  Win the wars on cancer *and* heart disease: optimize your cardiac risk factors

CHAPTER 19

HEART DISEASE IN KIDS: PREVENTION STARTS NOW!

THE BIG PICTURE

"For the first time in our nation's history, we are in danger of raising a generation of children who will live sicker and die younger than the generation before them. All the gains we have made in life expectancy are at risk."

These are the words of Senator Tom Harkin, chairman of the Senate Health, Education, Labor and Pensions Committee, elegantly summarizing the threat facing our youth. Home-cooked, healthy meals have been replaced by fast food. Riding bicycles with friends has given way to playing video games. Our technologically advanced, fast-paced society has created a population of overweight and obese children poised to suffer unprecedented levels of heart disease as adults.

Heart disease begins in childhood. This is the single most important message in this chapter. With our unhealthy diets and lack of exercise, we are setting our children up for lives that will be limited by obesity, diabetes, and heart disease.

This does not have to be the future. Fully 90 percent of heart disease is preventable. But early intervention is necessary. Securing our children's health requires a concerted effort by parents, grandparents, teachers, and everybody else who cares for them. The keys to prevention are understanding childhood factors that lead to heart disease and embracing a healthy lifestyle that minimizes the risk of heart disease.

In this chapter, you will find the knowledge to fulfill your most important obligation—ensuring the health and well-being of your children. We will share the evidence that coronary heart disease begins in childhood. We will then outline a plan for raising nutritionally savvy, active kids who will become heart-healthy adults. We will discuss the dangerous consequences of childhood obesity, and answer the controversial question "Should my son or daughter have a cholesterol test?"

CHILDREN: HEART PATIENTS IN WAITING

Although we had been treating Lauren Bradley's chest pain for ten years, we had never met her family until she arrived for her annual checkup with her two young kids in tow. Lauren's babysitter had car trouble, she explained, so the kids were with her this afternoon. Handing them a bag from McDonald's, she instructed the children to eat their dinners in the waiting room during her appointment.

Lauren reported that she was doing well. She had quit smoking (the main cause of the coronary heart disease that caused a heart attack at age forty-four). Medications controlled her cardiac chest pain, and she used her NordicTrack daily. She did her best on the diet front, although she confessed that fast food often fit best into her busy schedule. We congratulated her on her victory over cigarettes and told her that her numbers looked good: blood pressure, cholesterol values, and weight were all in the appropriate range. Escorting her out to the front of the office, we told her to schedule another appointment in twelve months.

When we opened the door to the waiting room, we were struck by the familiar smell of McDonald's. Eight-year-old Christy had just finished the french fries from her Happy Meal and was working on liberating her toy from its plastic wrap. Eleven-year-old Robert was working hard on a handheld Nintendo game. The kids looked up briefly as we came in, but then returned to their pursuits. Two things were immediately apparent: the kids had excellent powers of concentration, and they were both overweight.

Pausing at the door, we asked Lauren to come back in; we wanted to talk about her children. This caught her off guard. They were kids. Why would heart doctors want to talk about them?

We explained that her kids were on a path leading straight to obesity, diabetes, and heart disease. Lauren's own heart problems gave them a family history of cardiovascular problems. From what we could see, their diets were unhealthy and they were overweight. When we asked if they exercised or played outside, Lauren told us that they did "normal kid stuff," like working with their fingers on iPods, Nintendos, and Happy Meal toys.

"Isn't heart disease an adult problem?" Lauren asked. We answered, "Yes, but . . ." We wanted to help Lauren understand that adult heart disease begins in childhood.

Of course, Lauren did not want her kids to follow in her footsteps and become familiar with cardiologists when they were young adults. Luckily, it's always simpler to prevent disease than to treat it. We outlined a healthy diet for Lauren's kids, explaining that french fries can't be used to satisfy the daily vegetable requirement, and that soda has no place in kids' diets. While we are not against a good workout with the thumbs (we're no strangers to the BlackBerry and iPod ourselves), we reminded Lauren that every child needs at least one full hour of *real* exercise each day.

Things turned around quickly. Within six months, Lauren's kids were on the right track. In the afternoons, the kids and Lauren enjoyed exercising as a family and exploring bike paths at a nearby park. Both children had grown taller without gaining weight, putting them into normal weight ranges. And there had been few additions to Christy's collection of Happy Meal toys.

A fifteen-minute discussion with Lauren acted as a wake-up call for her children's heart health. An environment filled with unhealthy food and devoid of exercise had the kids on the path to cardiovascular disease. Sad to say, Lauren's kids are not unique. Today more than 90 percent of teenagers already carry at least one major cardiac risk factor.

It's time to put your kids on a different path. Like Lauren, you can make important changes to secure your children's health. Heart disease begins in childhood, and that is when prevention must start.

HEART MURMURS IN CHILDREN: SHOULD YOU WORRY?

When we were in medical school, nobody talked about kids' arteries or their cardiac risk factors. We learned to listen to children's hearts with a stethoscope to identify congenital heart disease—abnormal valves and connections in the heart that cause turbulent blood flow, which in turn creates the sound of a heart murmur. In the United States, each year 36,000 babies are born with a congenital heart defect. The most common congenital heart problem is a ventricular septal defect, a hole in the heart that usually closes within the first year of life. But while holes in the heart are relatively rare, audible murmurs are very common.

Should you worry if your pediatrician hears a heart murmur? The answer is almost always no. Many children develop murmurs at some point during childhood, most of which are benign. The pediatrician can usually tell that a murmur is not threatening simply by listening with a stethoscope. If there is any question, your doctor will order an echocardiogram to identify the cause of the murmur. In most cases, echocardiogram results allow parents to breathe a sigh of relief.

ADULT HEART DISEASE BEGINS IN CHILDHOOD: THE EVIDENCE

Many of the first clues to the childhood beginnings of adult heart disease arose from observations made during wartime. Doctors were surprised to find diseased arteries in 77 percent of the young soldiers killed in the Korean War. Military casualties from Vietnam produced similar results. These young men appeared physically fit and outwardly healthy, but their coronary arteries contained atherosclerotic plaques that would surely have led to heart problems later in life.

The progression of atherosclerosis follows a predictable pattern. The first visible change in an artery is a fatty streak, which forms as cells called macrophages absorb excess cholesterol and lipids and settle in the wall of the artery. Over the years, spurred by the presence of cholesterol and other lipids, additional macrophages, muscle cells, and lipids are deposited in the artery's wall, forming a raised fibrous plaque that narrows the artery and limits blood flow. At this stage, the disease is usually silent. But as more cholesterol and cells accumulate, the fibrous plaque becomes larger and develops a propensity to rupture. If the plaque ruptures, a blood clot forms at the site, completely blocking the artery and triggering a heart attack.

A landmark study called the Bogalusa Heart Study awakened doctors to the insidious early stages of heart disease. Scientists followed thousands of children for several decades with the goal of identifying childhood factors that lead to adult coronary heart disease. As one component of the research, investigators performed autopsies on all children who died, usually as the result of accidents. In total, they examined the hearts and arteries of 209 subjects who died between the ages of two and thirty-nine.

The findings from the Bogalusa study startled doctors. Fifty percent of the children, including some as young as three years old, had fatty streaks in their arteries, the first sign of atherosclerosis. Fibrous plaques, representing more advanced atherosclerosis, were common in ten-year-olds. Seventy percent of young adults had atherosclerosis involving both the aorta and the coronary arteries. The evidence was incontrovertible: coronary heart disease establishes a foothold in childhood.

Risk factors for heart disease in adults were already well known, but investigators wanted to determine whether these same risk factors posed threats to our children.

The answer was yes. The classic adult risk factors—elevated total and LDL cholesterol values, reduced HDL cholesterol, high blood pressure, obesity, diabetes, smoking, and physical inactivity—all contribute to the development of heart disease in children. These risk factors are synergistic in their negative impact, meaning that people with multiple risk factors develop more severe arterial disease. By age eighteen, sensitive testing reveals thickened and abnormal blood vessels in children with two or more risk factors.

Read the list of risk factors again. The majority are *not* genetically determined. In most cases, children begin to develop coronary heart disease as a result of modifiable risk factors related to diet, exercise, and lifestyle. Children with risk factors for coronary heart disease tend to maintain these characteristics as adults, prolonging the onslaught on their arteries' health and increasing the odds that they will develop significant heart disease.

But there are ways to break this cycle. If your child or grandchild currently suffers from obesity, elevated cholesterol, high blood pressure, and other classic risk factors, his or her fate is not preordained. In most children, the degree of vascular involvement is mild, and progression is slow. This opens the door to prevention and provides us with the opportunity to avert serious consequences.

As Lauren Bradley learned, we need to focus mostly on prevention, not treatment. Our goal must be to prevent injury rather than to stabilize damage. Every parent and grandparent should know the most important risk factors—childhood obesity, poor diet, inadequate exercise, and high cholesterol. Recognition of these risk factors is straightforward, and strategies for their correction are effective.

CANCER AND HEART DISEASE: LIGHTNING STRIKES TWICE

One in 600 children is a cancer survivor. After beating cancer, many of these kids don't receive regular checkups. This is a huge mistake; few parents recognize that the very treatment that cured the cancer can cause heart disease.

The primary offenders are radiation therapy to the chest and chemotherapy with a class of medicines called anthracyclines. Doctors frequently use chest radiation to treat childhood lymphomas. While the radiation often cures the cancer, it causes collateral damage to nearby tissues, including the heart. Radiation affects all components of the heart, including its lining, the coronary arteries, the valves, and the conduction system. The first symptoms of radiation damage, which usually don't appear until ten or more years after treatment, include chest pain, shortness of breath, and swelling of the legs.

The anthracyclines are a class of anti-tumor antibiotics that include doxorubicin (Adriamycin), daunorubicine (also called daunomycin), epirubicin, and idarubicin. In high doses, these agents can cause permanent damage to the heart muscle, producing a condition called dilated cardiomyopathy.

If you are a survivor of childhood cancer and were treated with radiation to the chest or with one of these chemotherapeutic agents, you should see a cardiologist for a physical examination and an echocardiogram. You should also see a cardiologist if you had childhood cancer but are not sure what treatment regimen you received. Identifying cancer-related heart issues early enables successful therapy and helps to prevent continuing damage. See your doctor—don't let lightning strike twice.

CHILDHOOD OBESITY IS EASY TO UNDERSTAND

The Obesity Epidemic

We can't escape the fact that we are an overweight society. Over the last thirty years, the percentage of overweight or obese adults has doubled. And we have set such a poor example for our kids that the increase in *their* weight has been even more staggering—and tragic.

The *Journal of the American Medical Association* reported that in 2007, 31.9 percent of children were overweight or obese. This is triple the number that were overweight or obese in 1980. Mississippi has the largest proportion of overweight kids (44 percent overweight or obese), while Utah has the smallest fraction (still, 23 percent of kids there are overweight or obese). Black and Hispanic teenagers face the greatest risk, with extreme obesity affecting 12 percent of black teenage girls and 11 percent of black teenage boys. The problem of childhood weight gain has reached epidemic proportions, and the associated health threats are a man-made disaster in the making. Obesity is the greatest threat to our children's hearts and lives today.

Diagnosing Obesity

How can you tell if your child is overweight or obese? The first step is obvious—look at your child. If your child looks overweight, he or she probably is. To confirm your diagnosis, either you or your pediatrician can easily determine the child's body mass index, or BMI (go to the CDC's website at http://apps.nccd.cdc.gov/dnpabmi to calculate the BMI and your child's percentile, which will tell you how your child's BMI compares to that of other kids of similar age). It is worth five minutes to get this information yourself—pediatricians only recognize a dangerous BMI in their patients about 50 percent of the time.

Experts agree that for children a normal BMI falls in the 5th through 84th percentiles. A child is classified as overweight if the BMI is in the 85th through 94th percentiles. If the BMI is in the 95th percentile or greater, the child is obese. It is important to realize, however, that not everybody with an elevated BMI has excess body fat. The old saying that muscle weighs more than fat is true. Therefore, very athletic and muscular people may have a high BMI and still be in excellent physical condition.

While some doctors will measure waist circumference and waist-to-hip ratio, or directly assess body fat, simple use of your eyes and your computer are all you need to screen for obesity.

Causes of Obesity

We have all heard individuals claim that their increased weight is caused by medical problems such as a hormone imbalance. Certain conditions such as decreased thyroid function can cause obesity, but they are relatively rare. Others argue that the obesity epidemic is attributable to genetic factors. But the facts refute this assertion. The number of obese kids has skyrocketed in the last thirty years, while our gene pool has remained relatively constant. So we cannot blame the explosion of obesity on genetics. Overall, less than 1 percent of overweight and obese children are afflicted with hormonal abnormalities, genetic factors, or other identifiable medical conditions.

The obesity epidemic is largely caused by diets packed with excess calories. Consider this statistic: consuming a single extra can of regular soda (120–140 calories) per day can result in a weight gain of twelve pounds over a one-year period.

Dramatic reductions in physical activity and increased screen time augment the problem. The risk of obesity is increased 12 percent for each hour of daily television a child watches. To make matters worse, the average child sees more than ten food commercials per day, most advertising fast food, soda, candy, and sugar-filled breakfast cereals. Meanwhile, images of Dora the Explorer, Shrek, and other animated characters adorn the packaging of unhealthy foods. The Federal Trade Commission reports that in 2006 companies spent $1.6 billion marketing food and beverages to children.

This relentless marketing lays the foundations for unhealthy behaviors. Although we protect our children by shielding them from pornography and violent images, we allow advertisers to manipulate them into making life-threatening decisions. Taking aim at one component of this problem, San Francisco now prohibits fast food chains from including toys with kids' meals that do not meet nutritional standards. New York legislators are trying to follow suit.

OBESITY IN THE GENES?

Your genetic makeup sets your general weight range. But what you eat and how much, along with your exercise pattern, determine where in this range you fall. The most commonly occurring weight-related gene is the FTO gene, nicknamed the "fatso gene" by some scientists. About two-thirds of people have at least one copy of this gene, with each copy of the gene associated with a three-pound increase in body weight among adults. A recent study revealed that when teens have this gene, one hour of daily moderate to vigorous exercise neutralizes the gene's impact on weight. In this case, genetics do not determine destiny.

Scientists have identified a small number of obesity genes that cannot be overcome with exercise and diet. In 1997, two massively obese Pakistani children were found to have a mutation in the gene responsible for leptin, a hormone that reduces appetite and is normally produced by fat cells. In these two children, this rare abnormal gene resulted in leptin deficiency, causing the children to consume enormous quantities of food and to become morbidly obese. Fortunately, treatment with synthetic leptin restored a normal appetite and resulted in dramatic weight loss.

In most people, lifestyle trumps genetics when it comes to determining weight. While we observe a clear association between parental and childhood obesity, shared lifestyles are more important than shared genes. We cannot choose our genes, but smart lifestyle choices can nearly always prevent or combat childhood obesity.

Obesity Hurts the Heart

Why should we care about the obesity epidemic? If a child appears otherwise healthy, do a few extra pounds really matter? Historically, a fat baby was considered healthy: free of disease and malnutrition. Most people believe that kids will grow out of it and baby fat will eventually disappear. So why are today's physicians and politicians so concerned about childhood obesity? The answer is that being overweight or obese is bad for all aspects of a child's health, particularly heart health.

Children who are overweight and obese have dramatic increases in their risk factors for heart disease, including unfavorable lipid profiles, diabetes, blood vessel dysfunction, inflammation, and high blood pressure. Yes, you read that correctly. Overweight kids get high blood pressure.

A recent study published in the *New England Journal of Medicine* investigated the relationship between a child's weight, his or her age, and the risk of future heart disease. The main finding: the older the obese child, the greater the risk of heart trouble as an adult. A thirteen-year-old boy who is about twenty pounds overweight has a 33 percent increase in the risk of developing a complication of coronary heart disease by the age of sixty. Dozens of other studies have confirmed that the overweight or obese child becomes the overweight adult heart patient. So don't wait for your child to "grow out of it." Recognize and treat overweight children early.

CHILDHOOD OBESITY AND DIABETES

Obesity causes diabetes, and diabetes causes coronary heart disease. One-half of heart attack victims have diabetes or a prediabetic condition. The obvious goal is the prevention of obesity and diabetes in children.

As we discussed in Chapter 2, there are two general types of diabetes. Patients with type 1 diabetes have an abnormality of the immune system that prevents the pancreas from making enough insulin. In people with type 2 diabetes, the pancreas does produce insulin, but cells are resistant to it. Type 2 is the kind of diabetes that is associated with obesity.

Twenty years ago, type 2 diabetes was called "adult-onset diabetes" and was almost unheard-of in children. Today it accounts for 20 to 40 percent of childhood diabetes, and 10 percent of obese adolescents have abnormal glucose metabolism that indicates a prediabetic condition. The health effects of diabetes can be devastating, including heart attacks, blindness, kidney failure requiring dialysis, and limb loss from amputation. Overall, diabetes shortens the average life span by thirteen years. Are we trying to scare you? You bet we are!

Avoiding type 2 diabetes requires preventing and treating obesity. Your first step: go to your refrigerator right now and remove all sodas that contain sugar. This will help your children avoid the excess sugar that contributes to obesity, metabolic syndrome, diabetes, and ultimately heart disease. Next, if you have an overweight child, make sure that your pediatrician has checked for diabetes or glucose intolerance, a prediabetic condition. The good news is that type 2 diabetes is reversible with weight loss produced by exercise and a healthy diet.

The bad health news generated by childhood obesity does not stop with heart disease and diabetes. Childhood obesity has a host of other alarming health consequences, including colorectal cancer, gallbladder disease, depression, gout, sleep apnea, gastroesophageal reflux, and orthopedic problems such as arthritis.

We cannot overstate the health risks of childhood obesity. *Childhood obesity doubles the risk of premature death.* For two hundred years, life expectancy in the United States has increased with each new generation. But because of the obesity epidemic, experts predict that this pattern will reverse itself within the next four decades. If the current trend continues, by 2050 average life expectancy in the United States will fall by two to five years.

Treatment

Treatment must begin early because the problem arises early. Half of children who become overweight or obese have accumulated excess body weight by the age of two—another reminder that the chubby infant is not a healthy infant. Ninety percent of overweight kids cross the BMI threshold by the age of five years. Without intervention, overweight and obesity become lifelong problems. One-third of obese preschoolers will become obese adults, while one-half of obese grade schoolers will maintain their obesity into adulthood.

These figures emphasize the importance of correcting obesity early. We know that about 50 percent of obese children become obese adults. The flip side of that coin is that 50 percent of obese children do *not* become obese adults. Finally, some good news: we have the opportunity to intervene, and treatment can be effective. In fact, treating obesity is far more successful in children than in adults, in large part because it is easier to change bad habits in children.

Treatment programs for truly obese children (those with a BMI in the 95th percentile or above) must be comprehensive, coordinated efforts that include the child, the parents, the rest of the family, the pediatrician, and a dietician or nutritionist. Treatment should include changes in diet, exercise programs, and counseling aimed at behavior modification. Some treatment programs can cost $50 to $250 per session, but many hospitals and schools offer less expensive or even free programs; ask your pediatrician about these opportunities. Lasting success almost always requires this kind

COLLEGE WEIGHT GAIN AND THE "FRESHMAN FIFTEEN"

It is a common observation that college students gain weight during their first year at school. Researchers from California Polytechnic State University found that each year of college is associated with an average weight gain of about two pounds; a fifteen- or twenty-pound weight gain is actually uncommon. But still, gaining two pounds per year can push normal individuals toward being overweight, and overweight students to obesity.

How can college students avoid this weight gain? Stanford researchers found that offering students a course on food and health resulted in a better diet. Scientists at the University of Michigan observed that dorm location is important. Students living in dorms with on-site dining halls ate more meals and gained more weight than those who had to walk to another building to get to the dining hall. They also found that students who lived closer to the gym exercised more often.

The "freshman fifteen" may be a myth, but college weight gain is real. In addition to teaching your children good habits while they're at home, continue to nudge them toward good decisions when they go away to school so they emerge from college both smarter *and* healthier.

of formal, multidisciplinary approach—a parent's decision to stop serving dessert won't by itself produce long-term success for obese children.

The goal is to get your child's BMI below the 85th percentile. As with Lauren Bradley's kids, this may be accomplished by keeping the child's weight steady as he or she grows. But if your health care team recommends weight loss, it is generally advisable for a child to lose no more than one pound per month.

The "magic formula" to losing weight is to cut calories while increasing exercise. If changes in diet and physical activity result in a net energy deficit, the child will lose weight. Your health care team will help you determine the right number of calories for your child. Staying within the calorie limit, vary the meal plan. Emphasize lean protein, low-fat dairy products, fruits, and vegetables. Keep portion sizes reasonable. Cut out sugar-filled sodas and juice drinks. But don't completely banish sweets—occasional desserts are fine.

Pay attention to snacks. Today, 98 percent of kids have snacks outside of regular meal times (compared to 74 percent in 1978). The average child snacks three times per day, representing 586 calories daily, compared to only 418 daily calories from snack foods in 1977. Limit snacks and replace high-sugar and high-calorie snacks with fresh fruit. Don't be tricked into choosing popular "100-calorie packs" of unhealthy food. An apple or an orange is a much better choice.

On the physical activity side of the equation, limit screen time to no more than one hour per day. Incorporate sports and exercise in your plan, particularly on weekends. Recent research demonstrates that children who live within 150 meters of heavy traffic are more likely to be obese, probably as a result of reduced physical activity. Parents living in cities or near traffic must therefore make special efforts to ensure physical activity; this may include visiting neighborhood parks or playgrounds or joining a YMCA close to home.

Achieving a normal weight in obese children takes time, often a year or more, but the payoff is big. Risk factors for coronary heart disease diminish. Cholesterol levels and blood pressure normalize and inflammation subsides. The child's emotional well-being is restored. Healthy eating and physical activity become habits for life. A healthy future replaces a life shortened by heart disease.

PREVENTION OF OBESITY AND HEART DISEASE

Primordial Prevention

Prevention is preferable to treatment. Preventing childhood obesity and its consequences requires early adoption of a heart-healthy lifestyle. Guiding children to healthy habits is one of the most important contributions a parent or caregiver can make to a child's welfare. Moving a step beyond prevention of heart disease, we want to help you prevent the risk factors that lead to heart disease. The idea that we can prevent development of risk factors themselves, well before they cause heart disease, is termed "primordial prevention."

Prevention must include changes in the dietary factors and sedentary behaviors which are toxic to health in general and to the heart in particular. Because children are relatively flexible in their attitudes and behaviors, successful intervention is achievable. The backbone of prevention rests in comprehensive efforts to ensure a healthy diet.

THE EARLIEST PREVENTION: PREGNANCY AND BEFORE

Believe it or not, prevention of heart disease in children should begin before birth and even before conception. Children born to mothers who were obese at the time of conception, or to those who gain too much weight during pregnancy, have double the risk of developing obesity and diabetes in adulthood, and are more likely to have high blood pressure and unfavorable lipid profiles.

Before becoming pregnant, a woman should optimize her weight. Once pregnant, it is critically important to avoid excessive weight gain. The Institute of Medicine has formulated recommendations for appropriate weight gain during pregnancy:

Mother's weight	Recommended weight gain in pregnancy
Normal	25–35 pounds
Overweight	15–25 pounds
Obese	11–20 pounds

Exercise during pregnancy helps expectant mothers to avoid excessive weight gain, and is perfectly safe. Studies have shown that babies whose mothers exercised during pregnancy have healthier hearts, and are more likely to be born at a healthy weight, than babies with sedentary moms.

Weight management after birth continues with breast-feeding. Breast milk is the ideal food for infants. Although breast milk is rich in saturated fat, studies suggest that breast-feeding decreases the risk of the child's future obesity and may reduce the risk of cardiovascular disease in adulthood. In addition, breast-fed infants do a better job of regulating their food intake than do those who are bottle-fed; when presented with a bottle later in infancy, a child who was breast-fed initially tends to stop drinking when satisfied, whereas babies that are exclusively bottle-fed usually empty the bottle. Breast-feeding should be continued for at least six months and ideally through the first year.

A Good Diet

What is the best diet is a matter of controversy. Both real and self-proclaimed experts have recommended a wide variety of diets for children. We are not going to force you to choose a specific diet or limit your child to particular foods. Instead, we will give you the knowledge you need to make smart decisions for your family. The guiding principles are not that complicated. Diets need to provide children with a variety of food choices and with adequate calories for growth and activity. This does not mean that you must count every calorie, but you do need a general idea of the number of daily calories that your child needs.

Recommended Caloric Needs According to Age		
	BOYS	GIRLS
1 year	900	900
2–3 years	1,000	1,000
4–8 years	1,400	1,200
9–13 years	1,800	1,600
14–18 years	2,200	1,800

Adjust these calorie recommendations according to your child's activity level. For example, if your teenage daughter is a competitive runner, she will need more calories in order to supplement the energy she expends at cross-country practice.

Caloric goals should be achieved with a nutritious, balanced meal plan. The American Heart Association's guidelines are easy to follow: Replace sugar- and salt-filled processed foods with fruits and vegetables. Emphasize whole grains and lean meats. Today most children do not consume enough fruits, vegetables, and whole grains.

Letting your child sprinkle half a teaspoon of sugar on fruit or a nutritious cereal provides far less sugar than a bowl of Froot Loops or Frosted Flakes. On the other hand, get rid of that other white stuff—salt. There is no need to keep a saltshaker on the table; it may set the stage for high blood pressure later in life.

Be careful when it comes to what your kids drink. Aside from milk, drinks should be non-caloric. One exception: you can give your child natural fruit juice if this is the only way to get him or her to take in fruit. But avoid sugar-sweetened sodas and juice drinks with added sugar. In addition, be careful with sports drinks, which contain sugar. An athlete needs hydration, electrolytes, and calories during competition, but your child does not need these while sitting down to dinner or a snack.

Good and Bad Choices

GOOD	BAD
Whole-grain cereals (may add fruit and half a teaspoon of sugar)	Sugary cereals
Chicken and fish	Hamburgers and hot dogs
Whole-wheat pasta with low-salt marinara sauce	Pizza
Sandwich: peanut butter and jelly, turkey with low-fat mayonnaise or mustard	Sandwich: bologna, salami, corned beef
Whole-grain bread	White bread
Almost *any* non-potato vegetable: broccoli, spinach, cauliflower	French fries
Fresh fruit (may sprinkle with half a teaspoon of sugar)	Cookies and cakes
Water, skim or 2 percent milk	Regular soda

Parents' big question is always "What is the role of fat in my child's diet?" There is legitimate cause for concern, as four out of five children exceed recommended guidelines for daily intakes of total and saturated fat. But it is a myth that children should eat a strict low-fat diet. Approximately 30 percent of a child's calories should come from fat.

You don't have to count how many grams of fat are in your child's diet. Instead, pay attention to the *types* of fat consumed. Trans fats should be excluded from the diet whenever possible. Traditionally found in processed baked goods, trans fats have been removed from most foods by manufacturers. In contrast, saturated fats are everywhere. Parents should limit saturated fat intake by avoiding processed lunch meats and minimizing other red meats, butter, and full-fat dairy products. After the first year of a child's life, dairy products should be low-fat. Children one to two years of age can have 2 percent milk, but after that skim milk is preferable.

Eating Away from Home

Parents and grandparents must work together to ensure a good diet. As children, we all enjoyed spending time with our grandparents. In addition

SCHOOL LUNCH: FRANCE VERSUS THE UNITED STATES

France is the first Western country to experience a leveling off of childhood obesity rates. Many attribute this victory to the French focus on food, particularly on lunch. For French children, lunch is important, occupying a full hour of the school day. A typical public school lunch in France has five well-balanced courses, including an hors d'oeuvre, salad or vegetable, main course, cheese board, and dessert. All eating is done in a structured format at the lunch table; there are no snack or soda machines in the school. Recognizing the importance of healthy eating, the French have resisted cutting school meal expenses in order to meet budgetary challenges.

In her anonymous blog, Fed Up with Lunch—The School Lunch Project (http://fedup withschoollunch.blogspot.com), Mrs. Q, an Illinois teacher, describes a decidedly different scene in American schools. She notes that American children have an average of thirteen minutes to consume their hot dogs, potato puffs, chicken nuggets, and other unhealthy foods. Unappetizing photos of these foods on her website illustrate what children in her school district receive for lunch. Mrs. Q even describes the intestinal distress caused by some entrees, such as the peanut butter and jelly sandwich on a graham cracker.

American parents, teachers, and politicians, recognize that school lunches represent a key opportunity to provide healthy food and to teach healthy habits and have started taking steps in this direction. But right now, we prefer the French school lunch.

---

to unconditional love, we were treated to sweets such as freshly baked cookies and brownies. It turns out that a grandparent's love is a good thing, but the accompanying calorie-dense treats create problems. A recent study of 12,000 English children showed that kids raised by grandparents full-time have a 34 percent increase in the risk of being overweight. Even part-time care by grandparents increases their risk of being overweight or obese by 15 percent. We encourage grandparents to pour on the love, but suggest that they impose some limit on the candy and sweets.

When eating at home, parents choose the meal. You don't have the same level of influence when children eat away from home, but you should not give up control completely when eating out. An occasional visit to McDonald's or Burger King is okay, but consider this statistic: a large fast-food meal contains as many as 2,200 calories, about the number of calories burned by running a full marathon. Most fast-food restaurants now have healthier choices, including grilled chicken sandwiches, fresh fruit, and low-fat milk.

When it comes to school lunches, be proactive. Review the menu in advance with your child, pointing out the best options. This can be a great moment to teach children which foods are healthy. If there are not enough healthy choices, engage other parents and voice your concerns to school officials. Healthy foods need not be expensive, and there is no reason that schools cannot provide appropriate fare for our kids.

Visit the school to see for yourself; younger children think it's cool when a parent shows up for lunch. Look for fruits and (not cooked-to-death) vegetables. Take note of processed foods. You and other parents can move the school and your children toward good choices.

OBESITY AND HEART DISEASE VERSUS ANOREXIA AND HEART DISEASE: TWO SIDES OF THE SAME COIN?

There is no debate. Excess calories and poor diet lead to obesity, increased risks of cardiovascular disease, and a host of other serious health issues. Healthy eating is instrumental in avoiding these problems. But we must be careful with both the food we serve and the message that we send our children. Misguided attempts to use a very-low-fat, very-low-calorie diet can stunt growth and harm multiple organ systems. Overeating and undereating are both dangerous.

If our children internalize the concept that fat and calories are bad, they run the risk of developing eating disorders such as anorexia. Anorexia, the third most common chronic health problem affecting teenage girls, can be fatal—primarily as a result of its effects on the heart. Cardiovascular complications affect 80 percent of anorexia patients and include heart rhythm abnormalities, dangerously low blood pressure, damage to the heart muscle, and sudden cardiac death. As we teach our children the elements of a healthy diet, we must ensure that they understand that fat and calories are not inherently bad. Let them know we don't want them to be thin. We want them to be healthy.

Exercise and Fun

Exercise complements a healthy diet. We recommend that all children enjoy at least one hour of physical activity every day of the week. The key word here is "enjoy." Kids like to play tag, roller-skate, ride bicycles, play tennis, and engage in a wide variety of sports. Today only 36 percent of children get an hour of exercise per day, with vigorous physical activity occupying an average of only twelve minutes. On the other hand, 37 percent of American kids watch at least two hours of television each day. These figures tell us where we can find the extra time to fit exercise into the schedule. Recalling his childhood playing outdoors in Brooklyn, former U.S. surgeon general C. Everett Koop recommends, "Turn off the video games, shut down the computer, unplug the television . . . and send your children outside for some good old-fashioned fun. One day they will thank you for it."

THREE SIMPLE HOUSEHOLD ROUTINES HELP PREVENT OBESITY

Researchers from Ohio State University studied the relationship between obesity and three simple routines in nearly 9,000 preschool children, 18 percent of whom were obese. The three household routines were: (1) family dinner more than five nights per week, (2) adequate sleep (more than ten and a half hours per weeknight), and (3) limited weekday screen time (less than two hours per day). Children exposed to all three of these simple routines had a 40 percent lower prevalence of obesity when compared to those who had none. These three routines provide a very simple prescription for preventing obesity—and for having better-rested kids and more family togetherness, too.

Limit screen time to an hour or less per day and encourage your children to exercise. Better yet, exercise with your kids. There is no reason that parents can't play tag, shoot some hoops, ride bikes with their kids, or throw a baseball around in the backyard.

Exercise is another topic that warrants parental involvement in the school curriculum. Only 54 percent of grade schools offer physical education, and only five states consistently require PE from kindergarten through twelfth grade. Fully 25 percent of schools have cut recess to save money and make more time for academic classes. Bucking this trend, some forward-thinking schools have hired "recess coaches" to ensure a recess filled with safe and enjoyable exercise. Physical activity and play should be regular components of your child's school day. If they are not, talk to teachers and administrators.

The relationship between physical activity and school goes beyond children's health; physically fit children do better academically. Researchers from UCLA assessed approximately 2,000 California children and found that kids who met or exceeded state fitness standards had higher test scores in math, reading, and language.

The precise mechanism by which fitness improves cognitive function is not known, but the relationship holds in adults as well. Studies show that adding daily physical activity to grade school curricula does not harm academic performance, in spite of the loss of formal teaching time. Both standard classroom instruction and athletic activity are important components of the school day.

EXERCISE IS FUN: THAT'S THE MESSAGE

A recent British study demonstrated that kids will exercise more if they focus on the fun of physical activity. Over a two-week period, 120 teens were randomly assigned to receive text messages concerning exercise. Those in the control group received a weekly message that was neutral ("What activity did you do today?"). Other teens received daily messages that focused on either the fun and enjoyment of exercise ("Physical activity can make you cheerful"), the health benefits of exercise ("Physical activity can keep your heart healthy"), or both the fun *and* the health benefits of exercise. Overall, physical activity improved by thirty-one minutes per week during the study. But the greatest increase in exercise occurred among previously inactive teens who were told that exercise is fun. They boosted their physical activity by an average of two hours per week. The message here is clear: the argument that "exercise is good for you" carries little weight with children, but kids will undertake physical activity if they believe that exercise is fun.

Smoking

We shouldn't even have to mention smoking. But 23 percent of high school students smoke, so we do have to make a comment. Don't smoke yourself, and make certain that your children don't smoke. Maintain a smoke-free home. If you live in an apartment, petition for your building to go smoke-free. Shared ventilation systems, ductwork, and walls mean that second-hand smoke from your neighbor can reach you and your children.

SECONDHAND SMOKE HURTS YOUR KIDS

Preventing your kids from smoking is a good thing. But *you* have to quit, too. A parent's smoking encourages children to model the lethal behavior and causes direct physical harm to children who inhale secondhand smoke. Kids exposed to secondhand smoke develop blood vessel dysfunction and thickening, two of the earliest signs of arterial damage. A recent study revealed that secondhand smoke increases blood pressure in children as young as five years old; smoking by mothers had a greater impact than by fathers, most likely because mothers smoke more in the home. These findings are no surprise, given that adults exposed to secondhand smoke have a substantial increase in their risk of cardiovascular disease.

Secondhand smoke may be even more damaging than the smoke inhaled by the smoker. Sidestream smoke, the smoke released from the burning end of the cigarette, contains several toxic substances in higher concentrations than the filtered smoke reaching the smoker's lungs. In addition to arterial damage, secondhand smoke increases the risks of asthma and respiratory infections in children and infants. You want to protect your children and ensure their health. You don't send your kids out to play in traffic, and you should not smoke around them. Do yourself and your children a favor—quit today!

CHOLESTEROL AND KIDS: WHAT YOU NEED TO KNOW

We all know that cholesterol influences the hearts of adults. And investigators have shown us that abnormal blood lipid values, particularly increased LDL cholesterol, set the stage for the beginnings of coronary heart disease in children. Should this finding worry you?

First, let's see how often kids have cholesterol issues. Total cholesterol and LDL cholesterol are elevated in 10 to 15 percent of children. In fact, by fourth grade, 13 percent of children have total cholesterol greater than 200 mg/dL, the upper limit of normal. As with other risk factors for coronary heart disease, elevated cholesterol levels tend to track into adulthood; put another way, without intervention, children with high cholesterol become adults with high cholesterol.

There is confusion concerning what constitutes normal lipid levels in children. Cholesterol and other lipid levels vary with age and development, but tend to reach adult-like levels by age two.

Cholesterol Levels in Children		
	TOTAL CHOLESTEROL (MG/DL)	LDL CHOLESTEROL (MG/DL)
Acceptable	< 170	< 110
Borderline	170–199	110–129
High	≥ 200	≥ 130

Kids under the age of two should not have a cholesterol test, as lipid levels are in flux during the first two years of life. In older children, doctors disagree about whether universal or targeted cholesterol screening is best.

Proponents of universal screening—routinely checking every child's cholesterol levels—point out that this is the surest strategy for identifying all kids with abnormal lipid levels, enabling early intervention to prevent heart disease. Commonly cited problems with universal screening include concern about labeling kids with minor lipid abnormalities as having a disease, the likely overuse of medicines such as statins for treatment, and expense.

For us, the primary problems with universal screening are that the findings will not change the therapy, and that the screening has no demonstrated benefits. If we screen all kids, we will find that 10 to 15 percent have modest elevations in cholesterol. We are not going to treat all of these kids with statins. We would recommend maintaining a good weight with a healthy diet and exercise. But we endorse these heart-healthy behaviors anyway, no matter what the cholesterol level. So universal screening would involve lots of blood tests, some expense, and no new action in most cases.

Instead, we favor selective screening based upon a child's family history to determine if a child has genetically determined high levels of LDL cholesterol, a condition called familial hypercholesterolemia. One in 500 kids has this condition, and they require aggressive medical treatment when they hit their teenage years. Without treatment, this silent killer will make itself known by middle age.

Every child with familial hypercholesterolemia has a parent or grandparent with the same condition. That parent or grandparent will have extremely high total and LDL cholesterol levels and will often have evidence of coronary heart disease or other vascular disease by middle age.

Triggered by such a positive family history, a fasting lipid profile will identify more than 90 percent of children with familial hypercholesterolemia. We recommend checking a child's lipid panel if a parent or grandparent has a total cholesterol of 240 or greater.

Children (and adults) with familial hypercholesterolemia are initially treated with lifestyle modifications, including a diet low in saturated fat and cholesterol and an exercise program. While these interventions help reduce total and LDL cholesterol, medications are almost always necessary to normalize values. Statins are the primary option for patients with familial hypercholesterolemia. They reduce cholesterol levels by 20 to 40 percent, rapidly restoring function of arteries' inner lining and reducing buildup of plaque. The controversy surrounding statins concerns the age at which children should begin taking the medicines.

The American Academy of Pediatrics recommends beginning statin treatment for hypercholesterolemia in kids as young as eight years old. We disagree. Although pediatricians wrote 2.3 million prescriptions for statins in 2009, there is not enough long-term data to confirm the safety of statins in children under the age of thirteen. We don't know the extent to which statin treatment influences growth and development, progression through puberty, and cognitive maturation in young children. New medicines— drugs that inhibit cholesterol absorption in the intestine—and future studies may influence our recommendations in the future. But right now, based upon the evidence, we would emphasize diet and exercise, and prescribe statins only in children over the age of thirteen.

SECURING THE FUTURE

In the United States, one person dies of cardiovascular disease every thirty-three seconds. During the twenty minutes that you were reading this chapter, forty people died of heart or cardiovascular disease—and thirty-six of those deaths were preventable. For most of the victims, the road to cardiovascular disease began in childhood.

Parents have both the opportunity and the obligation to ensure their children's heart health. This means ensuring a smoke-free environment that includes a healthy diet and emphasizes physical activity. The best way to establish these behaviors is to join your kids in a healthy lifestyle. Start today. Have some fun. Become healthier yourself. And secure your children's future.

RX: THE HEARTS OF CHILDREN

Prevent heart disease risk factors in children:

Model good behaviors for your children

- Heart-healthy diet
- Right number of calories
- Limit sugar-filled drinks and foods
- Avoid processed foods
- Fruits and vegetables at every meal

Check out the school lunch

Exercise at least one hour every day

Limit screen time to one hour per day

Recognize and treat overweight and obesity:

Extra baby fat is not good

Don't count on kids "growing out of" obesity

Develop a weight loss program with your pediatrician; you can't do it alone

Lipid and cholesterol screening:

Cholesterol screening in children only if a parent or grandparent has very high cholesterol

No statins before age thirteen

LOOKING FORWARD

CHAPTER 20

HEART HEALTH (AND REPAIR) IN THE FUTURE: *STAR TREK,* HERE WE COME!

THE BIG PICTURE

Heart disease is not going away. In spite of our ever-increasing understanding of it, and new, effective strategies for prevention, heart disease will remain our number one health problem for generations to come. But this sobering piece of information does not mean that we should give up the fight. We are making progress in our battle to prevent and treat heart problems, and we foresee tremendous advances over the next few decades.

What will heart care look like in five, ten, or twenty years? From a tiny, implantable total artificial heart that lasts a lifetime to the application of stem cells to repair damaged heart muscle, we are edging closer to dramatic changes in our ability to fix sick and damaged hearts. Today these sorts of therapies are promising components of an exciting R&D pipeline. In the not-too-distant future, they will enter the clinical mainstream, where they will extend and improve the lives of millions.

At the same time that we are creating advances in cardiac biotechnology to fix heart damage, we are also deciphering the genetic code with an eye toward determining whether a patient's heart problem is genetic, and if his or her children will suffer the same fate. Today we can pinpoint the genetic causes of only a few cardiovascular diseases—hypertrophic cardio-myopathy, Marfan syndrome, some abnormal heart rhythms, and a hand-ful of others. But what about coronary artery disease, the most common heart ailment? Where do genetics fit in?

A Google search would lead you to believe that it is a simple matter to predict your genetic risk of developing coronary heart disease. In fact, dozens of websites offer the "opportunity" to spend thousands of dollars to determine your genetic profile and disease risk. Companies that sell this kind of direct-to-consumer genetic testing provide information that is confusing, distressing, and, in practical terms, worthless. We will help you save money and prevent anxiety by explaining when genetic testing for heart disease is appropriate today, and where genetic technology may take us in the future.

For those who already have heart disease, automated electronic heart monitoring can help you avoid complications and maintain quality of life. If you know how to work an iPod or a BlackBerry, you can understand the latest and greatest in heart monitoring technology. The idea is akin to the gas gauge in your car, which tells you when it is time to stop at the gas station so you avoid the distress of running out of gas in the middle of nowhere. Scientists propose a similar paradigm for heart monitoring: early warning of a negative trend, prompting action that will avert illness and prevent hospital admission. Imagine a tiny sensor implanted in your heart that monitors your congestive heart failure and tells you when trouble is looming. An indicator might light up on your nightstand console, advis-ing you to avoid salt, decrease fluid intake, or call your doctor. Monitoring technologies that provide this sort of critical, real-time information are just a step or two away from widespread clinical use.

The future is high-tech and sleek, promising dramatic advances in heart care that will produce increased quantity and quality of life. Let's have a look deep into the crystal ball, unveiling cutting-edge research that will shape the next generation of cardiac care.

A WHOLE NEW HEART: WHAT ARE THE OPTIONS?

Today we are severely limited in our ability to repair the heart muscle once it has been damaged. When a person suffers a heart attack, muscle cells die, and a region of the heart stops contracting. In most cases, this decrease in heart function is permanent. If a person has enough heart damage from heart attacks, viral infections, heart valve disease, or other causes, heart failure may ensue. Today there are more than 5 million Americans who suffer from heart failure, and an additional 500,000 people develop the condition each year. Severe heart failure is often bad news; 50 percent of those affected die within five years. But doctors and scientists predict that game-changing advances will create a much brighter future for these patients.

Heart Transplantation

In theory, the ideal therapy for heart failure is to replace the damaged muscle with functioning muscle. We can do this by transplanting the heart. The first human heart transplant was performed in 1967, and while the early years of heart transplantation were plagued by complications and death, today patients do quite well after a transplant. Fifty percent of heart recipients live at least ten years after the transplant, representing a huge improvement over our early results.

Many of the early problems were caused by rejection of the transplanted heart. We continue to work on new medicines to prevent rejection, but today the biggest limitation to transplantation is the shortage of heart donors. Worldwide, surgeons perform about 3,500 heart transplants per year (2,300 of them in the United States, where nearly a hundred hospitals are accredited for heart transplantation). But at any given moment, there are more than 10,000 people on the waiting list for a new heart, and 10 to 15 percent of them will die before receiving one.

Today heart transplantation is an excellent option for patients with end-stage heart failure. But because donor hearts are such a scarce resource, transplants are offered to only the sickest patients and many others die before a heart becomes available. In addition, elderly people and those with other illnesses such as pulmonary disease, kidney dysfunction, severe diabetes, and strokes are not offered access to this therapy. What if we had an unlimited supply of new hearts to help these people? We replace human heart valves with valves from pigs, cows, and even horses. Why not extend this concept and transplant the entire heart from an animal into a human?

THE RACE TO PERFORM THE FIRST HUMAN HEART TRANSPLANT

Medical progress is often characterized as a race. There have been recent, highly publicized medical races to decode the human genome, develop the first medicine for erectile dysfunction, and design and implant the first drug-eluting coronary artery stent. But none of these ignited the public's imagination like the quest to perform the first human heart transplant.

By mid-1967, several heart surgery teams around the world were lined up at the starting gate, prepared to perform the world's first heart transplant. In Cape Town, South Africa, heart surgeon Christiaan Barnard won the race. On December 3, 1967, he implanted the heart of a young woman into Louis Washkansky, a fifty-four-year-old grocer with end-stage heart disease. Supported by a team of thirty nurses and doctors, Barnard focused anxiously on the operative field after completing the last stitch to sew the new heart into Washkansky's chest. When he saw the first beat, Barnard summed up the result of his efforts, boldly stating, "It works."

But success was short-lived. Washkansky died eighteen days later, succumbing to pneumonia that was caused in part by anti-rejection medicines necessitated by the transplant. Undeterred by this failure, surgeons flocked to the new, sexy procedure, which was featured on the cover of *Time*. Over the next year, 102 patients received heart transplants around the world. Results were dismal. Long-term survivors were rare. By the end of 1968, the enthusiasm was gone, and most surgeons discontinued their heart transplant programs.

But Norman Shumway, a Stanford heart surgeon, persisted. Shumway was the surgical pioneer who had taught Barnard how to perform a heart transplant. Backed by decades of research, Shumway and his team continued to refine both the transplant operation and, equally important, the complex medical care of the transplant recipient. Shumway made critical advances that enabled doctors to monitor and treat rejection of the new heart. Barnard may have won the race, but Norman Shumway, the true father of the field, completed the marathon to secure a place for heart transplantation in our medical armamentarium, extending the lives of thousands of heart patients.

Xenotransplantation: Using the Hearts from Different Species

The concept of cross-species transplantation, or xenotransplantation, is simple, but the biology is incredibly complex. Nevertheless, one enterprising surgeon took a shortcut to win this race, skipping more than a few critical steps in his rush to place an animal heart into a human. On October 26, 1985, the first xenotransplant was performed by Loma Linda heart surgeon Leonard Bailey, who placed a baboon heart into the chest of a newborn named Stephanie Fae Beauclair—known to the world as "Baby Fae."

Baby Fae was born with a condition called hypoplastic left heart syndrome, a cardiac birth defect that is uniformly fatal without surgery. Surgical repair of the defect is extremely challenging and risky, so some surgeons favor heart transplantation for these unfortunate babies. Bailey felt that obtaining a suitable donor heart—which would need to come from an infant of similar size—was unlikely. So he offered Baby Fae's parents an experimental procedure.

As with Barnard's first human heart transplant eighteen years earlier, the operation went well. The baboon heart started to beat immediately. The media frenzy was overwhelming, featuring footage of Baby Fae resting comfortably and feeding. But the best medicines could not stop Baby Fae's immune system from attacking and systematically destroying the heart that was keeping her alive. Within twenty days, Baby Fae died—another medical race both won and lost.

It is easy to look back and criticize the Baby Fae debacle. But it is more important to look forward and ask, "Is there a future for xenotransplantation?" Although scientists have made tremendous strides in understanding and treating organ rejection, to date Baby Fae is the sole recipient of a cardiac xenotransplant. Scientists are currently focusing on pigs as an organ source, genetically modifying their hearts with the goal of convincing the human immune system that the porcine heart "looks" human. Today, a pig heart can survive in a monkey for six months—better than Baby Fae's twenty days, but not good enough for routine use. We think it will be a long time before cross-species transplantation becomes a clinical reality. Summing up the enormous challenges associated with xenotransplantation, pioneering heart transplant surgeon Norman Shumway commented, "Xenotransplantation is, and always will be, the future."

The Total Artificial Heart: The Machine Takes Over

If we can't use a heart from a pig or a baboon, what about a completely man-made artificial heart to replace the damaged heart of the heart failure patient? This has been called one of the holy grails of medicine. The human heart is a pump about the size of your two hands clasped together. How hard could it be to create a machine that replicates its function?

In 1964 President Lyndon Johnson directed the National Institutes of Health to invest in an artificial heart program. Since that time, we have landed men on the moon, developed the smart phone, replaced typewriters with computers, and encircled the globe with GPS satellites that can determine your position on earth to within a few feet. But we don't have a workable permanent artificial heart—yet.

BARNEY CLARK: HIS ARTIFICIAL HEART, HIS SACRIFICE, AND THE ADVANCE OF SCIENCE

Sixty-one-year-old Seattle dentist Barney Clark was dying from heart failure when his heart surgeon, William DeVries, asked him if he was willing to become the first person to receive an experimental artificial heart as a permanent transplant. Near death, Clark understood that the operation would not restore him to normal life and that his chance of long-term survival was almost zero. But with an eye toward advancing our knowledge and helping others in the future, he said yes.

On December 2, 1982, DeVries removed most of Clark's heart and replaced it with the Jarvik 7 artificial heart. Attached to a refrigerator-sized console by power cables, the Jarvik 7 pumped enough blood to take over Clark's circulation.

Clark did well for a few days. Then problems emerged. First he required a second operation to repair the device. Then he suffered bleeding, strokes, and infections. He never left the hospital, eventually dying after 112 days of bewildering and extensive complications. But Clark's sacrifice led to new knowledge and engendered progress that would eventually save hundreds of lives.

Progress with artificial hearts has eclipsed work on xenotransplantation. By 2005, the FDA had approved two different total artificial hearts. One platform, the SynCardia Total Artificial Heart, is the modern version of the Jarvik 7. This device can pump nine liters of blood per minute (right now your heart is probably pumping five or six liters per minute) and has been implanted in nearly 1,000 patients with severe heart failure. It is used primarily as a bridge to transplantation, which means that the patient keeps the artificial heart until a donor heart becomes available. At that time, the artificial heart is removed in a second operation and the new heart is transplanted.

Eighty percent of people survive these two operations. However, this strategy has several limitations. Like Clark, today's artificial heart recipients are tethered to a large console by power cords that pierce the skin. They cannot leave the hospital for prolonged periods of time while they await a transplant. In addition, a variety of complications, including infection and bleeding, can slow progress and jeopardize results.

The second FDA-approved total artificial heart is designated for destination therapy, meaning that it is a permanent replacement for the patient's own heart. The AbioCor replacement heart weighs about two pounds (about three times as much as a human heart) and is powered by an external battery that transmits energy to the device through the skin. In theory, a patient could go home with this device in place; however, most patients are not discharged from the hospital. Experience with this heart is limited. There have been fewer than twenty implants, and the longest surviving patient lived for 512 days. However, it brings us a step closer to our goal of a permanent heart replacement.

Researchers are busily working to develop the next generation of artificial hearts. The goal is to produce a small, fully implantable device that will last five years or longer. It will not suffer from mechanical failure and will not cause blood clots that can lead to strokes. Devices with these features have already been implanted in animals, and early results look promising. Our prediction: unlike the search for the holy grail, the quest for a reliable total artificial heart will occur over decades, rather than centuries, and will come to a successful conclusion.

Ventricular Assist Devices: Replacing the Heart One Chamber at a Time

There is a very good intermediate mechanical step between the total artificial heart and a heart transplant, and this option is available today. As you recall from Chapter 15, a ventricular assist device is an implantable machine that can take over the pumping action of the right or left ventricle of the heart. This device is somewhat simpler than a total artificial heart, as it replaces only a single heart chamber. The procedure is fairly straightforward, and today this therapy is relatively commonplace.

In most patients, the left ventricular assist device (LVAD) is used as a bridge to transplantation. During the wait for a donor heart, the pump provides excellent blood flow, enabling the kidneys, liver, and other organs to recover from the ravages of heart failure. When a donor heart finally becomes available, the patient is a good candidate for heart transplantation.

Former vice president Dick Cheney is the most well-known LVAD recipient to date. Like most other recipients' devices, Cheney's device is a relatively bulky pump placed with standard heart surgery techniques, including an incision in the middle of the chest and use of the heart-lung machine. Major advances promise to make the next generation of ventricular assist devices look like Ferraris compared to Cheney's Pinto-like heart pump.

Currently in clinical trials, the latest ventricular assist devices are engineering marvels. The size of double-A batteries, these small pumps deliver two to three liters of blood per minute and can be placed with minimally invasive surgical techniques (no big incision through the breast bone). This sort of therapy will reduce the waiting list for heart transplants and will enable early therapy in patients who have moderate heart failure but not enough damage to warrant a heart transplant. These new devices will represent a dramatic shift in our ability to help the millions of current and future patients afflicted by heart failure.

FIXING THE HEART WITH STEM CELLS: TRANSPLANTING ONE CELL AT A TIME

"Within each of us lies a treasure-trove of renewable life that can be directed toward healing and revitalizing cardiac function."
— *Dr. Emerson Perin on the promise of stem cell therapy for heart patients*

Heart transplantation is limited by a donor shortage, and man-made pumps face technological challenges. Recognizing these hurdles, many scientists have turned to stem cell therapy to unlock the secrets that will enable us to cure heart disease. Stem cells are front and center in our imagination and plans for treating a wide variety of conditions, ranging from Alzheimer's disease to heart failure. Keenly aware of their promise, the media closely follow the stem cell field, covering dramatic scientific breakthroughs, disappointing setbacks in research progress, and political skirmishes over their use. Putting politics aside, the relevant medical question is "Can stem cells be used to repair a damaged heart?" The current answer is "Yes, but . . ." Before we add detail to this answer, let us give you a quick lesson in the biology of stem cells.

Stem Cells: The Three Types and What They Can Do

It is easy to understand the captivating medical promise of replacing damaged or diseased tissues and organs with new tissues derived from stem cells. But what are these magical cells and where do we find them?

Stem cells are immature, unspecialized cells that can be activated to differentiate, transforming into the specialized cells that make up the body's tissues (e.g., heart muscle, liver, kidney, blood vessels, etc.). Stem cells are present both in embryos and in adults. In the embryo, these cells are responsible for development of all of the different organs and tissues. In adults, stem cells are located strategically throughout the body, where they function as the body's internal repair system.

There are important differences between embryonic and adult stem cells. Embryonic stem cells are the "purest" type of stem cells. With the consent of fertility clinic donors, embryonic stem cells are derived from fertilized embryos that were not implanted for in vitro fertilization and were targeted for destruction. Embryonic stem cells can be induced to duplicate, creating cell lines. We say that embryonic stem cells are "totipotent," which means that they can become every sort of cell in the body—from hair to nerve cells to heart cells. This broad range of potential cell types is the great advantage of embryonic stem cells.

Adult stem cells are somewhat different. They are scattered throughout the tissues of our bodies, waiting—sometimes for years—for the signal to differentiate and divide to repair damage to the organ or tissue in which they reside. In most cases, adult stem cells are "progenitor" cells—they can replace or repair only their native tissue. So stem cells in muscle become muscle fibers, stem cells in the brain differentiate into nerve cells and their supporting structures, and stem cells in the heart replace heart and vascular cells. These adult, organ-specific stem cells generally replace cells and tissues lost by the normal wear and tear of daily life. In some tissues, such as those of the GI tract and bone marrow, stem cells are constantly differentiating and dividing. In others, including the heart and pancreas, stem cells are present but are rarely pressed into service to create new tissues.

While embryonic and adult stem cells occur naturally, scientists have recently created a third type of stem cell, "induced pluripotent stem cells." To make these cells, scientists take ordinary adult cells, such as skin cells, and genetically alter them to cause them to act like embryonic stem cells, reestablishing their ability to differentiate into many different cell types. Today, scientists are developing techniques to control this process so that they can dial in the cell type that they want. With this discovery comes the possibility that we will soon have a large, readily available source of versatile stem cells.

The three different types of stem cells—embryonic, adult, and induced pluripotent stem cells—present distinct advantages and challenges when it comes to their use for tissue and organ repair.

Stem Cell Types: Advantages and Challenges			
	EMBRYONIC STEM CELLS	INDUCED PLURIPOTENT STEM CELLS	ADULT STEM CELLS
Capacity to become any cell type	Yes	Yes	No
Easy to grow in culture with division outside of body	No	Yes	Yes
Likely to cause rejection by recipient (if cells not from same person)	Yes	Yes	Yes

Stem Cells: Do They Help?

Stem cells are part of both the future and the present. They have already entered the broad clinical arena in the form of bone marrow transplantation. During a bone marrow transplant, the recipient receives a stem-cell-rich mixture of cells that repopulates the bone marrow, establishing new dividing cells in cancer patients who have lost their own bone marrow cells as a result of the cancer or as a consequence of chemotherapy used to treat the disease. With their regenerative capacity, stem cells also hold promise in the treatments of Alzheimer's disease, Parkinson's disease, diabetes, arthritis, spinal cord injury, burns, and of course heart disease.

The target populations in heart disease are those patients who have heart damage, either from an acute heart attack or the long-standing heart muscle dysfunction of chronic heart failure. In both cases, the heart's pumping function is compromised. The plan is to introduce new cells to replace damaged and dysfunctional muscle cells. While the concept is straightforward, the science is extraordinarily complex.

The first few attempts at animal and human stem cell experiments have encountered daunting challenges. Stem cell therapy to treat heart disease requires more than simple delivery of these cells to the heart muscle. Questions abound, ranging from the best technique for getting stem cells to the heart (direct injection, intravenous injection, or injection into the coronary arteries) to the right type of stem cell for heart repair. The list of difficulties for stem cell therapy is long, but none of the challenges is insurmountable.

STEM CELL THERAPY: CHALLENGES

Identify the best type of stem cell for each problem

Create large number of these stem cells

Coax cells to differentiate into desired cell type

Create "friendly" environment so that cells survive in recipient instead of being rejected

Facilitate stem cell integration into surrounding tissue

Ensure that stem cells function appropriately for long periods of time

Prevent stem cells from "going wild" and growing into different types of tissues or even tumors

Preliminary data from more than a dozen studies offer encouragement for a future role of stem cells in the treatment of heart patients. In some studies, delivery of stem cells to damaged areas of the heart appeared to produce measurable benefits, including increased blood flow, small decreases in the damage caused by a heart attack, and small increases in heart function. In two recent studies, commercially available stem cell preparations were associated with slightly improved cardiac performance, decreased symptoms, and fewer abnormal heart rhythms in heart attack victims.

COMBINATION THERAPY: STEM CELLS AND LIPOSUCTION

You read correctly—there is a link between stem cells and liposuction. Scientists are always looking for new sources of stem cells. To date, most clinical trials of stem cell therapy have employed stem cells derived from bone marrow. Harvesting bone marrow is a major, somewhat uncomfortable medical procedure, and three tablespoons of bone marrow, the typical amount harvested, contains only about 25,000 stem cells. In contrast, it is easy to harvest 6 ounces of fat tissue from patients undergoing liposuction, and this yields millions of stem cells. Can stem cells from your love handles help your damaged heart? Preliminary data seem encouraging.

Dutch researchers injected fat-derived stem cells into the coronary arteries of ten heart attack victims. Six months after the heart attack, they had slightly better heart function and blood flow and less scarring than similar patients who received a placebo. This study is much too small to prove a benefit, but it does suggest possibilities.

So far, the demonstrated cardiac benefits of stem cells are small but encouraging. As we address the challenges associated with stem cell therapy, we will refine treatment procedures and strategies, and this will likely enhance the benefits. Along the way, we will figure out how stem cells actually work to treat disease. Once again, the science is not quite as simple as we thought. The idea that stem cells would differentiate into heart cells and help the heart beat more effectively may be incorrect. In experimental studies, only a small number of administered stem cells survive in the heart and become functional heart muscle cells—not enough to explain the observed cardiac benefits.

The most popular theory right now is that stem cells secrete chemicals that have a positive influence on neighboring native heart cells. These chemicals stimulate blood vessel growth, reduce inflammation, enhance healing, and may even induce the patient's own cardiac stem cells to divide and replace damaged muscle cells. In the next few years, we will refine our understanding of how stem cell therapy works, and this will help us to optimize the treatment.

Not all scientists share our belief in the promise of stem cell therapy. We recognize that there is considerable inconsistency in the results of stem cells trials in heart attack patients. But no medicine works in everybody, and periodic failures of a treatment should not cause us to discard the medicine or procedure. In addition, wide differences between the treatments tested—from type of stem cell to method of delivery—may explain inconsistent results. At this point, we do not know the right "recipe" for stem cell treatment of heart patients. But the scientist-cooks are in the kitchen, and we are optimistic that they will eventually create a recipe that will be a winner.

STEM CELLS, MAGNETS, AND NANOTECHNOLOGY

A child's magnet. That may be the answer to the question of how we get stem cells to go to the right place in the body and stay there. Researchers at Cedars-Sinai Medical Center harvested stem cells from rats and loaded them with tiny nanoparticles of iron. They then created heart attacks in the rats and injected the iron-containing stem cells into the heart muscle near the region of the heart attack. By holding a simple magnet over the animals' hearts for ten minutes, they attracted the iron in the stem cells, and were able to triple the number of stem cells that took up residence in the heart. With more stem cells in the heart, the size of the heart attack was diminished and heart function was improved. High-tech stem cells coupled with low-tech magnets may be one pathway to improving the reliability and effectiveness of stem cell therapy.

YOUR GENES, YOUR HEART, AND YOUR DESTINY

We all know that family history is an important risk factor for the development of coronary heart disease. But family history plays an even greater role in less common cardiac ailments, including Marfan syndrome, hypertrophic cardiomyopathy, and several heart rhythm abnormalities that cause sudden death; families with these conditions can often trace inheritance of the disease through multiple generations. The variable impact of family history on the risks of different types of heart disease provides key insights into the genetics of heart ailments.

The more we learn about the genetics of heart disease, the more complex the picture. There is no single "heart disease gene." The influence of genetic factors on the development of heart disease depends upon the specific heart problem and a host of environmental factors. As a consequence, the relationship between genes and heart health is far from straightforward.

The Genetic Map: What Do We Really Know?

Doctors and patients dream of employing the genetic map provided by the Human Genome Project to determine a person's risk of heart disease and create a personalized medical plan based on that information. The idea is appealing—based upon genetic analysis, each person gets a number, from 0 to 100, representing the lifetime risk of coronary heart disease. But to a heart doctor or geneticist, these concepts represent (currently) unattainable, almost romantic ideals. The development of coronary heart disease is related to both a variety of environmental factors and many different genes, and our understanding of these genes in particular, and human genetics in general, is incomplete.

How can this last statement be correct? The Human Genome Project was completed in 2003, and after thirteen years and $3 billion, the popular notion is that we now have all the answers. In fact, even though the Human Genome Project provided a great deal of information, it did not answer most of our questions about our genes. The Human Genome Project identified nearly all of our 20,000 to 25,000 genes (there are still a few to go) and determined the sequence of the 3 billion chemical base pairs, or building blocks, that make up human DNA. Remarkably, scientists found that 99.6 percent of these genetic sequences are identical between individuals; but with 3 billion DNA base pairs, this leaves 24 million sites of potential variation between people.

Every person has a unique genetic composition. Created by DNA analysis of only a few donors, the genetic map produced by the Human Genome Project does not represent *your* specific collection of genes. Furthermore, it does not tell us the function of each gene, its range of possible mutations, and the ways that its function and expression are controlled by other segments of DNA. So we have a DNA map, but we don't have the key to the map that guides us to a personalized health plan based on an individual's unique genes. Now you understand why it is premature to say that we have cracked the genetic code.

Nevertheless, an Internet search on "genetic testing" will lead you to the incorrect conclusion that scientists have all the answers. You will encounter dozens of companies that promise to reveal your personal risk of developing a wide range of health conditions, including coronary heart disease. The testing itself is sophisticated, screening hundreds of thousands, or even millions, of points of genetic variation. But these tests provide neither a complete map of your DNA nor your true risk of developing common diseases. After charges for $1,000 or more appear on your credit card bill, you will receive a list of conditions to which you are "predisposed." This is not quite the same as a "personalized health plan based upon your own genes."

Genetic Testing for Heart Disease: Where It Helps

In spite of the many gaps in our knowledge and the limitations of genetic testing, a person's genes can tell us a lot about the presence and risk of developing *certain types* of heart disease. We have the best handle on a group of relatively uncommon conditions that are influenced strongly by a small number of genes and, not surprisingly, clearly travel in families. As we mentioned earlier, this short list includes hypertrophic obstructive cardiomyopathy, Marfan syndrome, and three arrhythmia syndromes: right ventricular cardiomyopathy, long QT syndrome, and Brugada syndrome.

Each of these conditions is associated with sudden death, and each tends to be caused by a mutation in a single gene. Genetic testing for these diseases increases diagnostic accuracy, helps to guide therapy, and informs diagnosis and treatment for other family members. Of these, hypertrophic cardiomyopathy—a dangerous overgrowth of part of the heart muscle—is the best understood, and serves as an example of the proper application of genetic testing in today's cardiovascular care.

Many people with hypertrophic cardiomyopathy have a single genetic mutation, suggesting that screening for the condition might be pretty easy if you simply searched for the offending gene in each person. But there is a problem—hypertrophic cardiomyopathy patients don't all have the same

DIRECT-TO-CONSUMER GENETIC TESTING: BUYER BEWARE

Seeing a dollar sign (rather than a double helix) in your DNA, a host of companies have bypassed hospitals and doctors' offices, offering genetic testing directly to consumers via the Internet. More than 1,300 different genetic tests are available, including screens of approximately 100 genes that have been linked to heart disease. Some companies claim that their testing kits can both predict the risk of disease and guide the consumer toward personalized medicine, including foods, vitamins, and drugs suited to a particular genetic profile. But buyer beware.

We have already outlined the scientific limitations inherent in these tests. But there are other, equally important problems with these tests, including their regulation and interpretation. You know that the FDA determines when a medicine is safe and effective. Who regulates genetic testing, deciding whether the test is accurate and when it is ready for broad use? Nobody! Companies are free to make their claims with no oversight. While some genetic tests are validated, such as that for cystic fibrosis, others, including those promising to assess risks of coronary heart disease and diabetes, are not yet suited to become a part of routine clinical care. Furthermore, patients and even doctors frequently do not understand the results of these tests, and scientists are still arguing about the best ways to perform the tests and what the results mean. This is not the sort of "opportunity" that is worth thousands of dollars. In the future, well-designed and carefully validated—and cheaper—genetic testing will certainly help us evaluate and treat cardiovascular disease. But, for now, we recommend that most people spend their money elsewhere.

mutation in the same gene. To date, more than 900 different mutations in thirteen different genes have been identified in people with this condition. While the patients all "look" similar clinically—they have classic findings on an echocardiogram—they are often genetically different. Each family affected by hypertrophic cardiomyopathy tends to have its own unique, disease-causing mutation; geneticists call these "private mutations." At this point, we have characterized about two-thirds of the mutations that cause hypertrophic cardiomyopathy. Within a decade, we will probably reach 90 percent or more.

So the genetic basis of a relatively simple genetic disease that is passed from parent to child 50 percent of the time is actually quite complex. But we can still use genetically based targeted screening to help people with hypertrophic cardiomyopathy and their families.

Genetic screening begins by identifying the first person in a family who has a disease; this individual is called the "proband." This person should undergo genetic testing to determine the specific mutation that has caused the condition. In the case of hypertrophic cardiomyopathy, doctors can identify the disease-causing mutation 65 percent of the time. If this is successful, all first-degree relatives (siblings, children, parents) are screened to determine whether they carry the defective gene. This information is clinically useful. Family members who do *not* have the gene are reassured that they will most likely not develop the condition. On the other hand, those who are found to carry the gene for hypertrophic cardiomyopathy can be monitored and treated, helping to avoid serious complications.

Similar genetic testing is recommended for the families of people who suffer from Marfan syndrome, long QT syndrome, Brugada syndrome, and arrhythmogenic right ventricular cardiomyopathy. Given that the first symptom of each of these diseases can be sudden death, it is obviously important to secure the diagnosis before symptoms develop. Long QT syndrome is particularly notorious, as it has been linked to sudden infant death syndrome. In the future, the ability to screen for this condition will spare new parents the anguish of losing a child. Overall, these heart problems are relatively rare, with each affecting between 1 in 1,000 and 1 in 5,000 people, so genetic screening is recommended only if you have a family member who is affected. However, we believe that testing for cardiac conditions that cause sudden cardiac death will probably become routine in the future.

Genetic Testing:
The Problem with Coronary Heart Disease

So far, we have focused on a handful of relatively uncommon heart problems that are strongly influenced by genes. These represent the exceptions rather than the rule. Most common diseases, such as coronary heart disease, diabetes, and hypertension, are far more complex, affected by multiple genes, interactions between different genes, and a host of environmental factors. Undaunted by this complexity, scientists have worked tirelessly to explore the role of genetics in our biggest killer—coronary heart disease.

We know that we are not going to find a single gene that causes coronary heart disease. Dozens of genetic sites have been tied to coronary heart disease, with nearly a hundred genetic variations linked to LDL cholesterol levels alone. And these numbers are growing as research proceeds.

Recognizing that a variety of genes influence coronary heart disease, some scientists have grouped them together, testing the predictive power of multi-gene profiles. In the Women's Genome Health Study, investigators examined 101 genetic markers in 19,000 women and assessed their cardiovascular health over a twelve-year period. The authors found that standard risk factors—advanced age, smoking, high blood pressure, diabetes, cholesterol levels, and family history—strongly predicted development of cardiovascular disease, and the genetic markers for coronary heart disease added nothing. The authors concluded that genes alone rarely cause heart disease.

The primary goal of genetic testing—or any risk prediction model, for that matter—is to identify people at risk for a condition and enable them to take action to improve their future health. In the case of coronary heart disease, the idea would be to tailor prevention, lifestyle, and medical therapies to a person's individual biology, including the genetic makeup. Perhaps telling a person that his genes put him at higher-than-average risk of a heart attack might encourage a better diet, more exercise, and no smoking. Of course, we make these recommendations regardless of a person's genes. But the hope is that genetic information will give the person an extra push toward a healthier lifestyle.

Others have taken a different approach to the application of genetic testing in patients with coronary heart disease. One idea involves using genetic information to ascertain whether chest pain is coming from the heart and therefore merits further detailed cardiac investigation. Today, many people with chest pain undergo invasive cardiac catheterization to determine whether the pain is a result of coronary heart disease, and 30 percent of them are found to have normal arteries. What if we could use a person's genetic profile to help us determine whether cardiac catheterization is necessary? Right now, genetic testing is insufficient to rule out a cardiac cause of chest pain. But more advanced genetic tests may eventually help us decide who should and who should not undergo cardiac catheterization.

We would be remiss if we did not mention familial hypercholesterolemia, a genetic condition that affects 1 in 500 people and dramatically increases their risk of developing heart disease. People with this condition carry a mutation in the gene that encodes the cell-surface receptor for LDL cholesterol. Normally, the receptor helps to remove LDL cholesterol from the blood. In patients with familial hypercholesterolemia, faulty receptors fail to remove LDL from the blood, resulting in high circulating levels of LDL that lead to early onset of cardiovascular disease. If undiagnosed and untreated, people with heterozygous (one copy of the abnormal gene) familial hypercholesterolemia suffer premature coronary heart disease, with 60 percent of men and 30 percent of women developing coronary disease by age sixty. One out of every million people has two copies of the abnormal gene (homozygous familial hypercholesterolemia), resulting in extremely high cholesterol levels often exceeding 1,000 mg/dL. Most people with homozygous FH have a heart attack before reaching thirty years of age, sometimes as children or teenagers.

We know that most cases of familial hypercholesterolemia are caused by a genetic mutation on chromosome 19, and we have the ability to detect this mutation. So we have a well-characterized condition, an understanding of its genetic basis, the genetic testing necessary to confirm the diagnosis, and the appropriate medical therapy (statins) to treat the disease. Sounds like a perfect situation for genetic testing—except for one fact: we don't need genetic testing to diagnose this disorder. A simple family history and lipid profile will do the trick. If a person has an LDL cholesterol greater than 220, we can presume that familial hypercholesterolemia is present and treat the person with statins, diet, and other strategies to lower the cholesterol level. We also screen family members by taking their histories and measuring their cholesterol levels. This is a genetic disease, but just because we have a sophisticated and expensive test does not mean that we need to employ it. In many cases, good old-fashioned medicine—a medical history, physical examination, and routine blood tests—provides all of the information that we need.

Heart Valve Disease: Echocardiogram, Not Genetic Testing

What is the role of genes in the 300,000 people who go to the operating room for a heart valve operation each year? A person's genes do influence the development of heart valve disease, but at this point we do not recommend genetic screening for these conditions.

Mitral valve prolapse is the most common heart valve abnormality, affecting 2 to 3 percent of the population. Although familial forms do exist, in most cases this condition is not inherited. Similarly, aortic valve problems do not have a strong genetic basis. However, there is one exception. One percent of people are born with a bicuspid aortic valve, meaning that the heart valve has two flaps instead of three. Bicuspid aortic valves, which are identified by an echocardiogram, are prone to become narrowed (stenotic) or leaky (regurgitant) over time. In about 10 percent of cases, this valve abnormality clusters in families. If a family member has aortic valve disease caused by a bicuspid valve, we do recommend family screening—but with an echocardiogram, not a genetic test.

GENES AND THE MARLBORO MAN

Is smoking in your genes? This is an intriguing concept. If certain genes cause people to smoke, perhaps we can develop a way to modify the genes' effect and help people to stop smoking. Like heart disease itself, smoking tends to run in families. When parents smoke, there is a 50 percent or greater chance that children will take up the habit. But how much of this is shared genes versus shared environment?

Studies of more than 100,000 people have revealed that several regions on chromosome 15—in the neighborhood of the gene responsible for the nicotine receptor—influence smoking behavior. But the impact is small. The least favorable genetic profile in this area increases a person's tobacco consumption by only one cigarette per day. Scientists believe that years from now the best use of genetic information in smokers may be to guide the choice of program for smoking cessation. But we are still a long way from completely characterizing the role of genes in smoking addiction.

How Your Genes Will Guide Your Choice of Medicines

In addition to identifying people afflicted by or at risk for illnesses, genetic testing will one day be used to tailor medical therapy, telling us which patients are most likely to respond to particular medicines. This concept is already edging its way into medical practice. Scientists have demonstrated that a person's genetic profile helps to predict the response to the anticoagulant warfarin and the risk of developing rare but serious muscle damage from statin therapy. Genetic testing before administering these drugs may become commonplace in the future, depending in part on the outcome of a current, controversial test case concerning genetic testing for responsiveness to clopidogrel.

Clopidogrel is a medicine that reduces blood clotting by inhibiting platelet function. It is widely used in patients with cardiovascular disease and is particularly important when it comes to preventing blood clot formation in patients who have received cardiac stents. We have known for a long time that clopidogrel does not work until it is converted into an active metabolite by enzymes in the liver. It turns out that different people have different levels of function of these liver enzymes, and this characteristic is genetically determined.

Thirty percent of people have one copy of a gene that makes them a slow metabolizer of clopidogrel. In addition, 2 percent of people have two copies of this gene, rendering them very poor metabolizers. As a result, the drug is less effective at inhibiting platelet function. Some, but not all, observational studies suggest that such individuals have worse clinical outcomes—more heart attacks, strokes, and deaths. This increased risk appears to be highest in those undergoing cardiac catheterization and stent implantation, especially in the setting of a heart attack.

Based upon these preliminary observations, the FDA issued a black-box warning concerning decreased effectiveness of clopidogrel in those with two copies of the slow metabolizer gene. Some doctors began recommending genetic testing before giving the medicine, and it has become standard at some major medical centers. While we think that this approach may be useful in the future, it is premature today. Remember, genetic testing—like any medical testing—is appropriate only if the test results influence therapy and outcomes. At this time, we have not yet defined the change in therapy that represents a correct response to a positive clopidogrel slow metabolizer test.

Genetic Testing: Path to the Future

In the arena of cardiovascular disease, genetic testing currently plays a large role in the health of few, and a small role in the health of many. With continued research and discovery, this will change. In the case of rare but serious diseases such as hypertrophic cardiomyopathy and arrhythmia syndromes associated with sudden death, widespread and inexpensive screening will enable early identification and will save lives. With more common conditions such as coronary heart disease, the genetic profile will likely add to the broader risk profile but will not completely determine risk. Once conditions are identified, the genetic makeup will guide the choice of therapies, ensuring a personalized medical approach that fits the patient like a perfectly tailored suit.

Genetic testing raises three key questions that doctors and patients must answer while researchers work out the science: Who should be tested? What advice will the genetic test generate? Who will have access to the information? The answers to these questions must be spelled out in well-conceived, evidence-based guidelines. The government has already offered some help, passing the 2006 Genetic Information Nondiscrimination Act, which prohibits insurers and employers from discriminating based upon information derived from genetic testing. This is an important first step, but we have quite a ways to go. Widespread genetic testing for common diseases should not be undertaken until we have both the science to perform the tests and the wisdom to answer these questions.

BIG BROTHER IS WATCHING: MONITORING YOUR HEART

As we anticipate impressive advances in how we predict and treat heart disease, we also foresee huge improvements in the techniques we use to monitor the person with heart disease, enabling preventive therapy before problems develop. Think about combining an iphone and a blood pressure cuff, sending automatic electronic transmission of blood pressure data to your doctor in real time from your home. As we integrate different technologies, we will be able to recognize problems earlier and react more quickly, treating them before they cause irreversible damage or warrant hospital admission.

Electronic Monitoring: Pacemakers and Defibrillators Lead the Way

The convergence of medical and information technologies is progressing most rapidly with the development of new pacemakers and internal defibrillators. Since the 1970s, patients have been able to transmit information from their pacemakers over telephone lines. Initially, the transmitted information was limited, but today's pacemakers store megabytes of diagnostic data concerning both the patient's heart rhythm and device function. This information is easily transmitted over telephone lines or the Internet, enabling timely identification of heart rhythm abnormalities and device malfunction.

The capabilities of internal defibrillators are even more impressive than those associated with pacemakers. Many current defibrillators automatically transmit a daily data download via wireless transmission. If the daily transmission signals either an abnormal heart rhythm or device malfunction, the patient may receive an alarming—but potentially lifesaving—phone call. In one clinical study, this sort of daily monitoring reduced the number of doctor's visits and days in the hospital. If you or a family member has a defibrillator or pacemaker, ask about this sort of monitoring.

DEFIBRILLATORS GO WIRELESS

When heart failure patients receive an internal defibrillator, they get a generator that is a bit larger than an old-fashioned silver dollar and wire leads that travel through blood vessels from the generator to the inside of the heart. These wire leads are the Achilles' heel of the device. Placing them can cause complications, including injury to the heart, blood vessels, and lungs. In addition, the leads can fracture—one of the most common causes of heart device recalls. Why not eliminate these wire leads?

Recognizing the need for a wireless defibrillator, scientists have created an internal defibrillator that monitors and corrects heart rhythm without the placement of wires in the heart. The wireless defibrillator system includes just two components that are implanted under the skin. The implant does not require X-ray guidance for placement (no radiation exposure), and it takes only thirty minutes to put it in place. This simpler, less expensive, and less invasive procedure produces excellent outcomes; a study in the *New England Journal of Medicine* demonstrated that the new wireless defibrillator corrected serious abnormal heart rhythms in 98 percent of cases. Like your home computer and its Internet connection, future defibrillators and pacemakers will deliver the convenience of wireless technology.

Using Information Technology to Help the Heart Failure Patient

Doctors are particularly interested in leveraging information technology to improve the care of patients with heart failure. Managing such patients is challenging, as they often look healthy on the outside but may be teetering on the brink of an ambulance ride. A single bowl of chicken noodle soup, with its heavy salt load, can be enough to upset a patient's fluid balance and send him or her to the hospital. In the United States heart failure accounts for more than 1 million hospital admissions each year. During these visits, the patient is "tuned up," meaning that medicines are adjusted and the excess fluid that has collected in the lungs (causing shortness of breath) and in the ankles (causing swelling) is removed. Unfortunately, the fix is not permanent—one in four patients is readmitted to the hospital within twelve weeks.

Both doctors and commercial firms hypothesized that we could reduce hospital admissions in heart failure patients with more frequent assessment of their status at home. Instead of checking on them every few weeks at the doctor's office, we could gather daily information and intervene early when necessary. Recognizing the potential benefits of information and early intervention, entrepreneurs and medical device companies created a variety of home monitoring technologies, collectively called telemonitoring systems.

Telemonitoring technology enables daily (in some cases twice-daily) electronic transmission of patient data from home. The data include weight, heart rate, blood pressure, oxygen saturation, and presence of symptoms. In most instances, any value outside a preset range leads to notification of a doctor or nurse, who then contacts the patient to adjust therapy and try to avoid a hospital admission. For example, a two-pound weight gain over two days, which could be an early sign of fluid overload and impending shortness of breath, would alert a nurse or doctor to call the patient, who would advise fluid restriction and avoidance of salt, and possibly increase the patient's diuretic dose—all without a doctor's visit.

Several clinical studies suggest that home monitoring of heart failure patients decreases hospitalizations, emergency department visits, patient anxiety, and even mortality, while also improving quality of life. However, these purported benefits are controversial. A recent, widely publicized randomized controlled trial, in which half of the patients had telemonitoring and half had the usual care, showed no benefit to telemonitoring. Proponents of telemonitoring point out that the study had weaknesses, including an automated, voice-activated system for patient contact rather than direct contact with a nurse or doctor, and substantial attrition, with 45 percent of telemonitoring patients failing to use the system after six months.

Our take is that this sort of telemonitoring—limited assessment of symptoms, weight, and vital signs without direct caregiver contact—may be insufficient to make a difference in most heart failure patients. But that does not mean that the idea is worthless. Rather, we need to leverage the technology to get different, more meaningful information that we can really use to improve care of heart patients. This is where monitoring of the heart failure patient becomes truly high-tech.

Scientists have created a small sensor that can be placed inside a patient's heart to collect and transmit physiologic data that reflect that person's fluid balance. In a recent study of heart failure patients, this paper-clip-sized sensor was implanted in the pulmonary artery, where an increase in pressure is a very early sign of fluid overload in heart failure patients. This change is far more sensitive, and occurs earlier, than symptoms such as weight gain, shortness of breath, or swelling of the ankles. Using wireless technology, the sensor transmitted pulmonary artery pressure to a secure database, where doctors and nurses accessed the data and took preemptive action when necessary. The investigators reduced hospital admissions for heart failure by one-third over the course of a year. The senior investigator in this project commented that this represents one of the "first meaningful improvements in the management of heart failure in nearly a decade." We agree that the findings are promising, but urge caution. We need more research to determine precisely which patients might benefit from this type of device.

With wireless monitoring that can provide real-time physiologic data, we are poised to enter a new era in the management of heart patients. These sensors bring heart monitoring one step closer to the gas tank analogy, in which a light on the car dashboard tells you when the tank is low. Like glucose monitoring in diabetics, where the patient can obtain the data (blood sugar readings) and adjust the treatment (insulin dose) accordingly, we will soon have the ability to monitor a person's heart with similar precision.

WE HAVE AN APP FOR THAT

Patients are not the only ones who will soon be operating high-tech monitoring devices on a daily basis. Doctors and nurses are poised to add them to their daily activities as well. Hospitals can now download software that provides a real-time, ICU-like display of hospitalized patients' data on an iPhone, iPod Touch, or iPad. In addition, the system facilitates communication between members of a patient's medical team, ensuring that they all have the most current data as they make key decisions.

When a doctor gets a 2:00 a.m. call about a hospitalized patient who is in trouble, she can use this application to access patient data. The app can then be used to conduct a patient care conference, simultaneously engaging multiple caregivers who cannot get to the bedside; this feature should enhance team-based decision making, especially in rural areas that are not well served by specialists. The company that designed this app (AppPoint, from Airstrip Technologies) states that the platform supports multitasking and the on-the-go realities faced by physicians and nurses. It may also prove an invaluable aide for improving the care of hospitalized patients. And it's cool.

ADVANCES IN CARDIAC CARE: FIX THE PLUMBING AND HOME BY NOON

When it was developed in the 1950s, open heart surgery was hailed as a medical miracle. The idea that a surgeon could stop a person's heart, repair it, and then get the repaired heart to beat again defied expectations. Perhaps there was no heart problem that we could not fix.

Within a couple of decades, more than 1 million people were undergoing heart surgery each year. Results were excellent, with 99 percent of people surviving standard operations and most returning to normal life within a few weeks. Surgical techniques continued to improve, and minimally invasive and even robotic approaches to the heart's plumbing problems followed.

Heart surgeons and their teams have saved the lives of millions of patients. But today, the scope of heart surgery is changing rapidly as a result of advances in interventional cardiology. Innovative cardiologists and engineers have developed a variety of non-surgical techniques to fix structural problems in the heart. In most cases, these procedures depend upon gaining access to the heart by traversing the body's blood vessels with catheters, hollow tubes through which instruments and devices can be delivered and manipulated. The ability to work inside the beating heart via a catheter, introduced through a small incision in an arm or leg, is revolutionizing our approach to an increasingly wide variety of cardiac issues.

The most well-known interventional cardiology procedure is angioplasty with stent implantation for patients with plaque-filled arteries. Where bypass surgery reroutes blood flow around obstructing plaque, angioplasty with stenting involves working from the *inside* of the artery. Both techniques are effective, but today angioplasty with stenting is the most widely used intervention for patients with coronary heart disease. In 2006, there were approximately 1.1 million angioplasty procedures performed in the United States, versus only 250,000 bypass operations. Even though recent data support longer survival with surgery in certain patient groups, catheter-based, less invasive approaches are the patients' number one choice for managing coronary heart disease.

BIOABSORBABLE (DISSOLVING) STENTS

When a patient receives one of our latest drug-eluting coronary artery stents, he or she must take blood-thinning medicines for a year or more to prevent blood clots from forming in the metallic stent. What if we had a stent that dissolved after it did its job? This might eliminate the need for clopidogrel and other medicines. In addition, with today's permanent metal stents, long-term blood vessel function is decidedly abnormal; some believe that it is likely that arteries will function more normally over the long term if they are treated with dissolving, or bioabsorbable, stents. Such stents, constructed from biodegradable polymers, are now under investigation. Preliminary results look encouraging, although most experts predict that these stents will not completely replace metallic stents.

We have also developed non-surgical techniques to fix damaged heart valves. For the last five years, cardiologists and heart valve patients have been excited by advances in percutaneous, or non-surgical, replacement of the aortic valve. The traditional approach to most aortic valve problems is to open the chest, remove the old valve, and sew in a new one. In the 1990s investigators reasoned that it should be possible to develop an artificial heart valve that folds like an umbrella; this valve could then be threaded into the heart with a catheter under X-ray guidance and opened inside the failing native valve. If the new valve opened with enough force, it would both stay in place in the heart and collapse the patient's diseased valve. Some surgeons responded to this concept by saying, "Good luck with that. It will never work."

But it does work. More than 30,000 Europeans have received new aortic valves with this approach. In a recent North American trial, patients too sick for conventional surgery were randomly assigned to medical therapy or to receive a non-surgical valve. The outcomes were startling: those who received the non-surgical valve were 20 percent more likely to be alive one year after treatment when compared to patients who were treated with medicines alone.

Percutaneous aortic valves are not yet perfect. The risk of a stroke within thirty days of the procedure is about 5 percent, and in many cases there is a leak around the valve. In addition, we do not know how long these valves will last. As a result, the era of surgical aortic valve treatment, where we know the valves can last twenty years or longer, is not over yet. However, within a few years the option to forgo surgery but still have your aortic valve treated will be a clinical reality. Meanwhile, the non-surgical aortic valve has already been a boon for Doris Snyder, who received a valve at age 101 and celebrated her 102nd birthday shortly thereafter. Her next step is to plan her 103rd birthday party.

Technology is advancing a bit more slowly when it comes to fixing the mitral valve without surgery. The reason for this lag is that surgeons usually repair, rather than replace, the mitral valve. Valve repair is more challenging than valve replacement, requiring several different surgical maneuvers, and it is currently impossible to replicate all of these surgical steps using catheters. But, in some instances, a clothespin-like clip that holds the two parts of the leaking mitral valve together improves valve function enough to make people feel better. Elizabeth Taylor avoided invasive heart surgery by undergoing this experimental procedure.

Let's complete our discussion of new "plumbing" technology by returning to the beginnings of heart surgery. Many of the earliest open heart operations were performed on children, to close congenital holes in the heart. Most of these holes are septal defects, which permit inappropriate mixing of oxygenated and deoxygenated blood between the left and right sides of the heart, increasing the heart's workload. Today we can close these holes without surgery, using catheters to block the hole with devices that look a bit like open umbrellas. This technology means that many babies (and some adults with late recognition of the problem) can undergo a simple, low-risk procedure to fix a hole in the heart and be home the next day.

Plumbing Versus Prevention

As the march of technology continues, elegant, effective, less invasive procedures will dramatically reduce the need for open heart surgery and other "big" cardiac procedures. In many cases, we will soon be able to fix your broken heart in the morning and send you home in the afternoon. But even these approaches will have risks and limitations. And in the case of coronary heart disease, prevention will always be preferable to our best stent or operation. The best medical procedure is the one that you don't need to have.

EPILOGUE: PUTTING HEART DOCTORS OUT OF BUSINESS

In medicine, success does not occur by accident. Success begins with understanding and ends with action. Our understanding of heart disease increases every day. We know more about coronary heart disease than we do about the common cold. Each month medical journals fill hundreds of pages with new discoveries and insights into the workings of the heart and the causes and treatments of coronary heart disease. Some of our latest science even sounds like the stuff of science fiction. But as we have emphasized, understanding how to prevent coronary heart disease is *not* rocket science. Victory on this front is within our grasp, but we must act on all of the knowledge that we have gained. Previous medical success stories, such as the birth of antisepsis and clean surgery, demonstrate the profound lifesaving impact that comes from combining action with knowledge.

Have you washed your hands today? Do you carry a small bottle of Purell in your pocket? Would you shake hands with somebody who has just sneezed into his hand? Your predictable responses to these questions stem from your understanding that dirty hands can spread germs and cause illness. Today we recognize this as a simple but powerful concept. It even helped us to limit the spread of the H1N1 flu virus. But the role of cleanliness in preventing the spread of disease was not always so obvious. It took doctors centuries to understand the importance of hand washing, and the public's behavior lagged behind for decades more.

The story starts with surgery. In the mid-nineteenth century, half of all surgical patients died as a result of the procedure. Even a seemingly minor operation such as an appendectomy frequently ended in death. Infection and sepsis (an infection in the bloodstream) were the leading causes of these horrendous outcomes.

At the time, the accepted theory of "spontaneous generation" maintained that germs arose spontaneously from non-living material. But Louis Pasteur, a microbiologist and chemist, disagreed. Recognizing that germs in beer, wine, and milk could spoil the beverages, Pasteur extrapolated this idea to medicine and proposed that bacteria and viruses could also infect people and cause disease. This became known as the germ theory of disease. Pasteur encouraged doctors to wash their hands and sanitize their equipment before surgery.

Many doctors ignored him. But British surgeon Joseph Lister paid attention. When Lister began his practice of surgery, doctors believed that exposure to "bad air" was the cause of infection. Doctors did not wash their hands before operating or examining patients (they also wore their bloody, soiled gowns as badges of honor), and they unknowingly transmitted bacteria from one patient to the next as they moved through crowded hospital wards. Lister read Pasteur's description of the three methods to prevent infection: heat, filtration, and exposure to chemical solutions. While the first two were difficult to put into practice in the hospital and operating room, the use of antiseptic solutions held promise. Aware that carbolic acid could be used to remove odor from sewage, Lister used the chemical to clean surgical instruments, swab surgical wounds, and wash surgeons' hands.

With these practices, Lister's survival rates skyrocketed. In 1867 he published his work in the *Lancet,* and other surgeons began following suit. The risk of infection dropped dramatically. Years later, King Edward VII credited Lister with his survival from appendicitis. Today surgeons honor Lister as the father of sterile surgery. (The rest of the world knows of him through a mouthwash named in his honor.)

In the nineteenth century, fatal infections seemed insurmountable. But by pairing understanding with action, Pasteur and Lister led a change that has saved millions of lives. One hundred years later, we benefit from these men's efforts on a daily basis. Initially intended for doctors and nurses, the knowledge that Pasteur and Lister generated has affected all of our behaviors. We know that cleanliness and hand washing slow the spread of infection. Acting upon this knowledge has helped us to fight conditions ranging from the common flu to life-threatening surgical infections. The same paradigm applies when it comes to beating heart disease.

We don't yet have all of the answers concerning coronary heart disease, but we have enough to begin to act. Many of our colleagues claim that there are two types of people in the world: people who have coronary heart disease and people who are going to get it. To us, this view seems unduly pessimistic, but based upon our society's current trajectory, it may well be correct. Use the knowledge we have provided to change this trajectory. We know how hard it is to change entrenched habits. We are doctors, but we've been patients, too, and often find it difficult to follow our own doctors' instructions. After a long, hard day at work, it's difficult to imagine mustering up the energy even to lace up your running shoes, let alone to get in that much-needed half hour of exercise. Similarly, after a particularly stressful day at home with the kids, we recognize the lure of that carton of dark chocolate Häagen-Dazs in the freezer—you know, the one with your name written all over it. But these changes are well worth it.

{{{{{

We hope we have motivated you to begin making those changes in your life that will help you move in the right direction. Our goal is to create two new classifications of people: those who have been successfully treated for coronary heart disease, and those who have avoided it altogether.

If you follow our advice, our waiting rooms will empty out, and you just might put us out of business. Don't worry about us; we will gladly hang up our scalpels and stethoscopes if we can find a better way to lead you to a heart-healthy life.

In Chapter 1, we told you about a recent examination of Egyptian mummies. Using the latest high-tech CT scanners, scientists found evidence of heart disease in these 3,000-year-old "patients." Centuries from now, what will our descendants see when they perform a similar study on us? Accessed via the latest iPad-like device (iPad 4000), will the headlines read "Coronary Heart Disease in the Twenty-First Century: Everybody Had It"? Or will the findings produce a different headline: "The Disappearance of Coronary Heart Disease in the Twenty-First Century"? The answer to that question is up to us. Together, we have the opportunity to write this story.

ACKNOWLEDGMENTS

I want to thank my parents, Dr. Sheldon Gillinov and Lynda Gillinov. My father told me that there was no greater position of trust and responsibility than that of the surgeon standing poised over the sleeping patient, scalpel in hand. Understanding the focus and dedication required of my father in his role as a surgeon, my mother supported him by bringing boundless energy to the family front. My parents taught me that a career in medicine is a family undertaking.

These lessons and examples carry over into my own life. While I operate, rush to emergencies, and satisfy my desire to write, my wife, Lisa, supplies the love that fuels me and our family. Most important, Lisa focuses her love and attention on our three children, ensuring that they will grow up to become wonderful people. On that score, Stephen, Lauren, and Nicole are well on their way. With their support, my wife and kids make my careers as surgeon and author/speaker both possible and worthwhile.

I thank my teachers at Hawken School in Cleveland, Ohio, and at Yale University. I don't remember the trigonometry or ancient history they taught me, but I do know how to write clearly. Drs. Toby Cosgrove (Cleveland Clinic) and Duke Cameron (Johns Hopkins) taught me how to fix people's hearts and at the same time encouraged me to write and speak, helping me to hone both crafts.

This book is about evidence and truth. Steve Nissen is an incredible partner and a tireless advocate for patients everywhere. His knowledge is encyclopedic and his critical thinking unparalleled.

I thank all of those who have helped me by reading and editing my work. My readers include my wife, my parents, Laura Roberts, Cathy Kielar, Melanie Janka, Jeanne Ryan, Colleen Koch, Scott Linabarger, Paul Matsen, David Barr, Judy Pyle, Roger Joseph, Roy Jenkins, Marc Werner, John Liddicoat, Katy Brown Norris, Florin Sgondea, Sandy Bremec, Brian Kolonick, Betsy Stovsky, Megan Frankel, Cynthia Galbincea, Tom Rice, and Dan Stone. I also thank Brian Kohlbacher for his help with my speeches and presentations.

Karyn Toso, an English scholar and teacher and wife of my patient Gianni Toso (see Chapter 6), has served many roles—researcher, editor, and passionate advocate for making this book interesting and fun.

Alice Martell started as an adviser, agreed to become my agent, and along the way also became a friend. She is wonderful! Thanks to Sydny Miner, Anna Thompson, and the team at Crown for their editorial insight, enthusiasm, and support.

Finally, I thank all of my patients. You asked the questions. Here are the answers.

—Marc Gillinov, M.D.

I want to thank my extraordinarily patient wife, Linda Butler, who has supported me through many years of challenges from medical school to the present. Linda has made many sacrifices to support my career, sometimes going for extended periods without the vacations and family time most of her friends enjoy. No matter how daunting the task, I always know that I have her support and honest feedback to anchor my life.

I am grateful for the introduction to the science of medicine provided by my late father, Dr. Edward Nissen, who taught me the joy of approaching medicine from an academic perspective. He was a gynecologic oncologist whose dedication to his patients provided me with the inspiration to pursue medicine as a career. I am also indebted to my late mother, Shirley

Nissen, who stood by me during eight years as an undergraduate during the turbulent 1960s when I was uncertain about what direction to pursue.

I am also appreciative of the mentorship I have received during medical training, particularly from Dr. Anthony DeMaria, who encouraged me to pursue cardiology and taught me about critical scientific thinking and writing. Without his example, I might not have pursued cardiovascular medicine as a discipline. I had similar inspiration from Dr. Reginald Low, an exemplary cardiologist who taught me how to care for critically ill patients.

Finally, I would like to thank my extraordinary partner, Dr. Marc Gillinov, whose unwavering commitment kept this project on track, even when I stumbled. We are both fortunate to work at the Cleveland Clinic, where we receive incredible support from an institution committed to excellence in every aspect of medical practice. Alice Martell and the leadership at Crown mentioned by Dr. Gillinov provided us with exceptional support and guidance throughout this project.

—Steven Nissen, M.D.

INDEX

New Year's Eve, 177
New York City, stress of, 180
New York City Health
    Department, 117
Niacin, 61, 64, 196
Niaspan, 61
Nicotine, addiction to, 25
Nicotine replacement therapy,
    26
Night shift, 36
9/11 terrorist attacks, 178
Nitrates/nitrites, 102
Nitrates (nitroglycerin), 288,
    297, 304, 458–459
Noise pollution, as risk factor
    for CHD, 33
Non-Hodgkin lymphoma, 136
Northridge earthquake,
    California, 176–177, 178
NSAIDs (non-steroidal anti-
    inflammatory drugs),
    259, 384
NSTEMI, 304
Nuclear stress tests, 237–238,
    240, 249, 431
Nurses' Health Study, 173
Nutrition (see Diet and
    nutrition)
Nutrition Facts panel, 118
Nuts, 98, 106, 107

Oatmeal, 111
Obesity, 66–87 (see also Diet
    and nutrition)
    abdominal, 27, 63–64,
        71–72, 452
    armed forces and, 69
    bariatric surgery and,
        85–87
    body mass index (BMI), 66,
        70, 72–73, 85
    causes of epidemic, 73–78
    in children, 20, 471–473,
        475–483
    defined, 66
    diabetes and, 22, 67,
        480–481
    diet pills and, 83–85
    exercise and (see Exercise)
    financial costs of, 66, 70
    genetics and, 73, 478, 479
    household routines and, 489
    life expectancy and, 70, 481
    peer influence and, 74
    pregnancy and, 484
    prevalence of, 68–69
    as risk factor for CHD, 12,
        17, 27–28, 70–71, 140,
        450–453

screening for, 222–223
sleep and, 144
sleep apnea and, 36, 67
as socially contagious, 74
strategies to combat, 78–81
waist circumference and,
    27, 63–64, 72, 73, 478
Observational studies, 196,
    199–204, 215
Oculo-stenotic stenting reflex,
    305
Off-pump coronary artery
    bypass (OPCAB)
    grafting, 290, 322
Oleic acid, 94
Olive oil, 50–51, 60, 94–96,
    98, 106
Omega-3 fatty acids, 64, 98,
    103–106, 401–406
Omeprazole, 272
Open heart surgery (see Heart
    surgery)
Open-label trial, 206
Oral contraceptives, 260, 435,
    444
Orlistat (Alli, Xenical), 84
Ornish diet, 52, 79
Osteoarthritis, 71
Osteoporosis, 154, 193,
    408–409, 411
Ovarian cancer, 442
Overtime workers, 173
Overweight, defined, 66

Pacemakers, 338–340,
    346–350, 355–357, 388,
    520–521
Pacemaker syndrome, 348
Pain control, 319, 333–334
Palm oil, 98
Palpitations, 338, 342–343
Pancreas, 22
Panic disorders, 171
Partial sternotomy, 325
Pasteur, Louis, 530–531
Patient-controlled analgesia
    (PCA), 319
Peanuts, 107
Peer influence, obesity and,
    74
Penicillin, development of,
    376
Penn State University, 76
Pepperidge Farm, 117
PepsiCo, 78
Perceived justice at work,
    172–173
Percutaneous aortic valves,
    526

Perin, Emerson, 506
Periodontal/gum disease, as
    risk factor for CHD, 17,
    30–31
Peripartum cardiomyopathy,
    445–446
Pessimism, 170
Pet ownership, 185
PET (positron emission
    tomography) scans,
    238–239, 375
Pfizer, 62
Phentermine, 83, 84
Philbin, Regis, 289, 321
Physical education, 489–490
Physician's Desk Reference
    (PDR), 261
Phytosterols, 406
Pig valves, 324, 501
Plankton, 103
Plant stanols/sterols, 51, 107,
    406
Plaque formation, 15–16,
    45, 144, 147, 265, 410
    (see also Coronary heart
    disease [CHD])
Plavix, 134, 254, 268–272,
    280, 293–295, 304, 317,
    365, 519
Pneumonia, as cause of death,
    14
Policosanol, 407
Pollan, Michael, 77
Polychlorinated biphenyls
    (PCBs), 105
Polycystic ovarian syndrome,
    438
Polyphenols, 129
Polyunsaturated fats (PUSFs),
    51, 60, 98, 103–106, 107,
    452
Post-traumatic stress disorder,
    171
Postural hypotension, 281,
    381
Potassium, 113, 116, 280–281,
    382, 385
Poultry, 94
Power of Full Engagement,
    The (Schwartz), 186
Pradaxa, 274, 366, 367
Prasugrel (Effient), 270
Pravastatin (Pravachol), 53,
    54
Prayer, 189
Preeclampsia, 445, 447
Pregnancy, 438, 445–447, 484
Prehypertension, 221
Premarin, 441